The Echo Manual

Second Edition

The Echo Manual

Second Edition

Jae K. Oh, M.D.
Consultant, Division of Cardiovascular Diseases and Internal Medicine
Mayo Clinic and Mayo Foundation
Professor of Medicine
Mayo Medical School
Rochester, Minnesota

James B. Seward, M.D.
Director, Cardiovascular Ultrasound Imaging
and Hemodynamic Laboratory
Consultant, Division of Cardiovascular Diseases and Internal Medicine
Mayo Clinic and Mayo Foundation
Professor of Medicine and Pediatrics
Mayo Medical School
Rochester, Minnesota

A. Jamil Tajik, M.D.
Chair, Division of Cardiovascular Diseases and Internal Medicine
Mayo Clinic and Mayo Foundation
Thomas J. Watson, Jr., Professor in Honor of Dr. Robert L. Frye
Professor of Medicine and Pediatrics
Mayo Medical School
Rochester, Minnesota

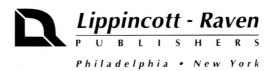

Lippincott - Raven
PUBLISHERS
Philadelphia • New York

Acquisitions Editor: Ruth W. Weinberg
Developmental Editor: Leigh Ann Simmons
Manufacturing Manager: Tim Reynolds
Production Manager: Cassie Moore
Production Editor: Rita Madrigal
Indexer: Elizabeth Babcock-Atkinson
Compositor: Maryland Composition
Publisher: Lippincott–Raven Publishers

Printed and Bound in China

9 8 7 6 5 4 3 2 1

Library of Congress Cataloging-in-Publication Data

Oh, Jae K.
    The echo manual / Jae K. Oh, James B. Seward, A. Jamil Tajik. —
2nd ed.
      p. cm.
    Includes bibliographical references and index.
    ISBN 0-7817-1205-X
    1. Echocardiograph—handbooks, manuals, etc. I. Seward, J. B.
    (James B.) II. Tajik, A. Jamil. III. Title.
    [DNLM: 1. Echocardiography handbooks. WG 39036e 1999]
RC683.5.U5037 1999
616.1'207543—dc21
DNLM/DLC
for Library of Congress
                                       98-19451
                                         CIP

To our families

Spouses

Terry H. Oh, Judith L. Seward, Zeest S. Tajik

Children

Phillip S. Oh
Kristin Seward Webert, J. Theodore (Ted) Seward
Jahangir K. Tajik, Jabeen (Nina) Tajik, Yasmin Tajik, Shabnam Tajik, Jamil K. Tajik

Contents

Preface

What a humbling experience to revise our own book! It has been four years since the publication of the first edition of *The Echo Manual*. The manual was well-received by students of echocardiography—echocardiologists, sonographers, and cardiology fellows—and was also translated into Italian and Portuguese. This enthusiastic response and the rapid, continuous progress in clinical applications of echocardiography prompted us to revise the *Manual*. Once we embarked on the revision process, we noticed that several chapters needed to be improved and expanded and that some new chapters needed to be added. As a result, the manual is thicker and has three more chapters: ''Assessment of Diastolic Function,'' ''Stress Echocardiography,'' and ''Contrast Echocardiography.'' All the figures were extensively revised and digitized, with the intention of eventually producing an electronic version of the *Manual*. Despite these changes, the *Manual* remains clinically oriented. We have tried to present echocardiography as the most comprehensive and definitive evaluation of cardiovascular structure, function, and hemodynamics. To achieve this, the text has been kept succinct and the figures have been created to provide a better understanding of the diagnostic role of echocardiography.

Many talented persons helped us with the revision. Roberta J. Schwartz (Supervisor), Virginia A. Dunt (Editorial Assistant), Dorothy L. Tienter (Proofreader), and O. Eugene Millhouse, Ph.D. (Editor) of the Section of Publications edited and processed the entire manuscript. Vernon P. Weber and Jeffrey R. Stelley, Echocardiography Laboratory technical coordinator and educational resource assistant, respectively, helped select and photograph the echocardiographic images digitally. Fred Graszer (Supervisor), Paul W. Honermann, and Diane M. Knight, computer artists in Visual Information Services, were responsible for the final production of all the figures. Jami A. Spitzer (medical secretary) typed the entire first draft of the manuscript and organized our correspondence with the publisher.

This second edition would not have been possible without encouragement and professional advice from Lippincott–Raven Publishers, who took over this book from Little, Brown and Company. We especially thank Ruth W. Weinberg, Acquisitions Editor, and Rita Madrigal, Production Editor, for their involvement in the coordination of this project.

Our sincere hope is that by presenting a comprehensive and practical approach to noninvasive assessment of cardiovascular morphology, function, and hemodynamics, our *Echo Manual* will help students, sonographers, and practiioners make optimal clinical use of echocardiography for the benefit of the patient.

Jae K. Oh, M.D.
James B. Seward, M.D.
A. Jamil Tajik, M.D.
Rochester, MN

Abbreviations Commonly Used in Text, Tables, and Figures*

A	Late diastolic filling due to atrial contraction
AO, Ao	Aorta
CHF	Congestive heart failure
CI	Cardiac index
CO	Cardiac output
DT	Deceleration time
E	Peak velocity of early diastolic filling
E/A	Ratio of E and A velocities
ECG	Electrocardiogram (-graphy)
EF	Ejection fraction
ERO	Effective regurgitant orifice
IVC	Inferior vena cava
IVRT	Isovolumic relaxation time
LA	Left atrium (-ial)
LV	Left ventricle (-icular)
LVOT	Left ventricular outflow tract
MV	Mitral valve
PFO	Patent foramen ovale
PHT	Pressure half-time
PISA	Proximal isovelocity surface area
PW	Posterior wall
RA	Right atrium (-ial)
RV	Right ventricle (-icular)
SV	Stroke volume
SVC	Superior vena cava
TEE	Transesophageal echocardiography
TTE	Transthoracic echocardiography
TVI	Time velocity integral
2D	Two-dimensional
VS	Ventricular septum

* The abbreviations are written out at first use in each chapter, table, and legend, except for LA, LV, RA, and RV, which are defined only here.

CHAPTER 1

Overview

ECHOCARDIOGRAPHY IN CARDIOVASCULAR DISEASES

Echocardiography is one of the most frequently used techniques for diagnosing cardiovascular diseases. It is non-invasive, and the equipment is portable. Echocardiography is so versatile, with clinical applications in the entire spectrum of cardiovascular disease, that it now is considered an *extension of the physical examination*. This diagnostic modality is unique in that it provides a comprehensive evaluation of the cardiovascular system, whereas most other diagnostic procedures address only a particular area of clinical concern. For example, in a patient with prolonged chest pain and nonspecific electrocardiographic findings, coronary angiography and nuclear imaging are useful if myocardial ischemia is the cause of the chest pain, but these modalities are usually not helpful if the patient has pericarditis, pulmonary embolism, or aortic dissection. In addition to its usefulness in confirming a clinical suspicion, one of the strengths of echocardiography is its ability to provide a diagnosis that may not be apparent to a clinician, because it can evaluate structural, functional, and hemodynamic abnormalities of the heart in one setting by using two-dimensional (2D), Doppler, and color-flow imaging via transthoracic and transesophageal windows (1–5).

Proper technical and cognitive skills are required for the optimal application of echocardiography and the interpretation of its results. It is an *operator-dependent* technique, more so than other cardiovascular techniques. The echocardiographic examination is most efficient and valuable if it is performed and interpreted by the clinician responsible for the patient. Usually, however, this is not practical, and most clinicians must rely on the examination and interpretation made by someone else. More objective and quantitative assessment of echocardiographic findings is therefore required, as opposed to subjective and qualitative interpretations. Echocardiography should be used as a *"definitive"* rather than a *"screening" diagnostic tool*. After a significant lesion that requires surgical treatment is identified by echocardiography, the patient should be able to receive that treatment without having to undergo other confirmatory diagnostic tests. To do so requires not only the expertise of an echocardiographer but also an understanding of the capabilities and limitations of echocardiography by other physicians involved in the care of the patient, including primary care physicians and surgeons. The most outstanding example is the evaluation of valvular and congenital heart diseases. Before the advent of Doppler echocardiography, all patients with severe aortic stenosis underwent hemodynamic cardiac catheterization before aortic valve replacement. Currently at our institution, fewer than 25% of such patients require invasive hemodynamic studies. Rarely is cardiac catheterization required for the diagnosis of congenital heart disease. To have clinical impact, a new diagnostic modality should replace an existing procedure, not be an additional procedure, and it should do so without increasing the cost or risk of the examination and without sacrificing the accuracy of the results. Echocardiography meets these criteria, and it has had considerable clinical impact on the diagnosis and management of various cardiovascular diseases.

DEVELOPMENT OF ECHOCARDIOGRAPHY

Cardiovascular Ultrasound Imaging and Hemodynamic Laboratory

Echocardiography uses *high-frequency ultrasound* (2.0 to 7.5 MHz) to evaluate the structural, functional, and hemodynamic status of the cardiovascular system. In 1954, Edler and Hertz (6) of Sweden were the first to record movements of cardiac structures, in particular, the mitral valve, with ultrasound. The reflected ultrasound pattern was so distinctive in patients with mitral stenosis that it became diagnostic, and the severity of mitral stenosis could be measured semiquantitatively by analysis of the M-mode echocardiogram. In the United States in the early 1960s, Joyner and Reid (7) at the University of Pennsylvania were the first to use ultrasound to examine the heart. Shortly afterward, in 1965, Feigenbaum and colleagues (8) at Indiana University reported the first detection of pericardial effusion with ultrasound and were responsible for introducing echocardiography into the clinical practice of cardiology. However, M-mode echocardiography produced only an "ice pick" view of the heart; 2D sector scanning, developed in the mid-1970s, allowed real-time tomographic images of cardiac morphology and function (1). The first phased array 2D sector scan at the Mayo Clinic was performed on March 17, 1977. Although the development of Doppler echocardiography paralleled that of M-mode and 2D echocardiography from the early 1950s, it was not used clinically until the late 1970s. Pressure gradients across a fixed orifice could be obtained reliably with blood-flow velocities measured by Doppler echocardiography (2,3,9). Numerous validation studies subsequently confirmed the accuracy of Doppler in the assessment of cardiac pressures. Therefore, the Doppler technique made echocardiography not only an *imaging* but also a *hemodynamic technique*. On the basis of the Doppler concept, color-flow imaging was developed in the early 1980s so that blood flow also could be visualized noninvasively (4).

Another major technological advance was the introduction of transesophageal echocardiography (TEE). In the United States (10), the clinical use of TEE became widespread in 1987. With M-mode, 2D, Doppler, and color-flow imaging with transthoracic and transesophageal windows, the application of echocardiography has been extended into numerous clinical areas, including the evaluation of diastolic function, stress echocardiography, intraoperative echocardiography, fetal echocardiography, contrast echocardiography, intravascular imaging, and vascular imaging. Tissue characterization and three-dimensional reconstruction are active areas of clinical investigation but have not become routine clinical procedures.

ECHOCARDIOGRAPHY AT THE MAYO CLINIC

An average of 150 echocardiographic examinations are performed daily at Mayo Clinic Rochester (Fig. 1-1). One-third of these examinations are for inpatients and two-thirds for outpatients. Stress echocardiographic, TEE, and intraoperative echocardiographic procedures account for about 20% of these procedures (10%, 7%, and 3%, respectively). About 15 additional examinations are performed daily off campus at various outreach sites by Mayo Clinic sonographers. Typically, a transthoracic echocardiographic (TTE) examination is initially performed by a sonographer or a cardiovascular fellow in training and requires 30 to 45 minutes. The findings are interpreted by a staff echocardiologist before the patient leaves the examination room. If more information is needed for optimal interpretation of the findings, the echocardiologist performs an additional examination. All echocardiologists at our institution are proficient in actual scanning and in operating the ultrasound units. The final interpretation of each examination is re-

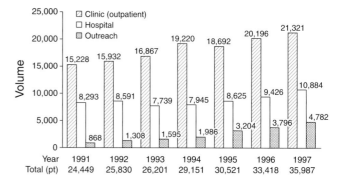

FIG. 1-1. The number of echocardiographic examinations performed at Mayo Clinic Rochester from 1991 to 1997. "Outreach" indicates the number of studies performed off campus at distant sites. *pt*, patients.

corded in the patient's medical record for the primary physician, and the findings are dictated and stored for the permanent record and review.

Stress echocardiography is performed by a group of sonographers, exercise technicians, and monitoring technicians. After completion of a stress test, digitized and videotape images are reviewed by a staff echocardiologist. TEE and intraoperative echocardiography are performed primarily by staff echocardiologists. With intraoperative echocardiography, anesthesiologists who have had echocardiographic training also are involved. Echocardiography may be performed by anyone who has technical or cognitive skills of level II or greater (defined below) during emergency situations. A team consisting of a sonographer and an echocardiologist is on call 24 hours a day to provide emergency coverage.

EXAMINATION

Echocardiography is an interactive procedure that involves an echocardiographer, a cardiac ultrasound unit, and a patient. To produce optimal echocardiographic images and signals, these three components of the examination should meet the requirements outlined below.

Operator

The person who performs echocardiographic examinations should have satisfactory cognitive and technical skills. Guidelines for clinical competence in performing echocardiography in adults were developed by the American College of Cardiology, American College of Physicians, and the American Heart Association (11) and are listed in Tables 1-1 and 1-2.

To obtain the necessary cognitive and technical competence for adult echocardiography, a guideline was established for the minimum training a physician should have (12). Echocardiographic training comprises three levels

TABLE 1-1. *Cognitive skills needed to perform echocardiography competently in adults*

Knowledge of the appropriate indications for echocardiography and its elements

Knowledge of the differential diagnostic problem in each patient and the echocardiographic techniques needed to investigate these possibilities

Knowledge of the alternatives to echocardiography

Knowledge of the physical principles of echocardiographic image formation and blood-flow velocity measurement

Knowledge of normal cardiac anatomy

Knowledge of the pathologic changes in cardiac anatomy due to acquired and congenital heart disease

Knowledge of the fluid dynamics of normal blood flow

Knowledge of the pathologic changes in cardiac blood flow due to acquired and congenital heart disease

Knowledge of cardiac auscultation and electrocardiography for correlation with the results of echocardiography

Ability to distinguish between an adequate and an inadequate echocardiographic examination

Ability to communicate the results of the examination to the patient, medical record, and other physicians

From ref. 11, with permission.

TABLE 1-2. *Technical skills needed to perform echocardiography competently in adults*

Technical proficiency with operation of ultrasonographic equipment and all controls affecting the quality of the received signals

Ability to position and direct the ultrasound transducer to obtain the desired tomographic images and Doppler-flow velocity signals

Ability to perform a complete standard examination, including all locally available elements of an echocardiographic study

Ability to record and recognize the electrocardiogram for correlation with the echocardiographic data

Ability to recognize abnormalities of anatomy and flow to modify the standard examination to accommodate perceived diagnostic needs

Ability to perform quantitative analysis of the echocardiographic study and to produce a written report

From ref. 11, with permission.

(Table 1-3). The *first level* (level I) is designed to provide an understanding of the basic principles and the indications for and applications and limitations of echocardiography. All cardiovascular-specialty trainees are expected to achieve this level of echocardiographic training. The first level (level I) of training requires 3 months dedicated solely to echocardiography. The trainee participates in the performance and interpretation of a minimum of 150 complete ultrasound imaging and Doppler hemodynamic examinations under the supervision of the laboratory director, designated faculty, and cardiac sonographers. This level does not qualify a trainee to perform echocardiography or to interpret echocardiograms independently. The *second level* (level II) of training requires 3 additional months. The trainee independently performs as well as interprets at least an additional 150 complete imaging and hemodynamic examinations. A trainee who has completed level II should be able to perform an echocardiographic and Doppler study that is diagnostic, complete, and quantitatively accurate but must be under the direction of a level III trained physician echocardiographer. The *third level* (level III) consists of 6

additional months of training, which is needed to qualify the trainee to direct an echocardiography laboratory. This level of training requires that an additional 450 personal examinations be performed in a patient population with a broad spectrum of adult-acquired and congenital heart disease. Special procedures in echocardiography (TEE, stress, contrast, and the other special areas of echocardiography) can be learned during level III training (i.e., after level II).

At the Mayo Clinic, a cardiology trainee spends 3 months of the first year of the fellowship program in the echocardiography laboratory to achieve level I training. During this 3 months, training is dedicated entirely to echocardiography. If the trainee wants to perform echocardiography independently or to direct an echocardiography laboratory, training for an additional 6 to 12 months as well as independent clinical research is required.

Because echocardiographic data acquisition usually is performed by a sonographer, the importance of the training of sonographers in echocardiography also should be recognized. Sonographer training depends on the person's background and should be under the supervision of a physician echocardiographer who has completed level III training. Technical skills similar to those outlined for physicians should be obtained by sonographers; however, the ultimate

TABLE 1-3. *Summary of training requirements for echocardiography*

| Level | Training (mo) | | No. of examinations | | TEE and special procedures |
	Duration	Cumulative	Minimal additional[a]	Cumulative	
I	3	3	150	150	No
II	3	6	150	300	No
III	6	12	450	750	Yes

TEE, transesophageal echocardiography.

[a] Performance and interpretation of the study.

From ref. 12, with permission.

responsibility for the interpretation of echocardiographic findings should rest with a physician who has the appropriate training (level II or III). The role of the sonographer during TEE and stress echocardiography varies depending on his or her qualifications and experience. This topic is discussed in subsequent chapters.

Instrumentation

All ultrasound units should be equipped with the basic requirements of M-mode, 2D sector scanning, Doppler, and color-flow imaging capabilities, although some portable units provide only M-mode and 2D imaging. However, the echocardiographer should optimize the examination by using the optimal transducer, knob settings, and transducer positions.

Diagnostic ultrasound requires a frequency of at least 2.0 MHz. As the sound frequency increases, the distance that the ultrasound beam penetrates the body decreases; therefore, the usual echocardiographic examination in adults begins with a 2.0- to 2.5-MHz transducer. However, image resolution improves with a higher frequency transducer (i.e., shorter wavelength). In a thin adult or pediatric patient, a 3.0- to 5.0-MHz transducer usually provides adequate penetration and also improves image resolution. Harmonic imaging is a newer way to improve image quality in technically difficult cases. Harmonic imaging was introduced initially to improve visualization of contrast bubbles, which create resonant ultrasound with frequencies that are a multiple of the transmitted frequency. For example, a second harmonic imaging transducer transmits ultrasound of 1.8-MHz frequency and receives a 3.6-MHz signal. Combined with trigger-response imaging (see Chapter 20), second harmonic imaging allows visualization of contrast in the myocardium. A similar technology also enhances the images of cardiovascular structure without the presence of contrast. This technology has been particularly helpful in regional wall motion analysis (see Fig. 7-6). In the TEE probe, a modification of an endoscopy probe with a higher frequency (3.5- to 7.5-MHz) transducer is used because the distance between the transducer and the cardiovascular structures is quite short and not interrupted greatly by other body tissues; therefore, penetration of the beam is not as significant an issue. In the Doppler examination, however, a lower frequency transducer is required to record high velocities because the measurable velocities are inversely proportional to the transmitted frequency (see Doppler equation in Chapter 6).

After a proper transducer has been selected, all the available ultrasound windows should be used. Gray scales and gains are controlled manually to minimize background noise and to maximize the delineation of cardiac structures. The depth of the fields can be controlled to provide the optimal image size. When a certain structure needs to be examined carefully, a ''zoom'' or regional expansion selection (RES) function can enlarge the selected portion of the image. Field depth is important during Doppler and color-flow imaging examinations because the *Nyquist limit* (i.e., the maximal velocity to be recorded without aliasing) is related to the depth of the examination: The shallower the field depth, the higher the Nyquist limit.

The setting of filters depends on the type of Doppler study being performed. When low-velocity flow is being measured with pulsed-wave Doppler echocardiography (e.g., mitral inflow or pulmonary venous flow velocities), the filter setting should be low, but when high-velocity flow is to be measured with continuous-wave Doppler echocardiography (e.g., aortic flow velocity in aortic stenosis), the filter setting should be high to eliminate the low-velocity flow signals. In color-flow imaging, the filter setting should be high to eliminate the noise artifacts near the cardiac walls. Theoretically, to obtain the highest available velocity by Doppler echocardiography, the Doppler beam should be parallel with the direction of the blood-flow jet (angle of θ should be 0); however, the error introduced by the angle of θ is acceptable as long as the angle is less than 20 degrees. Sometimes, an angle correction can overestimate the Doppler velocity; thus, it is rarely used in daily practice.

Color-flow imaging also depends on the gain and filter setting. It is important to make certain that the area of abnormal blood flow is not underestimated by a low gain setting or overestimated by a low filter setting, because the severity of valvular regurgitation or shunt flow depends on the area of abnormal blood flow detected with color-flow imaging. The optimal setting should be where the entire flow jet is displayed with minimal background noise. Usually it is best to start with maximal color gain to identify the largest area of abnormal blood flow and then to decrease the gain gradually to minimize the background noise without compromising the visualization of abnormal flow. It should be noted that the gain settings for 2D tissue imaging may affect color gains in flow imaging in some instruments.

Patient

Occasionally, because of emphysema, obesity, or a unique body habitus, the patient is a limiting factor in an echocardiographic examination. These features may preclude a meaningful TTE examination. Even with these limiting factors, however, echocardiographic images that are entirely uninterpretable are rare, and, in most patients, clinical questions can be answered with TTE. If a better image is required, the transesophageal (TEE) approach provides an alternative ultrasound window. Even in the ideal patient for TTE, visualization of certain structures such as the left atrial appendage, left main coronary artery, and descending thoracic aorta requires the transesophageal view. A patient's hemodynamic status may alter echocardiographic findings. Mitral regurgitation may become severe with higher blood pressure, and left ventricular systolic function becomes impaired with tachycardia. These variables should be considered in the interpretation of echocardiograms. Blood pressure needs to be measured and recorded on the screen at the beginning of each examination. Any symptoms or abnormalities in the electrocardiogram (e.g., paroxysmal atrial fibrillation or nonsustained ventricular tachycardia) during echocardiographic study should be reported to the responsible physician so that it can be correlated with the patient's presenting problem. It is also important to have a good electrocardiographic recording for optimal hemodynamic assessment.

REFERENCES

1. Tajik AJ, Seward JB, Hagler DJ, Mair DD, Lie J. Two-dimensional real-time ultrasonic imaging of the heart and great vessels: technique, image orientation, structure identification, and validation. *Mayo Clin Proc* 1978;53:271–303.
2. Hatle L, Angelsen B. *Doppler ultrasound in cardiology: physical principles and clinical applications*, 2nd ed. Philadelphia: Lea & Febiger, 1985.
3. Nishimura RA, Miller FA Jr, Callahan MJ, Benassi RC, Seward JB, Tajik AJ. Doppler echocardiography: theory, instrumentation, technique, and application. *Mayo Clin Proc* 1985;60:321–343.
4. Omoto R, Kasai C. Physics and instrumentation of Doppler color flow mapping. *Echocardiography* 1987;4:467–483.
5. Seward JB, Khandheria BK, Freeman WK, et al. Multiplane transesophageal echocardiography: image orientation, examination technique, anatomic correlations, and clinical applications. *Mayo Clin Proc* 1993;68:523–551.
6. Edler I, Hertz CH. The use of ultrasonic reflectoscope for the continuous recording of the movements of heart walls. *Kungliga Fysiografiska Sallskapets i Lund Forhandlingar* 1954;24:1–19.
7. Joyner CR Jr, Reid JM. Applications of ultrasound in cardiology and cardiovascular physiology. *Prog Cardiovasc Dis* 1963;5:482–497.
8. Feigenbaum H, Waldhausen JA, Hyde LP. Ultrasound diagnosis of pericardial effusion. *JAMA* 1965;191:711–714.
9. Holen J, Aaslid R, Landmark K, Simonsen S. Determination of pressure gradient in mitral stenosis with a non-invasive ultrasound Doppler technique. *Acta Med Scand* 1976;199:455–560.
10. Seward JB, Khandheria BK, Oh JK, et al. Transesophageal echocardiography: technique, anatomic correlations, implementation, and clinical applications. *Mayo Clin Proc* 1988;63:649–680.
11. Popp RL, Winters WL Jr. Clinical competence in adult echocardiography. A statement for physicians from the ACP/ACC/AHA Task Force on Clinical Privileges in Cardiology. *J Am Coll Cardiol* 1990;15:1465–1468.
12. Stewart WJ, Aurigemma GP, Bierman FZ, et al. Task Force 4: training in echocardiography. *J Am Coll Cardiol* 1995;25:16–19.

CHAPTER 2

Transthoracic Echocardiography

M-MODE AND TWO-DIMENSIONAL ECHOCARDIOGRAPHY

An echocardiographic examination begins with transthoracic two-dimensional (2D) scanning from four standard transducer positions: the parasternal, apical, subcostal (subxiphoid), and suprasternal windows. The parasternal and apical views usually are obtained with the patient in the left lateral decubitus position (Fig. 2-1A) and the subcostal and suprasternal notch views with the patient in the supine position (Fig. 2-1B). From each transducer position, multiple tomographic images of the heart relative to its long and short axes are obtained by manually rotating and angulating the transducer (Table 2-1), hence performing a multiplane examination (Fig. 2-2) (1–4). The long-axis view represents a sagittal or coronal section of the heart, bisecting the heart from the base to the apex. The short-axis view is perpendicular to the long-axis view and is equivalent to sectioning the heart like a loaf of bread ("bread-loafing"). Real-time 2D echocardiography provides high-resolution images of cardiac structures and their movements so that detailed anatomic and functional information about the heart can be obtained. Therefore, 2D echocardiography is the basis of morphologic and functional assessments of the heart. Quantitative measurements of cardiac dimensions, area, and volume are derived from 2D images or 2D-derived M-mode. In addition, 2D echocardiography provides the framework for Doppler and color-flow imaging. These standard long and short tomographic imaging planes are acquired as described in the following sections (1).

Parasternal Position

Examination is begun by placing the transducer in the left parasternal region, usually in the third or fourth left intercostal space, with the patient in the left lateral position (Fig. 2-1A). From this position, sector images can be obtained of the heart along its long and short axes.

Long-Axis View of the Left Ventricle

The long-axis view of the left ventricle (LV) is recorded with the transducer groove facing toward the patient's right flank and the transducer positioned in the third or fourth left interspace so that the ultrasound beam is parallel with a line joining the right shoulder to the left flank. The image thus obtained represents a section through the long axis of the LV (Fig. 2-3A). The image is oriented so that the aorta is displayed on the right, the cardiac apex to the left, the chest wall and right ventricle (RV) anteriorly, and posterior structures posteriorly on the image (Fig. 2-3B). Therefore, the long-axis view of the LV is displayed as a sagittal section of the heart viewed from the left side of a supine patient.

The long-axis view of the LV allows visualization of the aortic root and aortic valve leaflets. With the onset of systole, the leaflets open abruptly and come to lie nearly parallel to the aortic walls. The chamber behind the aortic root is the left atrial (LA) cavity. Usually, the left inferior pulmonary vein, appearing as a round structure, also can be seen immediately posterior to the lower part of the LA. The long-axis view allows good visualization of the anterior and posterior leaflets of the mitral valve and their chordal and papillary muscle attachments.

The coronary sinus, appearing as a small, circular echo-free structure, usually can be recorded in the region of the posterior atrioventricular groove. The LV outflow tract (LVOT), bounded by the ventricular septum anteriorly and the anterior leaflet of the mitral valve posteriorly, is well seen and normally is widely patent during systole.

Long-Axis View of RV Inflow

With the transducer in the same interspace (third or fourth) and with inferomedial tilt and slight clockwise rotation of the transducer, a long-axis view of the RV and right atrium (RA) is obtained. The image orientation of this view is such that the chest wall is anterior, the RA is on

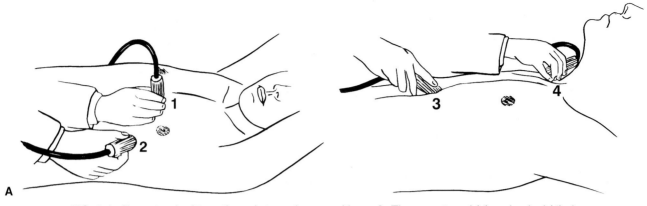

FIG. 2-1. Four standard transthoracic transducer positions. **A:** The parasternal (*1*) and apical (*2*) views usually are obtained with the patient in the left lateral decubitus position. The parasternal view usually is obtained by placing the transducer at the left parasternal area in the second or third intercostal space. The apical view is obtained with the transducer at the maximal apical impulse (usually slightly lateral and inferior to the nipple, but it may be significantly displaced further because of cardiac enlargement or rotation or both). These views may be imaged best during held expiration, especially in patients who have chronic obstructive lung disease. The apical view can be difficult to obtain in a thin young person, and the transducer may need to be tilted superiorly. **B:** The subcostal (*3*) and suprasternal notch (*4*) views are obtained with the patient in the supine position. For subcostal imaging, flexion of the patient's knees relaxes the abdominal muscles, and forced inspiration frequently improves the views. For suprasternal notch imaging, the patient's head needs to be extended and turned leftward so the transducer can be placed comfortably in the suprasternal notch without rubbing the patient's neck.

the right and posterior, and the RV apex is anterior and to the left side of the image. These views allow visualization of the RA cavity, the tricuspid valve, and the RV inflow up to the apex of the RV. This view is good for obtaining tricuspid regurgitation velocity.

TABLE 2-1. *Transducer positions and cardiac views*

Parasternal position
  Long-axis view
    LV in a sagittal section
    RV inflow
    LV outflow
  Short-axis view
    LV apex
    Papillary muscles (midlevel)
    Mitral valve (basal level)
    Aortic valve–RV outflow
    Pulmonary trunk bifurcation
Apical position
  Four-chamber view
  Five-chamber (or long-axis) view
  Two-chamber view
Subcostal position
  Inferior vena cava and hepatic vein
  RV and LV inflow
  LV-aorta
  RV outflow
Suprasternal notch position
  Long-axis aorta–short-axis pulmonary artery
  Short-axis aorta–long-axis pulmonary artery
  Long-axis aorta and superior vena cava

LV, left ventricle; RV, right ventricle.

Short-Axis Views

With the transducer placed in the parasternal position (third or fourth left intercostal space), the short-axis view of the heart is obtained by rotating the transducer clockwise so that the place of the ultrasound beam is approximately perpendicular to the plane of the long axis of the LV. The groove on the transducer is pointed superiorly facing the right supraclavicular fossa, and the beam is roughly parallel with a line joining the left shoulder to the right flank. With the transducer pointed directly posteriorly, a cross section is obtained of the LV at the level of the mitral leaflets. From this position, the transducer is tilted inferiorly toward the LV apex so that a transverse section of the ventricular apex is obtained. The images are displayed as if viewed from below (looking from the apex of the heart up toward the base). In this format, the cross-sectional view of the LV is displayed posteriorly and to the right side of the image and the RV is displayed anteriorly and to the left.

A cross section of the cardiac apex also can be obtained by placing the transducer directly over the point of maximal (apical) impulse (apical short-axis view). As the ultrasound beam is tilted superiorly, a cross section is obtained at the level of the papillary muscles. The papillary muscles, namely, the anterolateral and posteromedial, project into the LV cavity at approximately the 3 and 8 o'clock positions, respectively (Fig. 2-4).

With further superior tilting of the transducer so that it is nearly perpendicular to the chest wall, the ultrasound beam transects the body of the LV at the level of the mitral

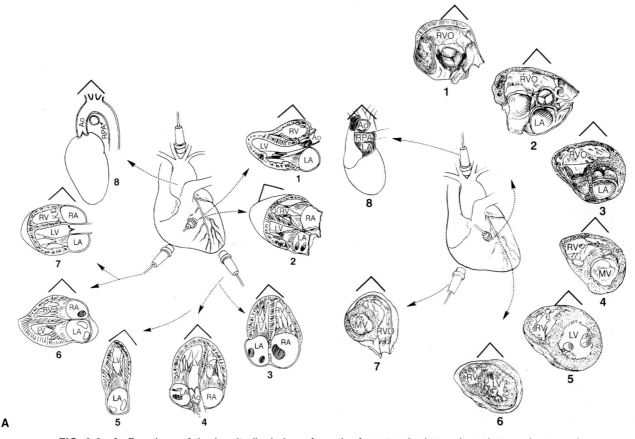

FIG. 2-2. A: Drawings of the longitudinal views from the four standard transthoracic transducer positions. Shown are the parasternal long-axis view (*1*), parasternal right venticular (*RV*) inflow view (*2*), apical four-chamber view (*3*), apical five-chamber view (*4*), apical two-chamber view (*5*), subcostal four-chamber view (*6*), subcostal long-axis (five-chamber) view (*7*), and suprasternal notch view (*8*). **B:** Drawings of short-axis views. These views are obtained by rotating the transducer 90 degrees clockwise from the longitudinal position. Drawings 1–6 show parasternal short-axis views at different levels by angulating the transducer from a superior medial position (for the imaging of the aortic and pulmonary valves) to an inferolateral position, tilting toward the apex (from level 1 to level 6 short-axis views). Shown are short-axis views of the right ventricular (*RV*) outflow (*RVO*) tract and pulmonary valve (*1*), aortic valve and left atrium (*LA*) (*2*), RV outflow tract (*3*), and short-axis views at the left ventricular (*LV*) basal [mitral valve (*MV*) level] (*4*), the LV midlevel (papillary muscle) (*5*), and the LV apical level (*6*). A good view to visualize the RV outflow tract is the subcostal short-axis view (*7*). Also shown is the suprasternal notch short-axis view of the aorta (*Ao*) (*8*). *RPA*, right pulmonary artery. (**B** from ref. 1, with permission.)

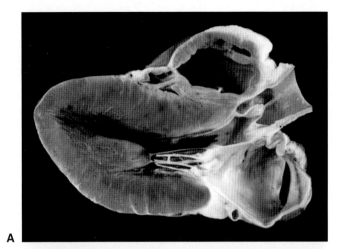

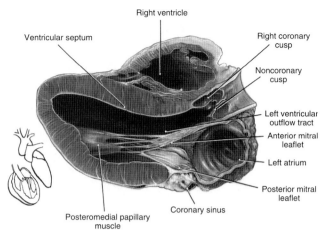

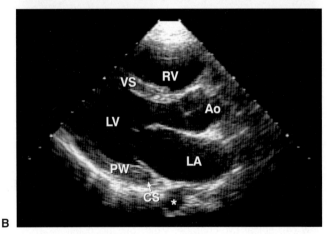

FIG. 2-3. A: Anatomic section of heart **(left)** with drawing **(right)**. B: Corresponding still-frame of two-dimensional echo-cardiographic image of parasternal long-axis view. The parasternal long-axis view allows visualization of the right ventricle (*RV*), ventricular septum (*VS*), aortic valve cusps, left ventricle (*LV*), mitral valve, left atrial (*LA*), and ascending thoracic aorta (*AO*). The coronary sinus (*CS*) may be seen as a small circular echo-free structure in the left atrioventricular groove. The descending aorta (*asterisk*) is also seen. *PW*, posterior wall. (**A** from ref. 1, with permission.)

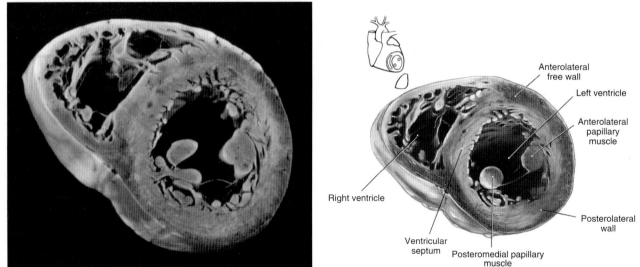

FIG. 2-4. Parasternal short-axis views: multiple tomographic planes obtained by angulating the transducer from the level of the aortic and pulmonary valves to the left ventricular (*LV*) apex. **A:** Anatomic section **(left)** of a parasternal short-axis view at the papillary muscle level and a drawing **(right)** that identifies the structures of the heart. **B:** Corresponding still-frame of a two-dimensional echocardiographic image in the parasternal short-axis view at the papillary muscle level. This view is particularly useful in measuring the LV cavity dimension and wall thickness and in assessing wall motion. *AL*, anterolateral papillary muscle; *PM*, posteromedial papillary muscle; *VS*, ventricular septum.

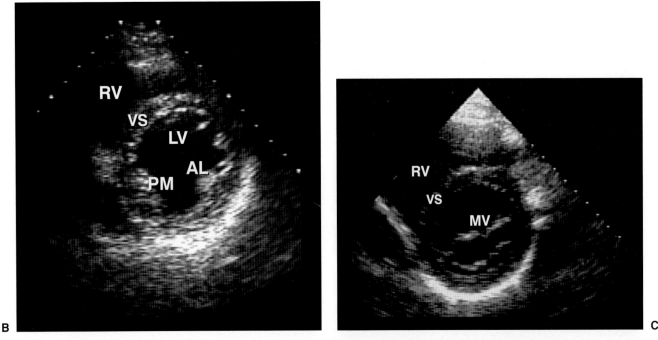

FIG. 2-4. *Continued.* **C:** Superior and rightward tilting of the transducer obtains a parasternal short-axis view at the basal level showing the mitral valve (*MV*). (**A** from ref. 1, with permission.)

leaflets. In this view, the mitral anterior and posterior leaf-lets are seen in cross section and, during diastole, look like a fish mouth; this view is good for measuring the mitral valve area in a patient who has mitral stenosis.

With further superior tilting of the transducer, the great arteries are sectioned transversely. At this level in normal subjects, the aorta appears as a circle with a trileaflet aortic valve that has the appearance of the letter ''Y'' during di-astole (Fig. 2-5). The right ventricular outflow tract (RVOT) crosses anterior to the aorta from the left to the right of the image, wrapping around the aorta; in cross sec-tion, it has a sausage-like appearance anterior to the circular aorta. The pulmonary valve is observed anterior to and to the right of the aortic valve. The origins of the right and left main coronary arteries also can be seen in this view.

Apical Position

This view is obtained with the patient turned in the left lateral decubitus position (Fig. 2-1A). The apical impulse is localized and the transducer is placed at or in the im-mediate vicinity of the point of maximal impulse. With the apical transducer position, a four-chamber view of the heart or a right anterior oblique equivalent view of the LV usu-ally is recorded. The notch on the transducer is placed pointing up or down, depending on whether the goal is to display the LV on the right or on the left side of the image, respectively. Because the views obtained with the apical transducer position represent long-axis views of the heart, particularly of the LV, it is desirable that the orientation of the image of these views be similar to that of the long-axis

view of the LV. For this reason, we have chosen to display the apical views with the LV on the left and the RV on the right sides of the image. For the four-chamber view, the ultrasound beam is directed superiorly and medially toward the patient's right scapula. This view displays all four chambers of the heart, the ventricular and atrial septa, and the crux of the heart (Fig. 2-6A). While recording the apical four-chamber view, we usually tilt the beam in a slightly anterior and posterior direction to scan a greater portion of the atrial septum. The image orientation is such that the apex is on the top and the atria are on the bottom. In the image, the RA and RV are on the right and the LA and LV are on the left, with the groove down (Fig. 2-6B). The continuation of ventricular and atrial septa is by means of a membranous connection. The left (*mitral*) atrioventricular groove normally is slightly higher than the right (*tricuspid*) atrioventricular groove. The anterior leaflet of the mitral valve inserts into the left atrioventricular sulcus and near the cephalic end of the membranous septum, whereas the septal leaflet of the tricuspid valve inserts near the mid-portion of the membranous septum. Therefore, the insertion of the septal leaflet of the tricuspid valve is somewhat in-ferior (5 to 10 mm in the hearts of older children and adults) to the insertion of the anterior mitral leaflet. This is an important anatomic distinction because it can be useful in identifying ventricular chambers.

In the apical view, the atrial septum usually can be seen in its entirety without any thinning or dropout if the ultra-sound beam is directed slightly anteriorly; however, drop-out of echoes does occur in its midportion, which is the region of the fossa ovalis, if the ultrasound beam is directed

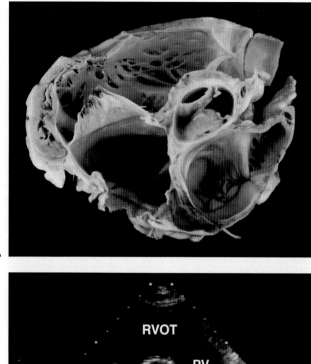

A

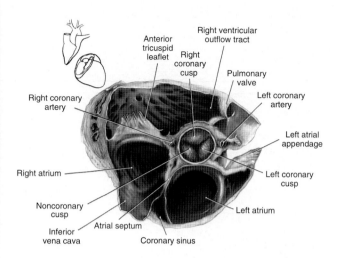

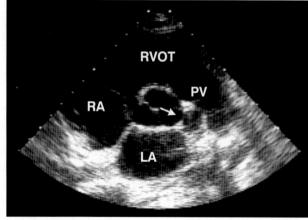

B

FIG. 2-5. With further superior tilting of the transducer, the short-axis view of the aortic valve is obtained. In this view, the right ventricular outflow tract (*RVOT*) and pulmonary valve are visualized. Below the aortic valve lies the left atrium (*LA*); the connection of all four pulmonary veins with the left ventricle (*LV*) is usually seen. **A:** Anatomic section (*left*) of the heart and drawing (*right*) of this view. **B:** Corresponding two-dimensional echocardiographic image. *Arrow* indicates the ostium of left main coronary artery. *PV*, pulmonary valve. (**A** from ref. 1, with permission.)

further posteriorly. This view also allows visualization of the emptying of the right and left inferior pulmonary veins into the LA.

With the same apical transducer position, the transducer is tilted further anteriorly to record the aortic root and valve in addition to the four chambers. The aortic root occupies the region where the crux of the heart was recorded in the previous section.

With further clockwise rotation of the transducer, the ap-

ical two-chamber view is obtained. These apical views are essential for analysis of regional myocardial contractility, and hence for stress echocardiography.

Subcostal Position

In certain patients, especially those who have chronic obstructive lung disease and emphysema, the usual precordial ultrasonic window may become obliterated because of

FIG. 2-6. A: Anatomic section **(left)** and drawing **(right)** of apical four-chamber view. **B:** Corresponding two-dimensional echocardiographic image of the apical four-chamber view. The apical view is obtained by placing the transducer in the immediate vicinity of or at the point of maximal apical impulse. The four-chamber view displays all four cardiac chambers, the ventricular and atrial septa, and the crux of the heart. It also should be noted that the insertion of the septal leaflet of the tricuspid valve is somewhat inferior to the insertion of the anterior mitral leaflet; this is an important anatomic distinction in the evaluation of congenital heart disease. **C:** By angulating the transducer in a clockwise rotation, the five-chamber, or long-axis apical, view allows visualization of the left ventricular (*LV*) outflow tract and the aortic valve. *AS*, anteroseptum; *AV*, aortic valve; *IL*, inferolateral wall. **D:** Further rotation of the transducer clockwise produces the two-chamber view, which is useful in visualizing the entire posterior or inferior (*Inf*) wall and in analyzing anterior (*Ant*) wall motion. *MV*, mitral valve. (**A** from ref. 1, with permission.)

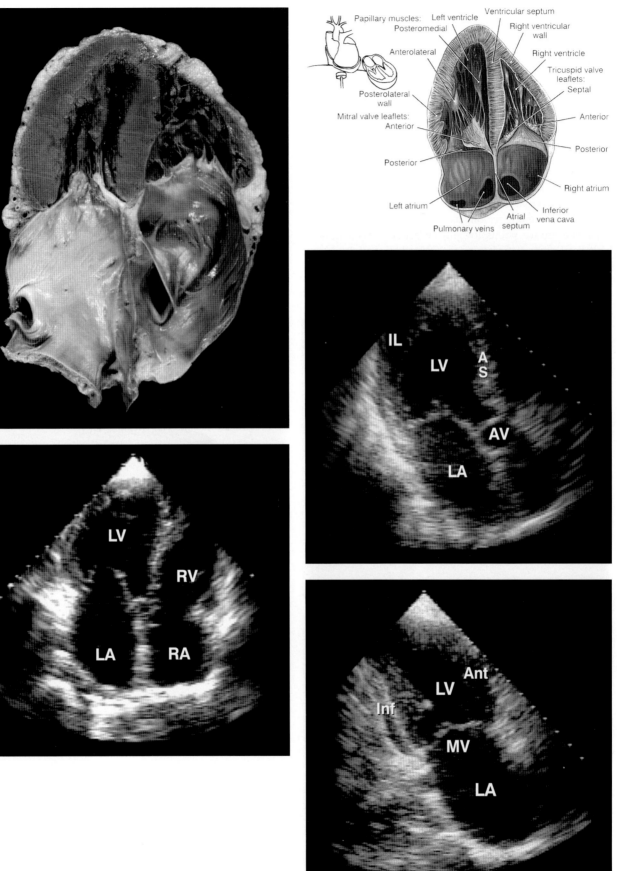

A

B

C

D

Papillary muscles:
Posteromedial
Anterolateral
Posterolateral wall
Mitral valve leaflets:
Anterior
Posterior
Left atrium
Pulmonary veins
Left ventricle
Ventricular septum
Right ventricular wall
Right ventricle
Tricuspid valve leaflets:
Septal
Anterior
Posterior
Right atrium
Inferior vena cava
Atrial septum

hyperinflated lungs. This situation necessitated a search for other locations for imaging the heart and led to the discovery of the subcostal region, a good ultrasonic window in such patients.

We begin the subcostal examination by placing the transducer in the midline or slightly to the patient's right, and the transducer groove is pointed down toward the patient's spine (Fig. 2-1B). The transducer head is tilted inferiorly and slightly toward the patient's right. With this position, the liver parenchyma, hepatic vessels, and short-axis view of the inferior vena cava are obtained. With slight superior tilt of the transducer, the drainage of the hepatic veins into the inferior vena cava can be identified. To record the inferior vena cava along its long axis, the transducer is rotated so that the groove points toward the patient's right flank. The hepatic veins again can be recognized by their draining into the inferior vena cava.

The transducer is tilted further superiorly so that it points roughly between the patient's suprasternal notch and the left supraclavicular fossa. Thus, a tomographic view of the heart is obtained that is nearly similar to the four-chamber view obtained from the parasternal position (Fig. 2-7), except that in this view the apices of the two ventricles can be visualized by tilting the transducer head slightly toward the patient's left. The two atria and especially the atrial septum are best visualized in this section. Although dropout of echoes of the atrial septum in the region of the fossa ovalis may be noted from parasternal and apical transducer positions, the atrial septum can be seen in its entirety from the subcostal position, and it appears intact in almost every examination, without any persistent dropout. Also, atrial septal motion can be well evaluated in this view. For image orientation of this view, we have followed the same format as that for the similar view from the parasternal position so

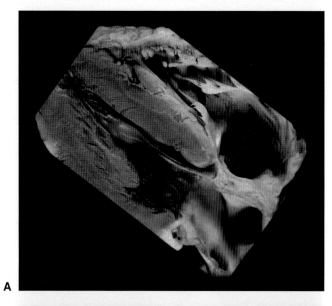

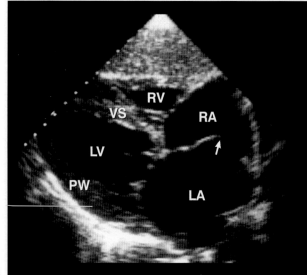

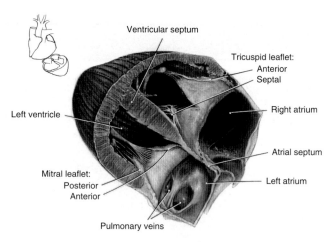

FIG. 2-7. Anatomic sections, drawings, and corresponding two-dimensional echocardiographic images in the subcostal view. **A,B:** Long-axis view.

that in the image the atria are displayed on the right and the cardiac apex on the left.

From this position, the transducer is rotated clockwise and tilted slightly superiorly to visualize the aorta and its relationship to the mitral valve and LV. In this tomographic section, a foreshortened view of the LV long axis is recorded. Both leaflets of the mitral valve and the aortic leaflets as well as the LVOT usually can be well visualized.

Further clockwise rotation and superior tilting of the transducer result in a cardiac cross section (Fig. 2-7C and D). In this view, the LV is visualized in the short axis, with portions of the mitral valve in its cavity. More importantly,

this view is used to show the long axis of the entire RVOT. The tricuspid valve orifice usually appears directly end on. On the video monitor, the heart appears upside down, with the RV inflow and RVOT along the right side of the image, the cross section of the left ventricle to the left, the hepatic tissue anterior, and pulmonary valve inferior.

Another important structure to scan routinely from the subcostal view is the abdominal aorta, which can be imaged accurately in most patients. A prospective study showed that the screening examination detected an occult abdominal aortic aneurysm in 6.5% of hypertensive patients older than 50 years (5).

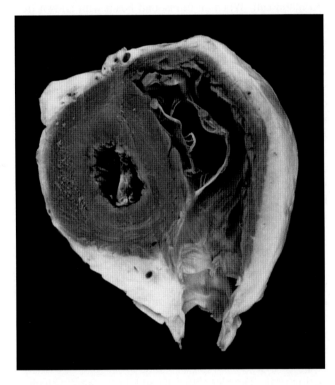

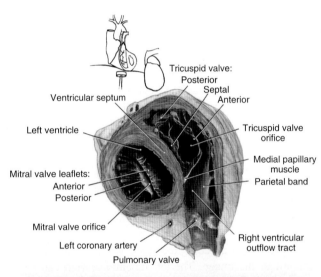

C

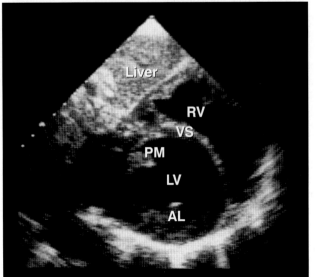

D

FIG. 2-7. *Continued.* **C,D:** Short-axis view. The subcostal view allows better definition of certain cardiac structures, such as the atrial septum, left atrium (*LA*) and right atrium (*RA*), right ventricular (*RV*) free wall, RV outflow tract and pulmonary valve, entrance of the inferior vena cava to the RA, hepatic vein, and abdominal aorta. This view may be the only satisfactory echocardiographic window for patients who have chronic obstructive lung disease and emphysema. *AL,* anterolateral papillary muscle; *PM,* posteromedial papillary muscle; *PW,* posterior wall; *VS,* ventricular septum. (**A** and **C** from ref. 1, with permission.)

Suprasternal Notch Position

For visualization of the left aortic arch in the long axis, the transducer head is positioned in the suprasternal notch (Fig. 2-1B), with the long axis of the transducer to the left and parallel with the trachea and the groove directed toward the right supraclavicular region. With this transducer position (Fig. 2-8A), the ascending aorta, aortic arch, origin of the brachiocephalic vessels, and descending thoracic aorta are visualized. Occasionally, leaflets of the aortic valve also can be seen in the aortic root. The orientation of the image of this view is similar to that seen with a lateral view of an angiogram; thus, the ascending aorta is on the left of the figure and the descending aorta on the right. The right pulmonary artery is visualized in the short axis posterior to the ascending aorta and beneath the aortic arch. Inferior to the right pulmonary artery, the LA can be recorded. For visualization of the long axis of the aorta in the presence of a right aortic arch, the transducer is rotated counterclockwise, with the groove directed toward the right breast.

The short axis of the aortic arch is obtained by rotating the transducer clockwise so that the groove is facing posteriorly toward the patient's trachea (Fig. 2-8B). In this view, the cross section of the ascending aorta appears superiorly and the right pulmonary artery, in its long axis, appears inferiorly. Occasionally, the first bifurcation of the right pulmonary artery can be visualized on the left of the image. By rotating the transducer slightly clockwise and by tilting it toward the patient's left and slightly anteriorly, the distal main pulmonary artery can be visualized. From this position, the left pulmonary artery occasionally can be seen by tilting the transducer posteriorly and to the left.

Inferior to the pulmonary artery is the LA cavity. Immediately beneath the distal part of the right pulmonary artery, the right superior pulmonary vein connects with the LA. The superior vena cava also can be recorded in this view, appearing as an echo-free space alongside the aorta on the left of the image. The left innominate vein can be visualized traversing superior to the aorta to its junction with the superior vena cava. With slight counterclockwise rotation and anterior tilt of the transducer, the long axis of the superior vena cava can be recorded alongside the long axis of the ascending aorta. In this view, the superior vena cava can be scanned to its junction with the RA. This same view of the superior vena cava occasionally can also be obtained with the transducer placed along the upper right sternal border.

M-mode echocardiography complements 2D echocardiography by recording detailed motions of cardiac structures. It is best derived with guidance from a 2D echocardiographic image by placing a cursor through the desired structure (Fig. 2-9). M-mode is used for the measurement of dimensions and is essential for the display of subtle motion abnormalities of specific cardiac structures. Methods for measuring cardiac dimensions from M-mode are shown in Fig. 2-10. Normal values for cardiac dimensions in adults are well established. Gender-specific reference M-mode values in adults were determined from a healthy subset of the Framingham Heart Study (6,7). These values are given in the Appendix.

DOPPLER ECHOCARDIOGRAPHY

Doppler echocardiography measures blood-flow velocities in the heart and great vessels and is based on the *Doppler effect*, which was described by the Austrian physicist Christian Doppler in 1842 (8). The Doppler effect states that sound frequency increases as a sound source moves toward the observer and decreases as the source moves away. In the circulatory system, the moving target is the red blood cell. When an ultrasound beam with known frequency (*fo*) is transmitted to the heart or great vessels, it is reflected by the red blood cells. The frequency of the reflected ultrasound waves (*fr*) increases when the red blood cells are moving toward the source of ultrasound. Conversely, the frequency of reflected ultrasound waves decreases when the red blood cells are moving away from the source. The change in frequency between the transmitted sound and the reflected sound is termed the *frequency shift* (*Δf*) or *Doppler shift* (= *fr* − *fo*). The Doppler shift depends on the transmitted frequency (*fo*), the velocity of the moving target (*v*), and the angle (*θ*) between the ultrasound beam and the direction of the moving target as expressed in the *Doppler equation* (Fig. 2-11):

$$\Delta f = \frac{2 \; fo \; \text{x} \; v \; \text{x} \; \cos \; \theta}{c}$$

where *c* is the speed of sound in blood (1,560 m/s). If the angle *θ* is 0 degree (i.e., the ultrasound beam is parallel with the direction of blood flow), the maximal frequency shift is measured because the cosine of 0 degree is 1. Note that as angle *θ* increases, the corresponding cosine becomes progressively less than 1, and this will result in underestimation of the Doppler shift (*Δf*) and, hence, peak velocity, because peak flow velocity is derived from *Δf* by rearranging the Doppler equation:

$$v = \frac{c}{2} \times \frac{\Delta f}{fo}$$

Blood-flow velocities determined by Doppler echocardiography are used in turn to derive various hemodynamic data (see Chapter 6).

The most common uses of Doppler echocardiography are in the *pulsed-* and *continuous-wave* forms (Fig. 2-12). Both modalities are necessary parts of a Doppler echocardiographic examination and provide complementary information. In the pulsed-wave mode, a single ultrasound crystal sends and receives sound beams. The crystal emits a short burst of ultrasound at a certain frequency [*pulse repetition frequency* (PRF)]. The ultrasound is reflected from moving red blood cells and is received by the same crystal. There-

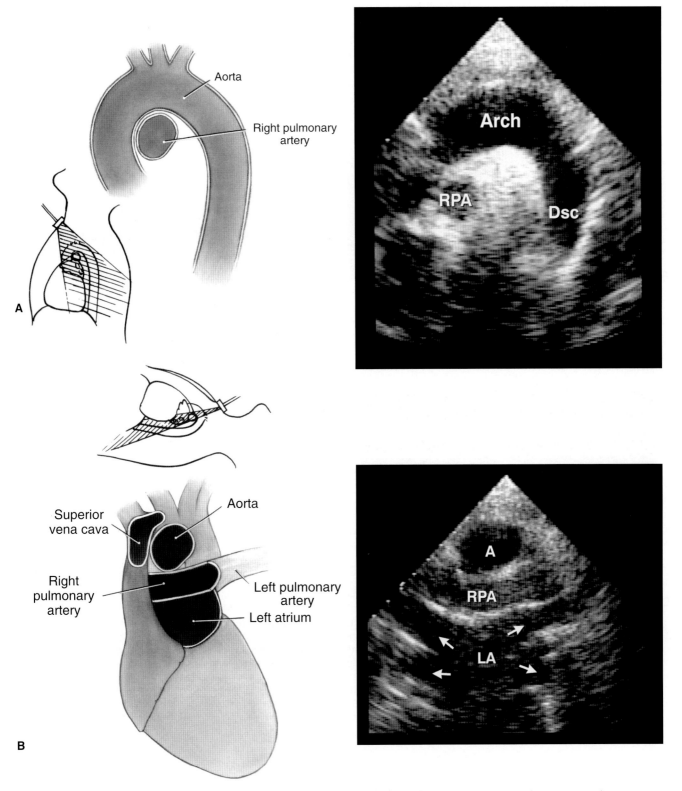

FIG. 2-8. Drawing and corresponding two-dimensional echocardiographic images of suprasternal notch long-axis **(A)** and short-axis **(B)** views. **A:** This transducer position allows visualization of the ascending aorta, aortic arch (*Arch*), origin of the brachiocephalic vessels, and descending thoracic aorta (*Dsc*). *RPA*, right pulmonary artery. **B:** The short-axis view of the aortic arch is obtained by rotating the transducer clockwise, which also allows visualization of the RPA in its long-axis format, located inferiorly to the aortic arch (*A*). Inferior to RPA is the left atrial (*LA*) cavity with connections of the four pulmonary veins (*arrows*). The superior vena cava is visualized by further clockwise rotation; it appears along the right side of the aorta.

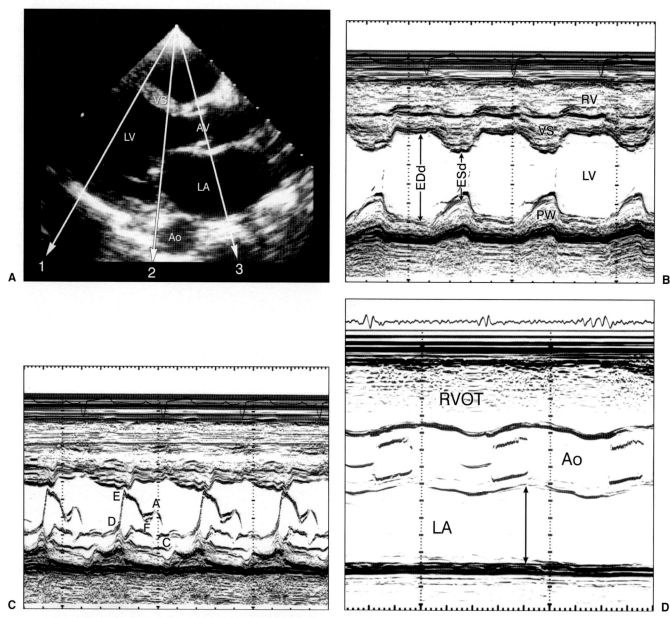

FIG. 2-9. A: An M-mode cursor is placed along different levels (*1*, ventricular; *2*, mitral valve; *3*, aortic valve level, in **A–D**) of the heart, with parasternal long-axis 2D echocardiographic guidance. **B–D:** Representative normal M-mode echocardiograms at the midventricular, mitral valve, and aortic valve levels, respectively. *Arrows* in **B** indicate end-diastolic (*EDd*) and end-systolic dimensions (*ESd*) of the left ventricle (*LV*). **C:** The M-mode echocardiogram of the anterior mitral leaflet: *A*, peak of late opening with atrial systole; *C*, closure of the mitral valve; *D*, end-systole before mitral valve opening; *E*, peak of early opening; *F*, middiastolic closure. The *double-headed arrow* in **D** indicates the dimension of the left atrium (*LA*) at end systole. *Ao*, aorta; *AV*, aortic valve; *PW*, posterior wall; *RVOT*, right ventricular outflow tract; *VS*, ventricular septum.

fore, the maximal frequency shift that can be determined by pulsed-wave Doppler is one-half of the PRF, called the *Nyquist frequency*. If the frequency shift is higher than the Nyquist frequency, *aliasing* occurs; that is, the Doppler spectrum is cut off at the Nyquist frequency, and the remaining frequency shift is recorded on the opposite side of baseline. Pulsed-wave Doppler measures flow velocities at a specific location within a "sample volume." The PRF varies inversely with the depth of the sample volume: The shallower the location of the sample volume, the higher the PRF and Nyquist frequency. In other words, higher velocities can be recorded without aliasing by pulsed-wave Doppler if the sample volume is closer to the transducer.

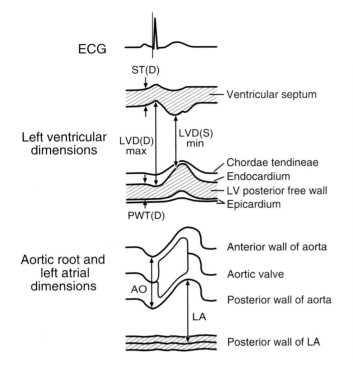

ECG

ST(D)

Ventricular septum

Left ventricular dimensions

LVD(D) max

LVD(S) min

Chordae tendineae
Endocardium
LV posterior free wall
Epicardium

PWT(D)

Aortic root and left atrial dimensions

AO

Anterior wall of aorta

Aortic valve

Posterior wall of aorta

LA

Posterior wall of LA

FIG. 2-10. Diagram of M-mode of the left ventricle (*LV*), aortic root, and left atrium (*LA*). The LV internal dimension (*LVD*) at end diastole (*D*) was measured at the onset of the QRS complex, and systolic (*S*) measurement was done at the maximal excursion of the ventricular septum, which occurs normally before the maximal excursion of the posterior wall. These measurements correspond, respectively, to the maximal (*max*) and minimal (*min*) internal dimensions between the ventricular septum and the posterobasal LV free wall endocardium. Septal thickness (*ST*) and posterior wall thickness (*PWT*) were measured at end diastole (*D*) at the onset of the QRS complex. The aortic root dimension (*AO*) was measured at the onset of the QRS complex from the leading edge to the leading edge of the aortic walls. The LA dimension was measured at end systole as the largest distance between the posterior aortic wall and the center of the line denoting the posterior LA wall. Their normal values are given in the Appendix. (From Gardin JM, Henry WL, Savage DD, Ware JH, Burn C, Borer JS. Echocardiographic measurements in normal subjects: evaluation of an adult population without clinically apparent heart disease. *J Clin Ultrasound* 1979;7:439–447, with permission.)

In the continuous-wave mode, the transducer has two crystals: one to send and the other to receive the reflected ultrasound waves continuously. Therefore, the maximal frequency shift that can be recorded by continuous-wave Doppler is not limited by the PRF or the Nyquist phenomenon. Unlike pulsed-wave Doppler, continuous-wave Doppler measures all the frequency shifts (i.e., velocities) present along its beam path; hence, it is used to detect and to record the highest flow velocity available. Continuous-wave Doppler usually is performed by using a nonimaging

transducer. This small transducer is more suitable for interrogation of a high-velocity jet from multiple windows. An image-guided continuous-wave examination may be necessary when the direction of blood flow is eccentric or the amount of desired blood flow is trivial. The characteristics and clinical applications of these Doppler modalities are summarized in Table 2-2. Their representative recordings are demonstrated in Fig. 2-13. Table 2-3 shows the mean and range of maximal velocities recorded from normal subjects by Doppler echocardiography.

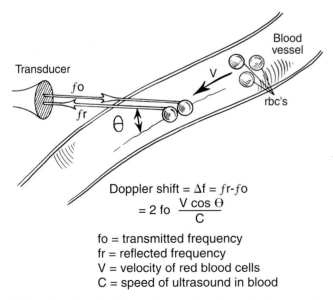

Doppler shift = $\Delta f = fr - fo$
$$= 2\, fo\, \frac{V \cos \theta}{C}$$

fo = transmitted frequency
fr = reflected frequency
V = velocity of red blood cells
C = speed of ultrasound in blood

FIG. 2-11. Drawing illustrating the Doppler effect (see text for explanation). *rbc's*, red blood cells.

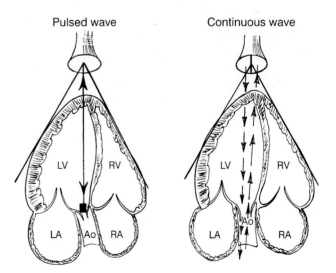

FIG. 2-12. Drawing of pulsed-wave and continuous-wave Doppler echocardiography from the apical view (see text for explanation). *Ao*, aorta.

TABLE 2-2. *Comparison of pulsed-wave and continuous-wave Doppler*

Pulsed-wave	Continuous-wave
Measures specific blood-flow velocity by placing the "sample volume" at the region of interest	Measures blood-flow velocities along the axis of the entire ultrasound beam (range ambiguity)
Maximal measurable velocity without aliasing is usually < 2 m/s	Able to measure high velocities ≤ 9 m/s
Performed by duplex transducer (two-dimensional and Doppler)	Performed by duplex as well as by nonimaging transducer
Suited for measuring low velocity at a particular intracardiac location	Suited for measuring peak velocities (i.e., gradients) across intracardiac orifices
Clinical applications: used for determining	Clinical applications: used for determining
LVOT velocity and TVI	Peak-flow velocity and TVI
Volume measurements	Valvular pressure gradient
Diastolic function/filling	Pressure half-time
Mitral inflow velocity	Dynamic LVOT gradient
Pulmonary and hepatic vein velocities	Pulmonary pressure
Location of flow disturbance	dp/dt
Mitral annulus velocity (DTI)	

LVOT, left ventricular outflow tract; TVI, time velocity integral; dp/dt, the rate of ventricular pressure rise obtained from mitral or tricuspid regurgitation Doppler signal. DTI, Doppler tissue imaging.

COLOR-FLOW IMAGING

Color-flow imaging, based on pulsed-wave Doppler principles, displays intracavitary blood flow in three colors (red, blue, and green) or their combinations, depending on the velocity, direction, and extent of turbulence (9). It uses multiple sampling sites along multiple ultrasound beams (*multigated*). At each sampling site (or *gate*), the frequency shift is measured, converted to a digital format, automatically correlated (*autocorrelation*) with a preset color scheme, and displayed as color flow superimposed on 2D imaging (Fig. 2-14). Blood flow directed toward the transducer has a pos-

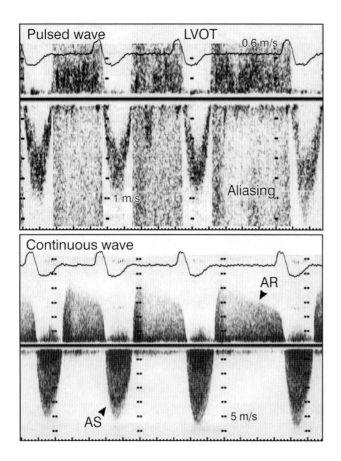

FIG. 2-13. Representative pulsed-wave and continuous-wave Doppler spectra from a 60-year-old patient who has aortic stenosis and regurgitation (*AR*). The pulsed-wave Doppler sample volume is placed at the left ventricular outflow tract (*LVOT*), and the Doppler spectrum shows systolic LVOT velocity and turbulent diastolic signal of aortic regurgitation recorded on both sides of the baseline. Although AR flow is toward the transducer, *aliasing* (velocity wraparound) occurs because of high velocity (4–5 m/s). Continuous-wave Doppler detects flow velocities all along its beam (LVOT and aortic valve) and is able to record high velocity. Systolic flow away from the transducer (spectrum below the baseline) represents flow across the stenotic aortic valve (*AS*) and diastolic flow is from AR. Peak AS velocity across the stenotic valve varies (5.0–5.5 m/s) because of atrial fibrillation.

TABLE 2-3. *Normal maximal velocities (m/s): Doppler measurements*

	Children		Adults	
	Mean	Range	Mean	Range
Mitral flow	1.00	0.8–1.3	0.90	0.6–1.3
Tricuspid flow	0.60	0.5–0.8	0.50	0.3–0.7
Pulmonary artery	0.90	0.7–1.1	0.75	0.6–0.9
LVOT	1.00	0.7–1.2	0.90	0.7–1.1
Aorta	1.50	1.2–1.8	1.35	1.0–1.7

LVOT, left ventricle outflow tract.
From ref. 8, with permission.

itive frequency shift (i.e., reflected ultrasound frequency is higher than the transmitted frequency) and is color-coded in shades of red. Blood flow directed away from the transducer has a negative frequency shift and is color-coded in shades of blue. Each color has multiple shades, and the lighter shades within each primary color are assigned to higher velocities within the Nyquist limit. When flow velocity is higher than the Nyquist frequency limit, color aliasing occurs and is depicted as a color reversal. With each multiple of the Nyquist limit, the color repeatedly reverts to the opposite color. *Turbulence* (i.e., blood moving in multiple directions with multiple velocities) is characterized by the presence of *variance*. The degree of the variance from the mean velocity can be coded as a variance color, usually a shade of green. Therefore, abnormal blood flow is easily recognized by combinations of multiple colors according to the directions, velocities, and degree of turbulence (Fig. 2-15). The width and size of abnormal intracavitary flows are used to semiquantitate the degree of valvular regurgitation or cardiac shunt.

Because the types and shades of color-flow imaging are determined by the direction and velocity of blood flow, color-flow imaging is an excellent way to visualize simultaneously all the intracavitary blood flow velocities. Color

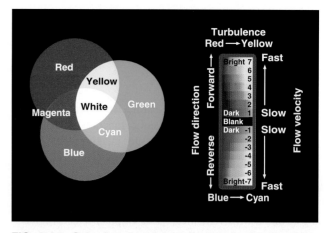

FIG. 2-15. Color-flow imaging is displayed using the three primary colors (red, blue, and green) and their combinations based on the velocity, direction, and turbulence of flow. (From ref. 9, with permission.)

M-mode helps to assess the timing and peak velocities of blood flow. Color-flow imaging is also an essential part of hemodynamic assessment. An important example is the calculation of flow rate at proximal isovelocity surface area (PISA) to determine mitral or aortic regurgitant volume and regurgitant orifice area (10). Blood flow converges toward a regurgitation orifice with accelerating velocities, forming multiple isovelocity hemispheric areas. When an isovelocity exceeds the Nyquist limit of a chosen (designated color) flow map, the color of the converging flow proximal to the regurgitant orifice changes from blue to red-orange or vice versa, depending on the direction of flow. As the Nyquist limit for proximal flow is lowered, the PISA is farther away from the regurgitant orifice (Fig. 2-16). The application of this method is discussed in Chapter 9. Color-flow imaging

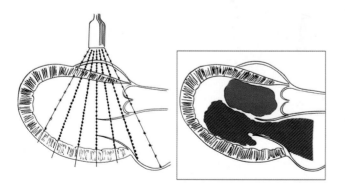

FIG. 2-14. Drawing illustrating how color-flow imaging is performed and displayed. *Dots* indicate multiple sampling sites (*gates*). The frequency shift measured at each gate is automatically correlated (*autocorrelation*) and converted to a preset color scheme (red for flow toward and blue for flow away from the transducer).

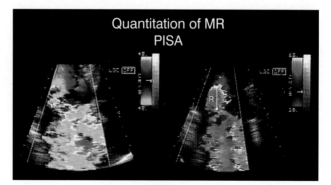

FIG. 2-16. Color-flow imaging of mitral regurgitation (*MR*) with two different aliasing velocities. **Left:** The aliasing velocity is 48 cm/s to either direction. The radius of the proximal isovelocity surface area (*PISA*) is small. **Right:** Zero baseline was shifted downward to make the negative aliasing velocity lower (28 cm/s). The color of blood flow proximal to the regurgitant orifice changed from blue to yellow-orange farther away from the orifice, which gives a larger PISA radius (*R*).

also is used in color M-mode of the mitral inflow for determination of diastolic function and the rate of flow propagation (see Chapter 5).

TISSUE DOPPLER

Movement and velocities of cardiac structures are related to underlying systolic and diastolic function of the heart. Tissue Doppler (or Doppler tissue imaging) provides a means for measuring and displaying cardiac wall motion velocities. Tissue velocities are lower (5 to 20 cm/s) than blood-flow velocities. Although tissue velocities with low frequency are filtered during conventional Doppler recording of blood-flow velocities, tissue Doppler rejects high frequencies to measure wall motion velocities. Tissue Doppler velocities can be recorded directly or can be autocorrelated to a color scheme. Isaaz et al. (11) were able to obtain a pulsed Doppler profile of the LV posterior wall, and this concept was expanded by McDicken et al. (12), who developed a prototype of color Doppler velocity display of myocardial wall dynamics. Since these reports, tissue Doppler imaging of normal and abnormal wall motion has been reported (see Chapter 4). Several investigators have used tissue Doppler to evaluate regional and global diastolic function in the setting of acute ischemia and diastolic heart failure (13), and it has been noted that mitral annulus velocity measured by tissue Doppler is an indicator of myocardial relaxation, relatively unaffected by preload or afterload (see Chapter 5). This property of mitral annulus velocity appears to be useful in estimating LA pressure in conjunction with mitral inflow E velocity. Further investigation is needed to establish the clinical application of this unique technology.

REFERENCES

1. Tajik AJ, Seward JB, Hagler DJ, Mair DD, Lie JT. Two-dimensional real-time ultrasonic imaging of the heart and great vessels: technique, image orientation, structure identification, and validation. *Mayo Clin Proc* 1978;53:271–303.
2. Bansal RC, Tajik AJ, Seward JB, Offord KP. Feasibility of detailed two-dimensional echocardiographic examinations in adults: prospective study of 200 patients. *Mayo Clin Proc* 1980;55:291–308.
3. Edwards WD, Tajik AJ, Seward JB. Standardized nomenclature and anatomic basis for regional tomographic analysis of the heart. *Mayo Clin Proc* 1981;56:479–497.
4. Henry WL, DeMaria A, Gramiak R, et al. Report of the American Society of Echocardiography Committee on Nomenclature and Standards in two-dimensional echocardiography. *Circulation* 1980;62:212–215.
5. Spittell PC, Ehrsam JE, Anderson L, Seward JB. Screening for abdominal aortic aneurysm during transthoracic echocardiography in a hypertensive patient population. *J Am Soc Echocardiogr* 1997;10:722–727.
6. Lauer MS, Larson MG, Levy D. Gender-specific reference M-mode values in adults: population-derived values with consideration of the impact of height. *J Am Coll Cardiol* 1995;26:1039–1046.
7. Vasan RS, Larson MG, Benjamin EJ, Levy D. Echocardiographic reference values for aortic root size: The Framingham Heart Study. *J Am Soc Echocardiogr* 1995;8:793–800.
8. Hatle L, Angelsen B. *Doppler ultrasound in cardiology: physical principles and clinical applications*, 2nd ed. Philadelphia: Lea & Febiger, 1985.
9. Omoto R, Kasai C. Physics and instrumentation of Doppler color flow mapping. *Echocardiography* 1987;4:467–483.
10. Enriquez-Sarano M, Sinak LJ, Tajik AJ, Bailey KR, Seward JB. Changes in effective regurgitant orifice throughout systole in patients with mitral valve prolapse: a clinical study using the proximal isovelocity surface area method. *Circulation* 1995;92:2951–2958.
11. Isaaz K, Thompson A, Ethevenot G, Cloez JL, Brembilla B, Pernot C. Doppler echocardiographic measurement of low velocity motion of the left ventricular posterior wall. *Am J Cardiol* 1989;64:66–75.
12. McDicken WN, Sutherland GR, Moran CM, Gordon LN. Colour Doppler velocity imaging of the myocardium. *Ultrasound Med Biol* 1992;18:651–654.
13. Fernandez MAG, Zamorano J, Azevedo J. *Doppler tissue imaging echocardiography*. Madrid: McGraw-Hill, 1998.

CHAPTER 3

Transesophageal Echocardiography

In 1987, transesophageal echocardiography (TEE) was introduced clinically in the United States (1). It has altered the diagnostic strategy for various cardiovascular diseases and, in many clinical situations, has replaced the need for other imaging techniques. The main reason for the clinical success of TEE is that it provides, with superb clarity and resolution, easily understandable images of cardiovascular abnormalities. Furthermore, TEE is relatively easy to perform and is without significant complications, even in the most critical patients. It has all the capabilities of transthoracic echocardiography (TTE), so that cardiac anatomy, function, hemodynamics, and blood flow can be evaluated reliably. Before the application of TEE, echocardiography was used as a screening tool in many clinical circumstances, and other techniques were used to substantiate a presumed echocardiographic diagnosis. Currently, definitive surgical repair of mitral valve regurgitation, aortic dissection, or removal of an intracardiac tumor occurs on the basis of a complete TEE examination (2–4). In this clinical context, TEE will continue to have a major role in the management of virtually all cardiovascular diseases. Today, approximately 5% to 10% of patients who undergo TTE need an additional examination with TEE. Since the first edition of this manual, the technology of TEE has matured, with multiplane imaging as the state-of-the-art transducer. Most of the discussion in this chapter is based on multiplane TEE. As in the first edition of *The Echo Manual*, TEE is discussed throughout as part of a comprehensive echocardiographic examination.

CLINICAL APPLICATIONS

The indications for 15,381 TEE procedures (excluding intraoperative TEE) performed at Mayo Clinic from November 1987 to May 1997 are shown in Table 3-1. The distribution of indications for TEE varies from institution to institution, depending on patient population. The most common indication at our institution has been the evaluation of a potential cardiac source of embolism. TEE is now considered essential in the evaluation of the mitral valve, left atrium (LA) or LA appendage thrombus, atrial septal defects (especially sinus venosus type), endocarditis and its complications, thoracic aortic lesions, and critically ill patients (5–10). Other clinical applications of TEE are discussed in detail in appropriate chapters.

PREPARATION AND POTENTIAL COMPLICATIONS

Although safe, TEE is a semiinvasive procedure that can be uncomfortable in unprepared patients. Patients should be informed about why TEE is performed, and the entire procedure should be explained, including rare side effects such as laryngospasm, transient throat pain, aspiration, hypotension, hypertension, tachycardia, and even the rare risk of death. The patient should fast for at least 4 hours before undergoing TEE, and a history of dysphagia or esophageal pathology should be evaluated before TEE (Table 3-2). If the patient has dentures, they should be removed. Every patient should have an intravenous access (preferably a three-way stopcock) for administration of contrast agent or medications.

Immediately before intubation of the transesophageal probe, lidocaine spray (10%) is used to anesthetize the posterior pharynx locally. Although lidocaine rarely causes a problem, locally administered lidocaine has been reported to cause central nervous system toxic effects in patients who have congestive heart failure or diminished liver function (11). Toxic methemoglobinemia also has been reported after use of a benzocaine spray. In that report, a patient had a methemoglobin level of 47.2% and oxygen desaturation after benzocaine spray. Treatment is with methylene blue, 1 mg/kg as a 1% solution administered over 5 minutes (12). A drying agent, glycopyrrolate (Robinul, 0.2 mg), minimizes oral secretions and the possibility of aspiration during the examination. Because glycopyrrolate is an atropine-like product, it may increase heart rate, especially in patients with atrial fibrillation. Use

TABLE 3-1. *Indications for transesophageal echocardiography at Mayo Clinic from November 1987 to May 1997: 15,381 procedures*

Indication	Procedures (%)
Source of embolism	42
Valvular disease	14
Native	10
Prosthetic	4
Suspected endocarditis	11
Precardioversion	6
Evaluation of aorta	5
Congenital heart disease	5
Intracardiac mass	2
Critically ill patient	1
Pulmonary hypertension	1
Other	13

TABLE 3-3. *Complications in 15,381 transesophageal echocardiographic examinations*

Complications	No. (%)
Hypoxia	99 (0.6)
Hypotension	78 (0.5)
Hypertension	37 (0.2)
PSVT	29 (0.2)
NSVT	10 (0.1)
Hematemesis	18 (0.1)
Laryngospasm	16 (0.1)
Esophageal tear	3 (<0.02)
Death	2 (<0.01)

PSVT, paroxysmal supraventricular tachycardia; NSVT, nonsustained ventricular tachycardia.

of the short-acting sedative midazolam (Versed), 1 to 10 mg (mean dose, 3.6 ± 2.3 mg), may be necessary to make the TEE examination more comfortable for the patient. This agent should be used with caution, however, in debilitated or elderly patients because of potential respiratory suppression. Midazolam can be reversed rapidly with flumazenil (0.2 mg intravenously). In young patients, meperidine hydrochloride (Demerol), 25 to 50 mg, also may be used to help alleviate the gag reflex and provide additional sedation. Prophylaxis for subacute bacterial endocarditis is not necessary or generally used even in patients with a prosthetic valve [13]. Occasionally, in a critically ill patient, it has been necessary to paralyze the patient if agitated. A nasogastric or endotracheal tube usually does not interfere with intubation of a TEE probe or with the acquisition of satisfactory images. Side effects and complications from 15,381 TEE examinations performed at the Mayo Clinic are shown in Table 3-3.

TABLE 3-2. *Preparation for transesophageal echocardiography*

Preparation
  Inquiry about history of dysphagia or esophageal abnormality
  NPO (fasting) for ≥ 4 hr
  Local anesthesia, lidocaine spray (10%)
  Intravenous access with three-way stopcock
Medications
  Drying agent 2–3 min before examination (optional); glycopyrrolate (Robinul, 0.2 mg intravenous)
Sedation
  Midazolam hydrochloride (Versed), 1–10 mg
  Meperidine hydrochloride (Demerol), 25–50 mg
  Paralyzing agent for agitated patient on mechanical ventilator
  Flumazenil (Romazicon), 0.2 mg, if needed for rapid reversal of midazolam hydrochloride

NPO, nothing by mouth.

INSTRUMENTATION

The TEE probe is a modification of a gastroesophageal endoscopy probe, with a 3- to 7.5-MHz ultrasound transducer at the tip (Fig. 3-1). It can be maneuvered to various positions in the esophagus and the stomach, from which the heart and other structures can be visualized. The width of the adult transducer tip is 10 to 14 mm and miniaturized to 4 mm for pediatric use. The multiplane transducer rotates 180 degrees. Rotation of the transducer usually is accomplished by a finger-pressure–sensitive switch at the proximal operator end. The scope tip also can be anteflexed or retroflexed or moved side to side by larger rotary knobs at the proximal end (Fig. 3-1). When performed electively, the examination begins with the patient in the left lateral decubitus position. The procedure room is equipped with oral suction, oxygen supply, pulse oximeter, and cardiopulmonary resuscitation capabilities. In critically ill patients for whom transfer is difficult, the examination is performed at the bedside. When the patient is mechanically ventilated, the TEE probe often is introduced with the patient supine.

We use a bite guard to protect the TEE scope unless the patient is edentulous. At scope introduction, the imaging surface of the transducer faces the tongue, which directs the ultrasound beam anteriorly toward the heart when the probe is in the esophagus. Normally, a digital technique is used for esophageal intubation. At probe introduction, the posterior portion of the tongue is pressed with the left index finger to minimize tongue movement, and the tip of the transducer is placed over the left index finger to a position at the center of the tongue. After the transducer is in the correct position, the left index finger is placed over the tip of the probe and pressed downward toward the tongue. The tip of the transducer is advanced smoothly and slowly posteriorly toward the esophagus. At that time, the patient is asked to swallow. The tip of the TEE transducer should be advanced into the esophagus without force or significant resistance. The tip of the scope is advanced about 30 cm from the incisors to obtain midesophagus views.

in preparing patients for TEE and in assisting the physician during the examination (14). The role of the sonographer or assistant in TEE is summarized in Table 3-4. In our laboratory, a registered nurse or nurse sonographer coordinates and assists with TEE examinations. Because of the semiinvasive nature of TEE, the skills of a registered nurse are preferred for closely monitoring the patient, that is, for obtaining vital signs; administering medications; inserting intravenous catheters; and using suction, oxygen, or other

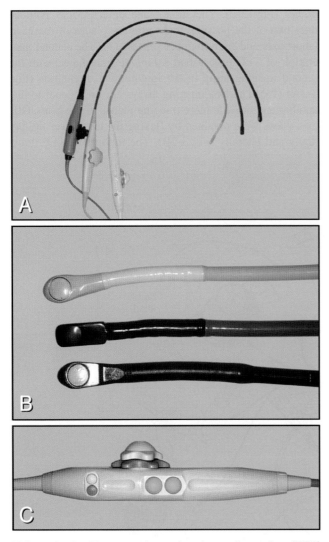

FIG. 3-1. A: Transesophageal echocardiography (TEE) probes from three different ultrasound units. **B:** Tip of multiplane TEE probes with a circular transducer that rotates. Note the different tip configurations of three different probes. **C:** Operator's end of a multiplane TEE probe; dials and knobs allow the operator to rotate the transducer and to manipulate the probe.

TRAINING OF PHYSICIANS AND THE ROLE OF SONOGRAPHERS

TEE complements the TTE examination. Therefore, it is mandatory that a physician who performs TEE has TTE competency [level II American Society of Echocardiography (ASE) training or greater], which includes personal performance of more than 300 surface echocardiograms. The physician also needs to learn esophageal intubation under the supervision of an endoscopist or other echocardiologists experienced in TEE procedure. We consider a minimum of 50 esophageal intubations necessary to provide adequate intubation training.

The sonographer or trained assistant has an essential role

TABLE 3-4. *Summary of the role of the sonographer/assistant in transesophageal echocardiography (TEE)*

Before procedure
  Preparation of equipment and supplies
    Assemble supplies
      Medications, normal saline flushes, and contrast medium
      Intravenous supplies (angiocatheter, three-way stopcock)
      Lidocaine spray and tongue blade
      Scope lubricant: lubricating jelly or viscous lidocaine
      Gloves, safety glasses, TEE probe, and bite block
    Maintain and check suction, oxygen, and basic life-support equipment
  Patient preparation
    Confirm that patient has had no oral intake for 4–6 hr before TEE
    Obtain brief history of drug allergies and current medications
    Explain procedure to patient
    Obtain baseline vital signs and monitor rhythm
    Remove patient's dentures, oral prostheses, and eyeglasses
    Establish intravenous catheter for administration of medications
    Place patient in the left lateral decubitus position with wedge support and safety restraints
    Assist patient during esophageal intubation, such as head position, breathing, and reassurance
  Drugs
    Endocarditis prophylaxis: American Heart Association recommendations
    Pharyngeal anesthesia: lidocaine 10% spray
    Drying agent: glycopyrrolate (Robinul)
    Sedative: midazolam hydrochloride (Versed), meperidine hydrochloride (Demerol)
During procedure
  Position and maintain bite block
  Monitor vital signs: rhythm, respiration, blood pressure, and oxygen saturation
  Use oral suction if necessary
  Have basic life-support equipment available
After procedure
  Assist patient during recovery period
  Remove intravenous catheter
  Instruct patient not to drive for 12 hr if sedation was used
  Record vital signs and patient's condition on dismissal
  Arrange for escort if patient is not completely recovered
  Clean scope with enzyme solution and glutaraldehyde disinfectant

Modified from ref. 14, with permission.

emergency equipment. A properly trained assistant can perform these functions except for the administration of intravenous medications.

COMPARISON OF MONOPLANE, BIPLANE, AND MULTIPLANE TEE

The first generation of TEE transducers was capable of producing only one tomographic imaging plane (mono-

plane) (Fig. 3-2). The monoplane device could produce only two of the possible three primary planes of the heart (short-axis and four-chamber planes) (1). The second generation of TEE probes had a *biplane* transducer, with the second imaging array in the longitudinal orientation (Fig. 3-3A) (15). The two imaging arrays are orthogonal to one another and provide more imaging planes of the heart. Off-axis views were obtained by flexing the transducer tip medially and laterally (Fig 3-3B). The multiplane TEE trans-

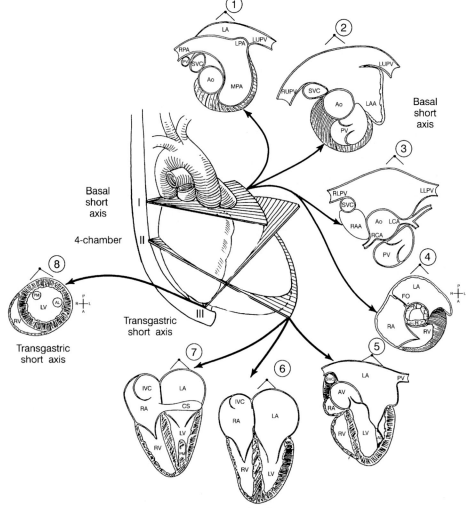

FIG. 3-2. Primary horizontal (cross-sectional) tomographic views from monoplane transesophageal echocardiography (TEE). Multiple tomographic planes are obtained by various transducer positions and angulation. Schematic images are shown with the transducer on the top. Basal short-axis planes (*I*) are obtained initially, usually with the transducer tip 25 to 30 cm from the incisors. Four-chamber planes (*II*) are obtained by retroflexion or slight advancement of the endoscope tip from position 1 (about 30 to 35 cm from the incisors). Transgastric short-axis planes (*III*) are obtained from the fundus of the stomach (35 to 40 cm from the incisors). *AL*, anterolateral papillary muscle; *Ao*, aorta; *AV*, aortic valve; *CS*, coronary sinus; *FO*, foramen ovale; *IVC*, inferior vena cava; *L*, left coronary cusp; *LAA*, left atrial appendage; *LCA*, left main coronary artery; *LLPV*, left lower pulmonary vein; *LPA*, left pulmonary artery; *LUPV*, left upper pulmonary vein; *MPA*, main pulmonary artery; *N*, noncoronary cusp; *PM*, posteromedial papillary muscle; *PV*, pulmonary valve; *R*, right coronary cusp; *RCA*, right coronary artery; *RLPV*, right lower pulmonary vein; *RPA*, right pulmonary artery; *RUPV*, right upper pulmonary vein; *SVC*, superior vena cava. (From ref. 1, with permission.)

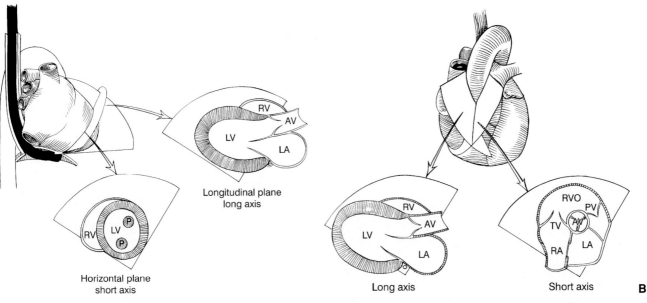

A

Longitudinal plane
long axis

Horizontal plane
short axis

Long axis

Short axis

B

FIG. 3-3. **A:** Drawing of horizontal and longitudinal transgastric views by transesophageal echocardiography (TEE). The transgastric short-axis view obtained with a horizontal array is displayed with a transducer artifact to the bottom of the video screen. The result is a view compatible with a parasternal short-axis view of the left ventricle (*LV*). From this orientation, switching to a longitudinal array results in a long-axis view of the LV. For optimal long-axis orientation of the scanning array, slight leftward or rightward flexion and rotation of the tip of the transducer may be necessary. Rotation of the scope medially images the right ventricle (*RV*) inflow. Anteflexion of the scope produces an apical long-axis equivalent view of the LV and aortic valve (*AV*) and mitral valve. **B:** Drawing of long- and short-axis tomographic views by the longitudinal plane of biplane TEE. The longitudinal array can be reoriented from the sagittal plane of the thoracic planes that are in the long axis or short axis of the heart. This manipulation requires leftward and rightward flexion of the tip of the endoscope from the neutral position. Leftward flexion results in a long-axis view of the heart, whereas rightward flexion orients the longitudinal plane into the short axis of the heart. *AV*, aortic valve; *P*, papillary muscle; *PV*, pulmonary valve; *RVO*, RV outflow; *TV*, tricuspid valve. (From ref. 15, with permission.)

ducer consists of a single array of crystals that can be rotated electronically or mechanically around the long-axis of the ultrasound beam in an arc of 180 degrees (Fig. 3-4). With rotation of the transducer array, the multiplane TEE produces a continuum of transverse and longitudinal image planes. In contrast to the biplane technology, multiplane TEE produces intermediate, transitional, and off-axis images more readily between the primary planes and considerably less lateral and medial flexion of the tip of the scope.

Multiplane TEE

Multiplane images are identified by an icon to indicate the degree of transducer rotation (Fig. 3-5). Such a designation helps the operator to understand the orientation of the ultrasound beam and to conduct the TEE examination more efficiently. The transverse esophageal plane is designated as 0 degrees. The longitudinal esophageal plane is designated as 90 degrees. The multiplane TEE transducer can be rotated in a continuum throughout 180 degrees, resulting in versatility of the examination and ease of understanding.

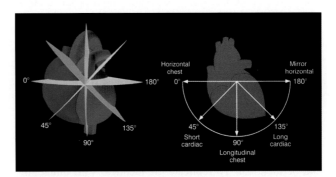

FIG. 3-4. Array rotations of selected degrees (0, 45, 90, 135, and 180 degrees) permit a logical sequence of standard transducer orientations and resultant images. Such a display helps the examiner acquire the desired views: 0-degree transverse orientation, which is horizontal to the chest at the midesophageal level; 45-degree short-axis orientation to the base of the heart from the midesophagus; 90-degree longitudinal orientation, which is in the sagittal plane of the body; 135-degree long-axis orientation to the heart from the midesophagus; and 180-degree rotation, which produces a mirror-image transverse plane. (From ref. 9, with permission.)

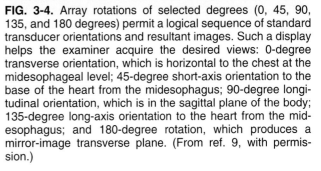

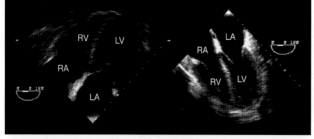

A

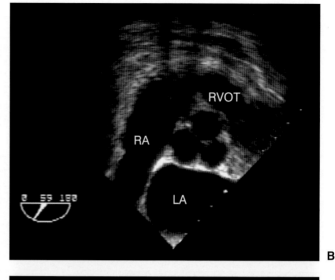

B

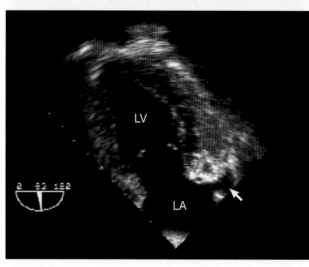

C

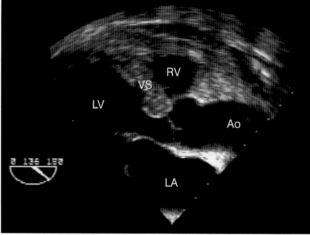

D

FIG. 3-5. Four multiplane transesophageal echocardiographic (TEE) images obtained by rotating the transducer array from 0 degrees to 135 degrees. The icon **(in the corner)** indicates the position of the transducer. **A:** 0 degrees, four-chamber view (with retroflexion of the transducer tip); two different image orientations on the screen are shown: apex-up **(left)** and apex-down **(right)** views. **B:** 59 degrees (45 to 60 degrees), short-axis view of the aortic valve. **C:** 90 degrees, two-chamber view (with leftward rotation of TEE shaft). *Arrow* indicates LA appendage. **D:** 136 degrees, long-axis view of the LV. *Ao,* aorta; *RVOT,* right ventricle outflow tract; *VS,* ventricular septum.

IMAGE ORIENTATION AND SPECIFIC VIEWS

Almost all views obtained by surface echocardiography can be duplicated by TEE. Because the same cardiovascular structures are imaged by both TTE and TEE, the anatomic correlations and image orientations should be maintained and be identical. To replicate the identical TTE image, the TEE electronic transducer artifact needs to be kept predominantly at the bottom of the displayed images throughout the multiplane TEE examination (16).

Primary Views

Four primary multiplane TEE views can be obtained (Figs. 3-6 and 3-7) by rotating the transducer array from 0 degrees to 135 degrees: (a) 0-degrees (transverse plane):

oblique view of basal structures; the four-chamber view or basal short-axis view can be obtained from this position by retroflexion and anteflexion of the transducer tip, respectively; (b) 45-degrees: short-axis view of the aortic valve; this image is similar to the transthoracic parasternal short-axis view at the level of the aortic valve; (c) 90 degrees: longitudinal transducer orientation, producing images oblique to the long axis of the heart; (d) 135 degrees: the true long axis of the LA and the left ventricle (LV) outflow tract (LVOT), analogous to the parasternal long-axis view.

Longitudinal Views

With the transducer array at 90 degrees, the plane is sagittal to the body and oblique to the long axis of the heart.

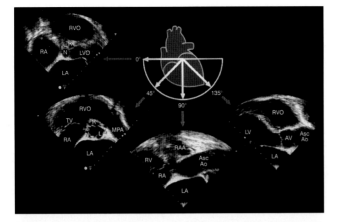

FIG. 3-6. Primary multiplane transesophageal views (0, 45, 90, and 135 degrees) are obtained by rotating the array indicator from left to right on the icon. The transducer is in midesophagus. At 0 degrees (transverse plane), an oblique view of the basal structures is obtained. At 45 degrees, a short-axis view of the basal structures [aortic valve (*L, N, R*)] is obtained. At 90 degrees (longitudinal plane), a long-axis view of the basal cardiac structures [ascending aorta (*Asc Ao*)] is obtained. At 135 degrees, the array is aligned with the long axis of the left ventricle (*LV*). *AV,* aortic valve; *L,* left coronary cusp; *LVO,* LV outflow; *MPA,* main pulmonary artery; *N,* noncoronary cusp; *R,* right coronary cusp; *RAA,* right atrial appendage; *RVO,* right ventricular outflow; *TV,* tricuspid valve; *VS,* ventricular septum. (From ref. 9, with permission.)

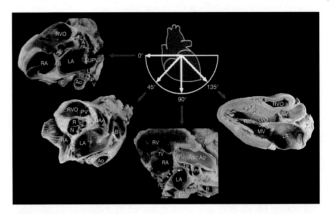

FIG. 3-7. Tomographic anatomy of the heart from midesophagus. The anatomic specimens are cut to correspond to the echocardiographic anatomy shown in Fig. 3-6. Specimens are presented from the perspective of 0-degree rotation of the imaging array **(left)** to 135 degrees rotation **(right)**. In an oblique short-axis cut at the base of the heart (0-degree rotation), the esophagus (*E*) is posterior and adjacent to the left atrium (*LA*). The image array is in the short axis of the body, and, consequently, the aortic valve (*AV*) cusps are cut obliquely. Frequently, the LA appendage (*LAA*) and left upper (*LUPV*) and lower (*LLPV*) pulmonary veins are visualized in this short-axis view. The right atrium (*RA*) is to the viewer's left; the right ventricular outflow (*RVO*) is anterior. In a short-axis view of the aortic valve (45 degrees rotation), note that aortic valve cusps (*L, N,* and *R*) are optimally displayed. The descending thoracic aorta (*Ao*) is cut obliquely. The RVO is anterior, and the esophagus is posterior. In a longitudinal scan (90 degrees rotation), the basal structures of the cardiac specimen, including the proximal ascending Ao (*Asc Ao*), are in the long axis of the body. The esophagus is posterior. A membranous atrial septum (*small arrows*) and patent foramen ovale (*large arrows*) are evident in this view. The right pulmonary artery (*RPA*) courses posterior to the ascending aorta. In a long-axis view of the LA (135 degrees rotation) (identical to parasternal long-axis view), the esophagus is posterior and adjacent to the LA. The AV, LV outflow (*LVO*), and body of the LV are viewed in long axis. The RVO is anterior. In this tomographic cut, the view of the heart is from the LV toward the ventricular septum (*VS*) and RV. *AS,* atrial septum; *B,* bronchus; *IVC,* inferior vena cava; *L,* left coronary cusp; *MV,* mitral valve; *N,* noncoronary cusp; *PM,* posteromedial papillary muscle; *PV,* pulmonary valve; *R,* right coronary cusp; *TS,* transverse sinus (a pericardial space separating the LA, RPA, Asc Ao, and RA); *TV,* tricuspid valve; *VS,* ventricular septum. (From ref. 9, with permission.)

Sequential leftward (counterclockwise rotation) and rightward (clockwise rotation) rotations of the probe shaft will develop a series of longitudinal TEE views (Figs. 3-8 and 3-9). These views include the following: (a) counterclockwise rotation of the scope, producing a two-chamber LV inflow view; (b) slight rightward rotation of the scope from the first view, producing a long axis of the right ventricle (RV) outflow tract; (c) further rightward rotation, producing a long-axis view of the proximal ascending aorta; and (d) still further rightward rotation of the scope, producing a long-axis view of the vena cava and atrial septum.

Transgastric Multiplane Views

With the transducer tip in the fundus of the stomach (about 40 to 45 cm from the incisors), the transducer array at 0 degrees produces the short-axis view of the LV and RV (Figs. 3-10 and 3-11). Anteflexion or slight withdrawal of the tip of the transducer will optimize the basal short-axis view of the ventricles, whereas retroflexion of the tip will result in a more apical short-axis view. Sequential rotation of the multiplane transducer provides the primary transgastric views of the LV: (a) 0 degrees, short-axis view of the LV and RV; (b) 70 to 90 degrees, longitudinal two-

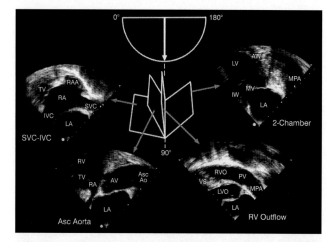

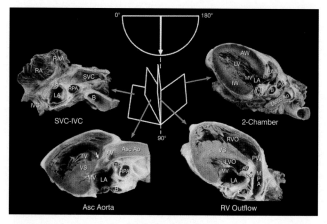

FIG. 3-8. Series of longitudinal echocardiographic views obtained with the tip of the transducer in midesophagus. By rotating the shaft of the scope to the patient's left (counterclockwise rotation of the shaft), an optimal image of the mitral valve (*MV*) and left ventricular (*LV*) inflow is produced. A sequence of longitudinal views is obtained by progressively rotating the shaft of the scope to the patient's right. (Note that the array is kept at 90 degrees throughout this maneuver.) The sequence presentation begins at the right in this illustration: (*1*) a two-chamber LV inflow view is obtained with the scope rotated to the left; (*2*) right ventricular (*RV*) outflow is depicted by a slight rightward rotation of the scope; (*3*) next, further rightward rotation (neutral position) results in a long-axis view of the proximal ascending aorta (*Asc Ao*); and (*4*) a long-axis view of the cavae and atrial septum is obtained by further rightward rotation of the scope. *AV*, aortic valve; *AW*, anterior wall; *IVC*, inferior vena cava; *IW*, inferior wall; *LVO*, LV outflow; *MPA*, main pulmonary artery; *PV*, pulmonary valve; *RAA*, right atrial appendage; *RVO*, RV outflow; *SVC*, superior vena cava; *TV*, tricuspid valve; *VS*, ventricular septum. (From ref. 9, with permission.)

FIG. 3-9. Midesophageal longitudinal tomographic anatomic sections cut to correspond to the echocardiographic presentation in Fig. 3-8. Anatomic views are described from the viewer's right to left. In a two-chamber view, the esophagus is posterior to the left atrium (*LA*), which is the primary chamber visualized along with the left ventricle (*LV*). Mitral valve (*MV*) inflow is demonstrated best in this view. The LA appendage (*LAA*) is imaged in the anterior LA. The view of the specimen is from the LV toward the chambers on the right side of the heart. In a long-axis view of the RV outflow (*RVO*), the section is oblique to the body of the heart but in the long axis of the RVO, pulmonary valve (*PV*), and proximal main pulmonary artery (*MPA*). The posteriorly located LA is adjacent to the esophagus. In a long-axis view of the proximal ascending aorta (*Asc Ao*), the LV and aortic valve (*AV*) are cut obliquely. This view is best for visualizing the membranous ventricular septum (*VS* and *arrow*). The right pulmonary artery (*RPA*) is posterior to the ascending aorta. In a long-axis view of the superior (*SVC*) and inferior (*IVC*) venae cavae, the specimen is viewed from the left toward the free wall of the RA. The right atrial appendage (*RAA*) is anterior in the RA cavity. The right pulmonary artery (*RPA*), transected in short axis, courses posterior to the SVC. The posteriorly located LA is adjacent to the esophagus. *AS*, atrial septum; *AW*, anterior wall; *B*, bronchus; *Desc Ao*, descending thoracic aorta; *IW*, inferior wall; *LCA*, left main coronary artery; *LPA*, left pulmonary artery; *LVO*, LV outflow; *Pul V*, left lower pulmonary vein; *TS*, transverse sinus; *TV*, tricuspid valve. (From ref. 9, with permission.)

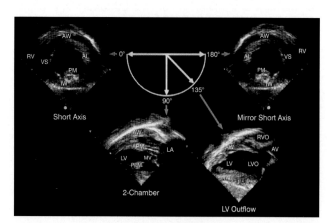

FIG. 3-10. A series of multiplane transgastric echocardiographic views. With the tip of the transducer anteflexed in a stable transgastric position, the array can be rotated to obtain the following sequence of short- and long-axis views: (*1*) short-axis left ventricular (*LV*) and right ventricular (*RV*) array at 0 degrees (transverse plane); (*2*) two-chamber LV array at 70 to 90 degrees (longitudinal plane) with a slight leftward rotation of the scope; (*3*) long-axis left ventricular outflow (*LVO*) array at 110 to 135 degrees, which best visualizes the LVO and aortic valve (*AV*) (a good view to obtain Doppler velocity from LVO and the aortic valve); and (*4*) mirror-image short-axis view by overrotation of array, a mirror-image (right-left reversal) short-axis view results. If the transducer shaft is rotated rightward (clockwise), chambers and structures on the right side of the heart are visualized (not shown). *AL*, anterolateral papillary muscle; *APM*, anterior papillary muscle; *AW*, anterior wall; *IW*, inferior wall; *MV*, mitral valve; *PM*, papillary muscle; *PPM*, posterior papillary muscle; *RVO*, RV outflow; *VS*, ventricular septum. (From ref. 9, with permission.)

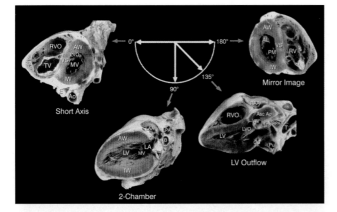

FIG. 3-11. Transgastric short- and long-axis tomographic anatomic specimens cut to correspond to the views in Fig. 3-10. In a short-axis midventricular view (0-degree rotation), the anatomic specimen is viewed from the apex toward the base. The esophagus (*E*) is posterior and adjacent to the inferior wall (*IW*) of the left ventricle (*LV*). The LV is to the viewer's right, and the right ventricle (*RV*) is to the viewer's left. The RV outflow (*RVO*) and LV anterior wall (*AW*) are viewed anteriorly. The thoracic aorta (*Ao*) is posterior and to the left of the esophagus (viewer's right). In a two-chamber view (70 to 90 degrees of rotation), the LV and left atrium (*LA*) are in the same long-axis tomographic cut. This view is excellent for assessing the mitral support apparatus and LV wall motion. In an LV outflow view (110 to 135 degrees of rotation), the aortic valve (*AV*) and LV outflow (*LVO*) are cut in the long axis. The esophagus is posterior to the LV IW. In a mirror-image short-axis view (180 degrees of rotation), the anatomic specimen is viewed from the base toward the apex. It represents the bisected apical half of the cardiac specimen shown at 0-degree rotation. *AL*, anterolateral papillary muscle; *Asc Ao*, ascending aorta; *AW*, anterior wall; *B*, bronchus; *CS*, coronary sinus; *LAA*, LA appendage; *LPA*, left pulmonary artery; *MV*, mitral valve; *PM*, posteromedial papillary muscle; *Pul V*, pulmonary vein; *RAA*, right atrial appendage; *RPA*, right pulmonary artery; *T*, trachea; *TS*, transverse sinus; *TV*, tricuspid valve; *VS*, ventricular septum. (From ref. 9, with permission.)

chamber view of the LV; and (c) 110 to 135 degrees, transgastric view of the LVOT.

Pulmonary Artery Bifurcation

To visualize the bifurcation of the pulmonary artery, the tip of the transducer needs to be withdrawn to a level slightly higher than the LA. With the transducer array at 0 degrees, the main pulmonary artery and the proximal bifurcation of the right and left pulmonary arteries are visualized (Fig. 3-12). By rotating the transducer shaft counterclockwise, only the very proximal portion of the left pulmonary artery can be visualized. By rotating the transducer shaft clockwise, the long axis of the right pulmonary artery and the short axis of the superior vena cava and the right upper pulmonary vein are viewed adjacent to the ascending aorta. This is the best view for vi-

sualizing an anomalous connection of the right upper pulmonary vein with the superior vena cava (6).

Pulmonary Veins

The best methods for consistently visualizing the pulmonary veins are the following two maneuvers. For the right pulmonary veins, set the transducer array to 45 to 60 degrees (oblique short-axis view of the aortic valve) and rotate the shaft of the transducer to the patient's extreme right (clockwise rotation of the transducer shaft); this allows the right upper and lower pulmonary veins to be visualized simultaneously, which appear as a "y" configuration, where they enter the LA (Fig. 3-13B). For the left pulmonary veins, set the transducer array to about 110 degrees and rotate the shaft of the transducer to the patient's extreme left (counterclockwise rotation of the shaft of the transducer) to visualize simultaneously the left upper and lower pulmonary veins (Fig. 3-13B). The connection of the pulmonary veins with the LA also is visualized from the transverse view with the transducer behind the LA. The upper pulmonary veins are easier to see, but the lower veins also are seen by slightly advancing the probe from the position used for the upper pulmonary veins.

LA Appendage

With the transducer behind the upper portion of the LA, the basal short-axis view (0- to 45-degree array position) and the longitudinal view (90 degrees) show the crescent-shaped LA appendage (Fig. 3-14). The LA appendage is normally multilobed. The LA also is visualized from the two-chamber view, with the transducer array at 90 degrees and rotated counterclockwise (Fig. 3-5C).

Thoracic Aorta

The anatomic relationship between the thoracic aorta and the esophagus is intimate (Fig. 3-15). The proximity between these two structures allows superb visualization of the aorta by TEE. The proximal part of the aortic arch and the distal portion of the ascending aorta may not be accessible with transverse imaging because of the interposed trachea, but the longitudinal view and multiplane TEE usually allow complete visualization of the entire thoracic aorta. The multiplane TEE examination of the aorta is as follows (Fig. 3-15). With the transducer in the midesophagus, set the array at 0 degrees (transverse plane). The descending thoracic aorta is to the patient's left and posterior to the esophagus; thus, from the probe position for cardiac imaging, rotate the shaft of the scope to the patient's left until the short axis of the midthoracic aorta is visualized. Advance the scope to visualize the lower thoracic and the upper abdominal aorta. Withdraw the scope to visualize the upper thoracic aorta. With the transducer array at 90 degrees, the longitudinal view of the aorta is well seen. It

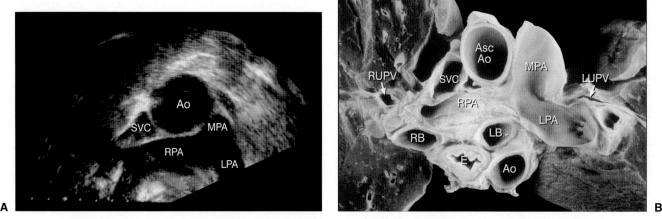

FIG. 3-12. A: Echocardiographic view of the bifurcation of the pulmonary artery. With the array at 0 degrees (transverse plane), the scope is withdrawn to the level of the bifurcation of the pulmonary artery (image shown is a composite wide-field view for optimal illustration of anatomy). The transesophageal transducer is posterior to the right pulmonary artery (*RPA*). Note the excellent visualization of this artery, including its bifurcation into upper and lower branches. Anteriorly, the ascending aorta (*Asc Ao*) and superior vena cava (*SVC*) are visualized in the short axis. In this image, only a small portion of the proximal left pulmonary artery (*LPA*) is visualized. *MPA*, main pulmonary artery. **B:** The corresponding anatomic section shows the bifurcation of the pulmonary artery. The esophagus (*E*) lies between the right (*RB*) and left (*LB*) bronchi, adjacent to the thoracic Ao, and posterior to the RPA. Frequently, the LB obscures visualization of the LPA. The Asc Ao, cut in the short axis, lies between the MPA and the SVC. Note the right upper pulmonary vein (*RUPV*) medial to the SVC. *LUPV*, left upper pulmonary vein. (From ref. 9, with permission.)

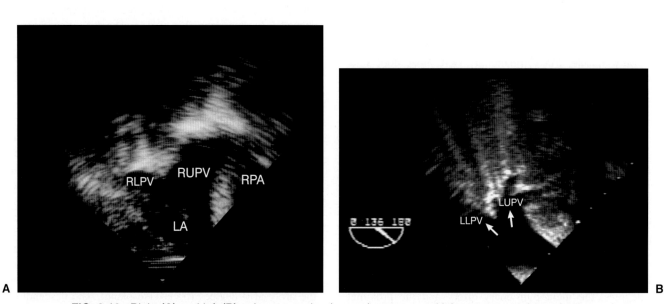

FIG. 3-13. Right **(A)** and left **(B)** pulmonary veins (*arrows*) seen on multiplane transesophageal echocardiography (see text for details). *LLPV*, left lower pulmonary vein; *LUPV*, left upper pulmonary vein; *RLPV*, right lower pulmonary vein; *RPA*, right pulmonary artery; *RUPV*, right upper pulmonary vein.

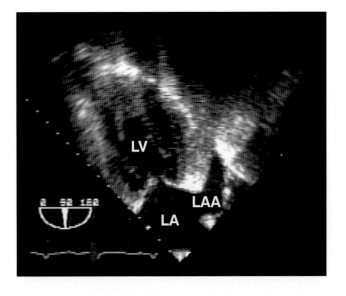

FIG. 3-14. Longitudinal transesophageal view demonstrating the left atrial appendage (*LAA*).

may be possible to visualize the takeoff of the left subclavian, the left carotid, and the innominate arteries.

Coronary Arteries

The proximal portions of the coronary arteries are normally seen with TEE. The left coronary is best visualized from the transverse basal short-axis view (0 degrees). The left main coronary artery is located immediately below the level of the LA appendage. From the transverse LA appendage view, the probe needs to be withdrawn slightly to demonstrate the left main coronary artery and its bifurcation into the left anterior descending and the circumflex coronary arteries (Fig. 3-16). The proximal right coronary artery is best visualized in the longitudinal plane, arising from the anteriorly located right aortic sinus (135 degrees), about 1 to 2 cm above the aortic valve (Fig. 3-16B). Anomalous coronary arteries, coronary aneurysms, and coronary fistulas can be diagnosed with TEE (see Chapter 7).

PITFALLS

TEE has improved the visualization not only of cardiovascular structures previously seen with TTE but structures

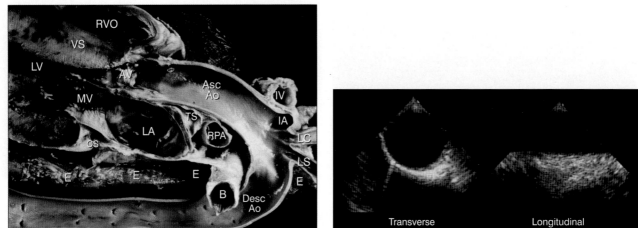

FIG. 3-15. A: Anatomic specimen demonstrating the proximity between the esophagus (*E*) and the aorta (*Desc Ao*). The bronchus (*B*) is between the esophagus and the proximal portion of the aortic arch. **B:** Transverse (0-degree) and longitudinal (90-degree) images of the normal descending thoracic aorta. *Asc Ao*, ascending aorta; *AV* aortic valve; *CS*, coronary sinus; *IA*, innominate artery; *IV*, innominate vein; *LC*, left carotid artery; *LS*, left subclavian artery; *MV*, mitral valve; *RPA*, right pulmonary artery; *RVO*, right ventricular outflow; *TS*, transverse sinus; *VS*, ventricular septum.

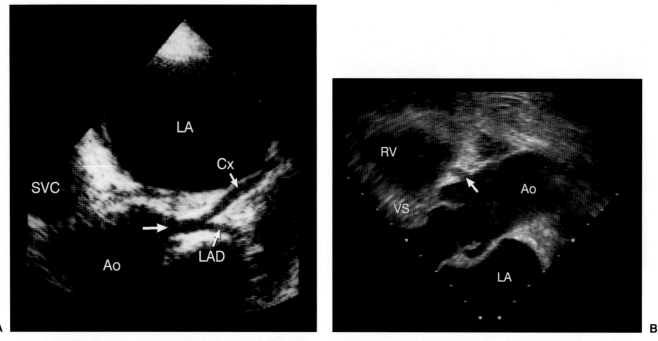

FIG. 3-16. A: Transverse view above the aortic valve showing the left main (*large arrow*) coronary artery and its bifurcation into the circumflex (*Cx*) and left anterior descending (*LAD*) coronary arteries. **B:** Long-axis view of the aorta (*Ao*) showing the ostium of the right coronary artery *(arrow)*. (See Chapter 7 for transesophageal imaging of abnormal coronary arteries.) *SVC,* superior vena cava; *VS,* ventricular septum.

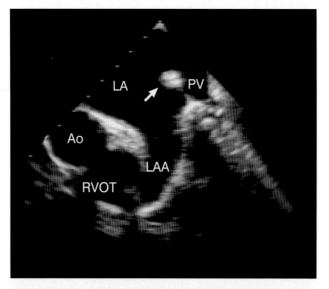

FIG. 3-17. Basal short-axis view showing a bulbous (*arrow*) structure (which resembles a Q-tip), separating the left upper pulmonary vein (*PV*) from the left atrial (*LA*) appendage (LAA). It is a normal structure. *Ao,* aorta; *RVOT,* right ventricular outflow tract.

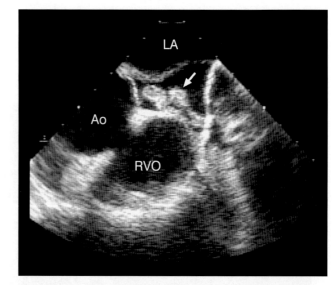

FIG. 3-18. Basal short-axis view showing soft-tissue masses (*arrow*) in a space between the left atrium (*LA*) and aorta (*Ao*). The space is the transverse sinus. The soft-tissue masses are either fibrin material in pericardial effusion or the tip of the LA appendage. *RVO,* right ventricular outflow.

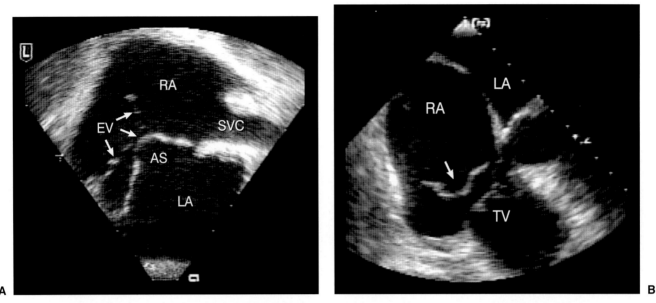

A

B

FIG. 3-19. A: Longitudinal view (90 degrees) with the probe shaft turned clockwise (rightward), showing a linear density in the right atrium (*RA*). It is the eustachian valve (*EV*). **B:** Four-chamber view showing a linear density (*arrow*) in the RA. It is another manifestation of the EV, but in this patient it was obstructive. *AS*, atrial septum; *SVC*, superior vena cava; *TV*, tricuspid valve.

that were not well appreciated on TTE. Understanding the unfamiliar but normal structures will minimize misinterpretation of TEE findings (17). Previously unrecognized normal structures seen with TEE are the most frequent reasons for referral of TEE images for interpretation from physicians beginning to perform TEE. TEE images frequently asked to be interpreted are shown in Figs. 3-17 to 3-20. Imaging of the heart by TEE may be impaired by a large hiatal hernia, pneumopericardium, or mechanical valve prosthesis.

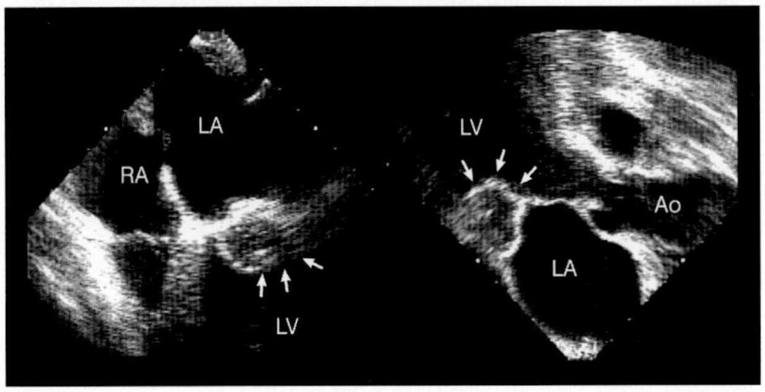

FIG. 3-20. A large mass (*arrows*) in the left atrioventricular groove seen from both the four-chamber and long-axis views. This appearance is typical of excessive mitral annulus calcification, a benign transesophageal echocardiographic finding. *Ao*, aorta.

REFERENCES

1. Seward JB, Khandheria BK, Oh JK, et al. Transesophageal echocardiography: technique, anatomic correlations, implementation, and clinical applications. *Mayo Clin Proc* 1988;63:649–680.
2. Erbel R, Engberding R, Daniel W, Roelandt J, Visser C, Rennollet H. Echocardiography in diagnosis of aortic dissection. *Lancet* 1989;1:457–461.
3. Freeman WK, Schaff HV, Khandheria BK, et al. Intraoperative evaluation of mitral valve regurgitation and repair by transesophageal echocardiography: incidence and significance of systolic anterior motion. *J Am Coll Cardiol* 1992;20:599–609.
4. Hoffmann R, Flachskampf FA, Hanrath P. Planimetry of orifice area in aortic stenosis using multiplane transesophageal echocardiography. *J Am Coll Cardiol* 1993;22:529–534.
5. Amarenco P, Cohen A, Tzourio C, et al. Atherosclerotic disease of the aortic arch and the risk of ischemic stroke. *N Engl J Med* 1994;331:1474–1479.
6. Pascoe RD, Oh JK, Warnes CA, Danielson GK, Tajik AJ, Seward JB. Diagnosis of sinus venosus atrial septal defect with transesophageal echocardiography. *Circulation* 1996;94:1049–1055.
7. Karalis DG, Bansal RC, Hauck AJ, et al. Transesophageal echocardiographic recognition of subaortic complications in aortic valve endocarditis: clinical and surgical implications. *Circulation* 1992;86:353–362.
8. Sohn DW, Shin GJ, Oh JK, et al. Role of transesophageal echocardiography in hemodynamically unstable patients. *Mayo Clin Proc* 1995;70:925–931.
9. Seward JB, Khandheria BK, Freeman WK, et al. Multiplane transesophageal echocardiography: image orientation, examination technique, anatomic correlations, and clinical applications. *Mayo Clin Proc* 1993;68:523–551.
10. Manning WJ, Silverman DI, Gordon SP, Krumholz HM, Douglas PS. Cardioversion from atrial fibrillation without prolonged anticoagulation with use of transesophageal echocardiography to exclude the presence of atrial thrombi. *N Engl J Med* 1993;328:750–755.

11. Sharma SC, Rama PR, Miller GL, Coccio EB, Coulter LJ. Systemic absorption and toxicity from topically administered lidocaine during transesophageal echocardiography. *J Am Soc Echocardiogr* 1996;9: 710–711.
12. Grauer SE, Giraud GD. Toxic methemoglobinemia after topical anesthesia for transesophageal echocardiography. *J Am Soc Echocardiogr* 1996;9:874–876.
13. Steckelberg JM, Khandheria BK, Anhalt JP, et al. Prospective evaluation of the risk of bacteremia associated with transesophageal echocardiography. *Circulation* 1991;84:177–180.
14. Mays JM, Nichols BA, Rubish RC, O'Meara KW, Koverman PA. Transesophageal echocardiography: a sonographer's perspective. *J Am Soc Echocardiogr* 1991;4:513–518.
15. Seward JB, Khandheria BK, Edwards WD, Oh JK, Freeman WK, Tajik AJ. Biplanar transesophageal echocardiography: anatomic correlations, image orientation, and clinical applications. *Mayo Clin Proc* 1990;65:1193–1213.
16. Freeman WK, Seward JB, Khandheria BK, Tajik AJ, eds. *Transesophageal echocardiography*. Boston: Little, Brown and Company, 1994.
17. Khandheria BK, Seward JB, Tajik AJ. Critical appraisal of transesophageal echocardiography: Limitations and pitfalls. *Crit Care Clin* 1996;12:235–251.

CHAPTER 4

Assessment of Ventricular Systolic Function

Evaluation of ventricular systolic and diastolic functions is an essential part of all echocardiographic examinations. Two-dimensional (2D) echocardiography allows visualization of the endocardial thickening of ventricular walls, by which global and regional ventricular functions are assessed. Determination of global systolic function is based on changes in ventricular size and volume. Regional (or segmental) wall motion analysis is fundamental in evaluating coronary artery disease and in performing stress echocardiography. Diastolic function is assessed mainly by Doppler echocardiographic analysis of mitral inflow, tricuspid inflow, and pulmonary vein, hepatic vein, and superior vena cava flow velocities, but it needs to be interpreted in conjunction with clinical and 2D echocardiographic findings. Both systolic and diastolic functions change as a disease process regresses or progresses (by natural history or treatment). The treatment strategy for a patient's condition is affected by systolic and diastolic functions. Hence, echocardiography is useful for monitoring serial changes in systolic and diastolic functions in response to treatment and for following the progression of a patient's underlying cardiovascular disease. This chapter discusses the measurement of cardiac dimensions, area, volume, mass, and systolic function. Their normal values are listed in the Appendix. Chapter 5 discusses the technique, interpretation, and applications of the assessment of diastolic function are discussed.

DIMENSIONS AND AREA

In our laboratory, representative left ventricular (LV) dimensions usually are measured from 2D-guided M-mode echocardiograms of the LV at the papillary muscle level using the parasternal short-axis view. When no significant regional wall motion abnormalities are present, the LV dimensions measured from the papillary muscle of the LV can be used to calculate LV ejection fraction (LVEF) (Fig. 4-1). Thicknesses of the ventricular posterior wall and the ventricular septum are measured from the same M-mode echocardiogram (see Fig. 2-10). These values are used to calculate LV mass. The long-axis and short-axis dimensions of the ventricle can be obtained directly from systolic and diastolic frames of 2D parasternal long-axis and short-axis views and also apical views (Fig. 4-2). The American Society of Echocardiography recommends the quantitative method by 2D echocardiography for determining the linear dimensions, area, and volume of the LV cavity (1). After a satisfactory 2D echocardiographic image has been obtained to optimize endocardial definitions, measurements of the dimensions, area, volume, and mass are obtained. The normal values are listed in the Appendix. Representative LV cavity areas are determined from the short-axis view at the level of the papillary muscle, from which fraction area changes are calculated, but changes in the apical segment are not accurately reflected.

Measurements of LV dimension are used to calculate the ejection fraction (EF) and are clinically useful for detecting LV dilatation and for follow-up of patients who have valvular regurgitation or a cardiomyopathy. Detection of right ventricular (RV) dilatation may be the first clue for RV pressure or volume overload. RV dimension is measured by M-mode echocardiography from the parasternal long-axis view. Subjectively, RV dilatation is better appreciated from the parasternal short-axis or apical four-chamber view. By convention, the size of the left atrium (LA) is determined from the parasternal long-axis view, but the LA size may be underestimated because this chamber may enlarge longitudinally. Therefore, LA size should also be measured from apical views (from the tip of the mitral valve to the posterior wall of the LA). LA area and volume are best measured from two apical orthogonal views, either by planimetry or by automated border detection (Fig. 4-3) (2). LA size is an important determinant of LA pressure, diastolic function, and prognosis (3,4).

VOLUME

The volume of the LV is measured from the dimension and area obtained from orthogonal apical views (four-chamber and two-chamber views). The LV volume then is calculated by the *modified Simpson method* or disk sum-

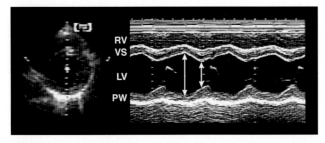

FIG. 4-1. Two-dimensional-guided M-mode echocardiogram of the left ventricle (*LV*) at the papillary muscle level. The LV end-diastolic internal dimension (*long double-headed arrow*) measured at the onset of QRS is 65 mm, and the LV end-systolic internal dimension (*short double-headed arrow*) is 40 mm. Therefore,

$$\text{LV ejection fraction (LVEF)} = \frac{65^2 - 40^2}{65^2} \times 100 = 62\% \text{ (uncorrected)}$$

If apical contractility is normal,

$$\begin{aligned}
\text{corrected LVEF} &= 62\% + [(100 - 62) \times 15\%] \\
&= 62\% + 6\% \\
&= 68\%.
\end{aligned}$$

PW is the posterior wall, and *VS* is the ventricular septum.

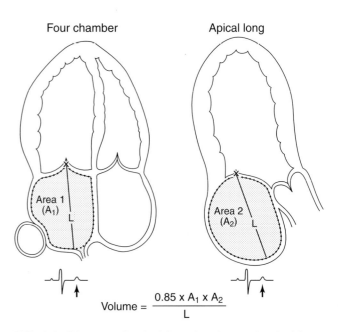

FIG. 4-3. Diagram of apical four-chamber and apical long-axis views of the left atrium (*LA*) showing how to measure LA size and volume. (Courtesy of Mary Ann Capps.)

$$\text{Volume} = \frac{0.85 \times A_1 \times A_2}{L}$$

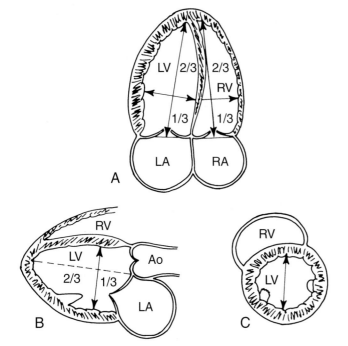

FIG. 4-2. Measurement of ventricular dimensions. **A:** The major long-axis measurement is obtained from the apical four-chamber view from the apical endocardium to the plane of the mitral valve. The minor short axis is measured from one-third the length of the long axis from the base and orthogonal to it. **B:** By using these same criteria, the long and short axes can be measured from the parasternal long-axis view, but this view rarely shows the true apex of the LV. **C:** The short axis is measured from the parasternal short-axis view at the level of the tip of the papillary muscle. *Ao*, aorta. (From ref. 1, with permission.)

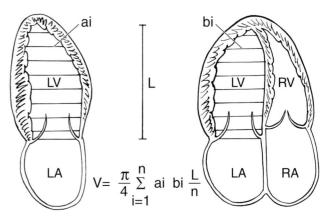

$$V = \frac{\pi}{4} \sum_{i=1}^{n} ai \; bi \; \frac{L}{n}$$

FIG. 4-4. Diagram of two orthogonal apical views to illustrate modified Simpson rule in calculation of the left ventricular (*LV*) volume. In this method, the LV is divided into a number (*n*) of cylinders or disks of equal height. The height of each cylinder is determined by the number of cylinders; *height* = L/n. The volume of each cylinder is calculated from the two diameters of the cylinder (*ai* and *bi*):

$$V = \pi \times \frac{ai}{2} \times \frac{bi}{2} \times \frac{L}{n} = \frac{\pi}{4} (ai \times bi) \times \frac{L}{n}$$

where *L* is the length of the long axis of the LV. (Modified from ref. 1, with permission.)

mation method (Fig. 4-4). If only one apical view is available, a single-plane area length method is used. LV endocardial borders can be traced manually (Fig. 4-5) or detected automatically using *acoustic quantification* (AQ) or integrated backscatter information (Fig. 4-6) (5).

ACOUSTIC QUANTIFICATION (AUTOMATED BORDER DETECTION)

AQ is based on the automated detection of the blood–tissue border by using integrated backscatter analysis (6–8). Because the difference between the amplitude of integrated backscatter from the myocardium and the blood is substantial, large changes in the amplitude of the integrated backscatter signal represent the blood–tissue border. Therefore, the blood–tissue border is recognized by a ''threshold'' change in amplitude, and these borders are marked with colored dots. The colored dots superimposed on 2D echocardiographic images represent the LV endocardial border (Fig. 4-6A and B).

The area of blood-containing cavity within a region of interest (ROI) is determined continuously during the cardiac cycle in real time. If the LV cavity is selected as the ROI, the change in LV cavity area or volume with systolic contraction is calculated instantaneously, conveniently providing LVEF (Fig. 4-6C and D).

Thus, AQ is an attractive concept for determining the area, volume, and EF of the LV. The accuracy of this system has been validated against other established methods.

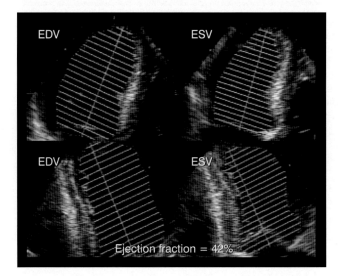

FIG. 4-5. Still frames of two orthogonal views [apical four-chamber **(top)** and apical two-chamber **(bottom)** views] to calculate the left ventricular (*LV*) volume and ejection fraction using a modified Simpson method. End-diastolic (*EDV*) and end-systolic (*ESV*) frames illustrate 20 cylinders (disks) of equal height. When the endocardial border and the long-axis (vertical line to the short-axis lines) are identified, a fixed number of cylinders are created, and the volumes of the cylinders are summed to estimate ventricular volume.

The main limitation of the AQ system is its *dependency on echocardiographic gain* and image quality. An increased echo density or artifact in the cardiac cavity is interpreted as ''tissue,'' and this affects the accuracy of the method. The definition of the lateral wall is less adequate than it is for other segments of the LV, and it needs to be adjusted by lateral gain.

AQ also has been used to evaluate changes in LA size, compliance of the aorta, and the diastolic filling pattern. Despite the initial enthusiasm for this method, however, it has not become a routine method for evaluating systolic and diastolic function in our laboratory.

Mass

The two methods of calculating LV mass from 2D echocardiography are the *area length method* and the *truncated ellipsoid method* (6). Both methods require the short-axis view of the LV at the papillary muscle level and the apical four-chamber and two-chamber views at end-diastole (Fig. 4-7). Myocardial mass is equal to the product of the volume and the specific gravity of the myocardium, 1.04 or 1.05 g/mL. Built-in software in the ultrasonographic unit can make both methods available so that the mass is calculated automatically after all the variables have been entered. LV mass also can be estimated from 2D-guided M-mode measurements of LV dimension and wall thicknesses at the papillary muscle level. Without measuring the major axis of the LV, LV mass is obtained from the LV short-axis dimension and a simple geometric cube formula. According to Devereux and associates (9), the following equation provides a reasonable determination of LV mass in grams:

$$1.04 \ [(LVID + PWT + IVST)^3 - LVID^3] \times 0.8 + 0.6$$

where *LVID* is the internal dimension, *PWT* is the posterior wall thickness, *IVST* is the interventricular septal thickness, 1.04 = specific gravity of the myocardium, and 0.8 is the correction factor. All measurements are made at end-diastole (at onset of the R wave) in centimeters.

Values for the upper LV mass index (LV mass in g/m^2 body surface area) determined with the above formula at the Mayo Clinic are shown in the Appendix.

The correlation between LV mass measured with 2D echocardiography as recommended by the American Society of Echocardiography, with M-mode echocardiography, and determined at autopsy was reasonable (10). If the papillary muscles were included in the measurement of LV mass, diastolic 2D methods overestimated autopsy values of LV mass. If the papillary muscles were excluded, the systolic area length method showed the best agreement with autopsy-determined LV mass. Further progress in echocardiography technology undoubtedly will allow a simpler and more reliable method for determining LV mass. Until that time, however, the 2D-derived M-mode method is a reasonably reliable measurement of LV mass despite interobserver and temporal variability (11).

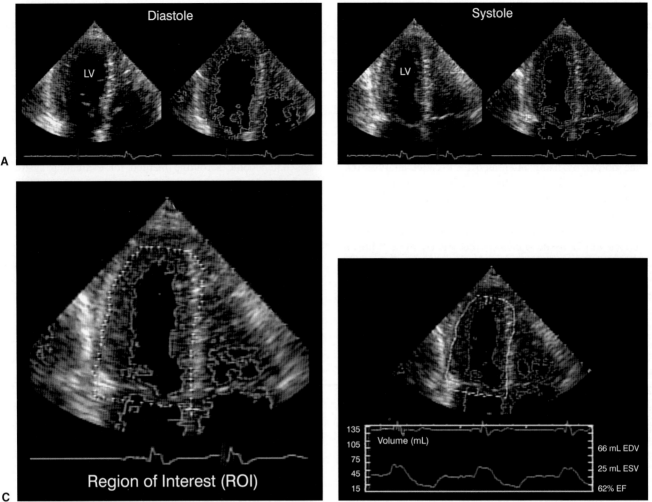

FIG. 4-6. A,B: Ultrasound backscatter differs markedly between the myocardium and intracavitary blood pool. Therefore, the endocardial border is defined where a greater than preestablished threshold difference in backscatter is identified. The borders are identified and dotted. Connection of the endocardial dots creates an endocardial border in real time throughout the cardiac cycle. **C:** An area of interest is identified by selecting the region. Because we are interested in the volumetric change of the left ventricle (*LV*), the LV cavity was chosen as the region of interest (*ROI*). **D:** From the real-time automatic border detection of the LV endocardium, LV volume changes are instantaneously determined to provide end-diastolic volume (*EDV*), end-systolic volume (*ESV*), and ejection fraction (*EF*).

GLOBAL SYSTOLIC FUNCTION

The three variables used most frequently to express LV global systolic function are (a) fractional shortening, (b) EF, and (c) cardiac output. Fractional shortening is a percent change in LV dimension with systolic contraction and can be calculated from the following equation:

$$\text{Fractional shortening} = \frac{\text{LVED} - \text{LVES}}{\text{LVED}} \times 100\%$$

where *LVED* is the LV end-diastolic dimension, and *LVES* is the LV end-systolic dimension.

EF represents stroke volume as a percent of end-diastolic LV volume; hence, its determination requires measurement of LV volume.

$$\textit{Stroke volume} = \textit{EDV} - \textit{ESV}$$

$$\text{EF} = \frac{\text{EDV} - \text{ESV}}{\text{EDV}} \times 100\%$$

where *EDV* is the end-diastolic volume, and ESV is the end-systolic volume.

Most of the current echocardiographic units have the capability of measuring volume by tracing the LV endocardial surface (manually or by automated edge detection). The American Society of Echocardiography recommends the modified Simpson method to estimate ventricular volume from two orthogonal apical views (1) (Figs. 4-4 and 4-5). Quinones and colleagues (5) proposed a simplified method

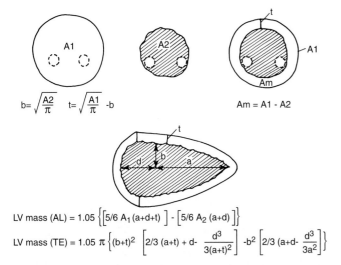

$$b = \sqrt{\frac{A2}{\pi}} \quad t = \sqrt{\frac{A1}{\pi}} - b \quad\quad Am = A1 - A2$$

LV mass (AL) = 1.05 $\left\{ \left[5/6\ A_1\ (a+d+t) \right] - \left[5/6\ A_2\ (a+d) \right] \right\}$

LV mass (TE) = 1.05 $\pi \left\{ (b+t)^2 \left[2/3\ (a+t) + d - \frac{d^3}{3(a+t)^2} \right] - b^2 \left[2/3\ (a+d - \frac{d^3}{3a^2} \right] \right\}$

FIG. 4-7. Top: Diagram of the left ventricular (*LV*) short axis at the level of the papillary muscle tip demonstrating epicardial and endocardial perimeters that are traced to calculate myocardial thickness (*t*), short-axis radius (*b*), and areas (*A1* and *A2*). Note that the papillary muscles are excluded (left within ventricular cavity) when measuring these perimeters. Two methods of computing LV mass use the short axis in this manner. **Bottom:** LV mass by area length (*AL*) and truncated ellipsoid (*TE*). Where *a* is the long or semimajor axis from widest minor axis radius to apex, *b* is the short-axis radius and is back-calculated from the short-axis cavity area, *t* is the myocardial thickness back-calculated from the short-axis epicardial and cavity areas, *d* is the truncated semimajor axis from the widest short-axis diameter to the mitral annulus plane.

for determining EF by measuring the internal dimensions of the LV.

$$EF = (\%\Delta D^2) + ([1 - \Delta D^2]\ [\%\Delta L])$$

where $\%\Delta D^2 = \dfrac{LVED^2 - LVES^2}{LVED^2} \times 100\%$

$\%\Delta D^2$ = the fractional shortening of the square of the minor axis, and

$\%\Delta L$ = the fractional shortening of the long axis, mainly related to apical contraction: 15% for normal, 5% for hypokinetic apex, 0% for akinetic apex, −5% for dyskinetic apex, and −10% for apical aneurysm.

The equation has two components: fractional shortening of the square of the minor axis and fractional shortening of the long axis. LVED and LVES can be measured as an average of three short-axis dimensions at the basal, mid (papillary muscle), and apical levels using a pair of calipers on the video screen or from a midlevel short-axis dimension assuming a uniform contraction of minor axes. Because it is difficult to measure the fractional shortening of the long axis, empirical values are assigned according to apical wall motion. An example of estimating LVEF from the midlevel short-axis view is shown in Fig. 4-1.

Cardiac output is the product of stroke volume and heart rate. Stroke volume is determined either by 2D volumetric measurement, as in calculation of EF, or by the Doppler method (see Chapter 6).

REGIONAL FUNCTION

LV regional wall motion analysis usually is based on grading the contractility of individual segments (1,8). There are various LV segmental models, depending on how the LV is subdivided. For the purpose of standardized analysis, the LV is *divided into three levels* (basal, mid, and apical) and *16 segments* (Fig. 4-8) (1). The basal and mid (papillary muscle) levels are each subdivided into six segments, and the apical level is subdivided into four segments. All 16 segments can be visualized from multiple tomographic planes of surface echocardiography. With transesophageal echocardiography, regional wall motion analysis is performed best with a multiplane probe. Transesophageal views analogous to transthoracic apical four- and two-chamber views are obtained with horizontal and longitudinal views (transducer array at 0 degrees and 90 degrees, respectively), with the transducer tip in the midesophagus area (about 30 cm from the teeth). When the transducer crystal is rotated to 120 to 135 degrees from the horizontal plane (at 0 degrees), an imaging plane similar to that of the parasternal long-axis view is produced. Transgastric imag-

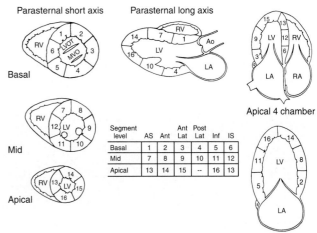

FIG. 4-8. Sixteen-segment model for regional wall motion analysis proposed by the American Society of Echocardiography. The left ventricle (*LV*) is divided into three levels (basal, mid or papillary muscle, and apical). The basal (segments 1–6) and mid (segments 7–12) levels are each subdivided into six segments, and the apical level is subdivided into four segments (segments 13–16). All 16 segments can be visualized from multiple tomographic planes. According to contractility, each segment is given a wall motion score. Segment 13 (apical septum) should be used only once, depending on coronary artery anatomy. Also, it should be noted that there is no apical segment of the posterolateral wall. *Ao*, aorta; *LVOT*, LV outflow tract.

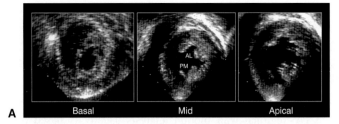

FIG. 4-9. A: A series of left ventricular (*LV*) short-axis views obtained by transgastric imaging with the multiplane transducer array at 0 degrees. Apical short-axis view is obtained by retroflexion or slight advancement of the transducer tip, and the basal short-axis view is obtained by anteflexion or slight withdrawal of the tip from the position to obtain a short-axis view at the mid (papillary muscle) level. *AL*, anterolateral papillary muscle; *PM*, posteromedial papillary muscle. **B:** When the transducer array is rotated to 90 degrees, transgastric imaging provides a long-axis view of the LV, although the true apex may not be seen by this view.

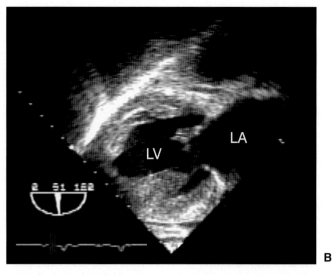

ing in the horizontal plane (0-degree transducer array) provides a series of short-axis views similar to parasternal short-axis views (Fig. 4-9A). Rotation of the transducer to 90 degrees provides a long-axis view of the LV (Fig. 4-9B).

A numeric scoring system has been adopted based on the contractility of the individual segments. In this scoring system, higher scores indicate more severe wall motion abnormality (1, normal; 2, hypokinesis; 3, akinesis; 4, dyskinesis; 5, aneurysmal). A *wall motion score index* (WMSI) is

derived by dividing the sum of wall motion scores by the number of visualized segments; it represents the extent of regional wall motion abnormalities. A normal WMSI is 1.

WMSI = Sum of wall motion scores/Number of visualized segments

WMSI has been correlated with the extent of myocardial ischemia and infarction determined by perfusion imaging and autopsy (12) (see Chapter 7). WMSI ≥1.7 usually indicates a perfusion defect of ≥ 20%.

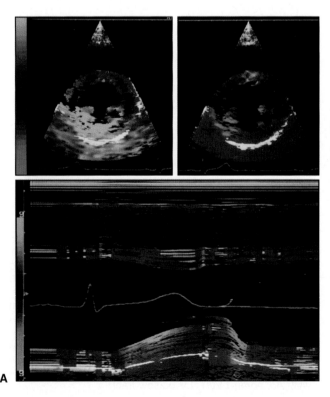

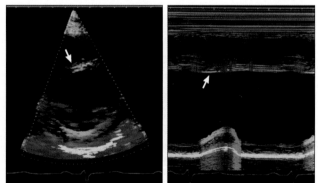

FIG. 4-10. A: Top: Tissue Doppler images, parasternal short-axis view, of the left ventricle (*LV*) in a healthy subject. **Top left:** During midsystole, the anteroseptal wall appears *bright blue* and the posterior wall *bright red*, indicating good contraction toward the center of the ventricle. **Top right:** In early diastole, the anteroseptal wall appears to be *bright red* and the posterior wall *bright blue,* indicating movement away from the center of the ventricle. **Bottom:** M-mode tissue Doppler imaging in the same subject. **B:** Tissue Doppler image, parasternal short-axis view, of the LV in a patient with anteroseptal myocardial infarction. **Left:** During midsystole, the anteroseptal wall shows no color (*arrow*), indicating akinetic wall motion. **Right:** The M-mode tissue Doppler image also shows no color at the septal wall during systole (*arrow*). (From ref. 14, with permission.)

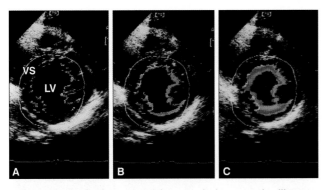

FIG. 4-11. A–C: Sequential frames during systole, illustrating a progressive color-encoded display of the inward movement of the endocardium by color kinesis. *VS,* ventricular septum. (From ref. 16, with permission.)

DOPPLER TISSUE IMAGING (TISSUE DOPPLER) AND COLOR KINESIS FOR WALL MOTION ANALYSIS

McDicken and colleagues (13) developed a technique (tissue Doppler) to image the velocities of the myocardium with the use of the color-flow method. The myocardium is color-coded according to the direction and velocity of its motion (Fig. 4-10). The conventional color-flow Doppler system was modified to detect low wall motion velocity. The color-flow imaging of wall motion velocity is superimposed on the 2D echocardiographic images. From the parasternal view, normal LV anterior wall movement during systole is color-coded *blue* (away from the transducer) and the posterior wall is color-coded *red* (toward the transducer). Akinetic segments show *no color* because wall motion velocity is zero. Wall motion velocity over time can be demonstrated by the M-mode. The reliability of Doppler tissue imaging in measuring wall motion velocity was validated in normal subjects, and a different color pattern was noted in patients with regional wall motion abnormalities (14). The clinical role and practicality of this new method are being investigated.

Color kinesis provides a real time color-coded display of LV endocardial motion on sequential frames of 2D echocardiographic images (15,16). A color is added to pixels that are identified as having changed from blood to tissue in systole, which results in color maps of sequential endocardial motion (Fig. 4-11). This method may be limited by poor endocardial definition and translational motion of the heart.

Although these two new developments are promising, they currently are not substitutes for standard 2D echocardiography in the evaluation of regional wall motion.

REFERENCES

1. Schiller NB, Shah PM, Crawford M, et al. Recommendations for quantitation of the left ventricle by two-dimensional echocardiography. American Society of Echocardiography Committee on Standards, Subcommittee on Quantitation of Two-Dimensional Echocardiograms. *J Am Soc Echocardiogr* 1989;2:358–367.
2. Gutman J, Wang YS, Wahr D, Schiller NB. Normal left atrial function determined by 2-dimensional echocardiography. *Am J Cardiol* 1983;51:336–340.
3. Appleton CP, Galloway JM, Gonzalez MS, Gaballa M, Basnight MA. Estimation of left ventricular filling pressures using two-dimensional and Doppler echocardiography in adult patients with cardiac disease: additional value of analyzing left atrial size, left atrial ejection fraction and the difference in duration of pulmonary venous and mitral flow velocity at atrial contraction. *J Am Coll Cardiol* 1993;22:1972–1982.
4. Gottdiener JS, Reda DJ, Williams DW, Materson BJ, for the Department of Veterans Affairs Cooperative Study Group on Antihypertensive Agents. Left atrial size in hypertensive men: influence of obesity, race and age. *J Am Coll Cardiol* 1997;29:651–658.
5. Quinones MA, Waggoner AD, Reduto LA, et al. A new, simplified and accurate method for determining ejection fraction with two-dimensional echocardiography. *Circulation* 1981;64:744–753.
6. Vandenberg BF, Rath LS, Stuhlmuller P, Melton HE Jr, Skorton DJ. Estimation of left ventricular cavity area with an on-line, semiautomated echocardiographic edge detection system. *Circulation* 1992;86:159–166.
7. Stewart WJ, Rodkey SM, Gunawardena S, et al. Left ventricular volume calculation with integrated backscatter from echocardiography. *J Am Soc Echocardiogr* 1993;6:553–563.
8. Shiina A, Tajik AJ, Smith HC, Lengyel M, Seward JB. Prognostic significance of regional wall motion abnormality in patients with prior myocardial infarction: a prospective correlative study of two-dimensional echocardiography and angiography. *Mayo Clin Proc* 1986;61:254–262.
9. Devereux RB, Alonso DR, Lutas EM, et al. Echocardiographic assessment of left ventricular hypertrophy: Comparison to necropsy findings. *Am J Cardiol* 1986;57:450–458.
10. Park SH, Shub C, Nobrega TP, Bailey KR, Seward JB. Two-dimensional echocardiographic calculation of left ventricular mass as recommended by the American Society of Echocardiography: correlation with autopsy and M-mode echocardiography. *J Am Soc Echocardiogr* 1996;9:119–128.
11. Gottdiener JS, Livengood SV, Meyer PS, Chase GA. Should echocardiography be performed to assess effects of antihypertensive therapy? Test-retest reliability of echocardiography for measurement of left ventricular mass and function. *J Am Coll Cardiol* 1995;25:424–430.
12. Oh JK, Gibbons RJ, Christian TF, et al. Correlation of regional wall motion abnormalities detected by two-dimensional echocardiography with perfusion defect determined by technetium 99m sestamibi imaging in patients treated with reperfusion therapy during acute myocardial infarction. *Am Heart J* 1996;131:32–37.
13. McDicken WN, Sutherland GR, Moran CM, Gordon LN. Colour Doppler velocity imaging of the myocardium. *Ultrasound Med Biol* 1992;18:651–654.
14. Miyatake K, Yamagishi M, Tanaka N, et al. New method for evaluating left ventricular wall motion by color-coded tissue Doppler imaging: *in vitro* and *in vivo* studies. *J Am Coll Cardiol* 1995;25:717–724.
15. Lang RM, Vignon P, Weinert L, et al. Echocardiographic quantification of regional left ventricular wall motion with color kinesis. *Circulation* 1996;93:1877–1885.
16. Lau YS, Puryear JV, Gan SC, et al. Assessment of left ventricular wall motion abnormalities with the use of color kinesis: a valuable visual and training aid. *J Am Soc Echocardiogr* 1997;10:665–672.

CHAPTER 5

Assessment of Diastolic Function

Congestive heart failure is one of the most common cardiac problems in adults. Approximately 400,000 new cases are diagnosed annually in the United States. In two-thirds of the patients, the syndrome of congestive heart failure is due to the combination of systolic and diastolic dysfunction of the left ventricle (LV), and in the other one-third, the primary cause of heart failure is *diastolic* dysfunction, with preserved LV systolic function.

In 1982, Kitabatake et al. (1) introduced pulsed-wave Doppler recording of transmitral blood flow velocities to assess diastolic filling of the LV. During the last 15 years, this method has been validated and refined and is the main clinical modality for noninvasively evaluating diastolic filling patterns (2–4). With Doppler echocardiography, the recorded flow velocities across the atrioventricular valves and in the central veins are used to assess filling patterns and to estimate indirectly LV filling pressures.

Normal diastolic function allows adequate filling of the ventricles during rest and exercise without abnormal increase in diastolic pressures. Adequate diastolic filling ensures normal stroke volume, according to the Frank-Starling mechanism. LV filling consists of a series of hemodynamic events (Fig. 5-1) that are affected by numerous intrinsic and extrinsic factors (Table 5-1). *The initial diastolic event is myocardial relaxation,* an active energy-dependent process that causes pressure to decrease rapidly in the LV after the end of contraction and during early diastole. When LV pressure falls lower than left atrium (LA) pressure, the mitral valve opens, and rapid early diastolic filling begins. *Under normal circumstances, the predominant determinant of the driving force of early diastolic filling is the elastic recoil and the rate of relaxation of the LV;* LA pressure is less important. Normally, approximately 80% of LV filling occurs during this phase. As a result of rapid filling, LV pressure increases and momentarily may exceed LA pressure, and this loss of positive driving force results in deceleration of mitral flow velocity. A positive transmitral pressure gradient and flow are created again by atrial contraction during late diastole, accounting for 15% to 20% of LV filling in normal subjects.

For each person, the proportion of LV filling during the early and late diastolic phases depends on elastic recoil (*suction*), the rate of myocardial relaxation, chamber compliance, and LA pressure. The status of these variables is the result of the interaction among the cardiac disease process, the baseline diastolic properties, and the volume status. The LV filling pattern is the result of the transmitral pressure gradient produced by these various factors. With Doppler echocardiography, diastolic filling is analyzed from recordings of mitral flow velocity that represent the transmitral pressure gradient and from pulmonary venous flow velocity that represents LA filling (Fig. 5-2) (1–7).

DOPPLER FLOW VELOCITIES

How to Record Mitral and Pulmonary Venous Flow Velocities

1. Transducer position: *The ultrasound beam needs to be parallel with the direction of blood flow* to obtain the optimal flow signal. Because of the location of the papillary muscles, normal mitral inflow is directed toward the mid-to-distal portion of the posterolateral wall of the LV, which is approximately 20 degrees lateral to the apex (Fig. 5-3). With dilatation of the LV, as in patients with dilated cardiomyopathy, the heart becomes more spherical, which results in mitral inflow being directed progressively more laterally and posteriorly (6). Hence, the optimal transducer position is approximately 20 degrees lateral to the apex in normal subjects and more lateral in those with LV enlargement. An optimal transducer position for recording flow velocities in the pulmonary veins varies depending on which view and which vein is to be interrogated. Usually, an apical four-chamber view is used to record flow velocities from the right upper pulmonary vein. Color-flow imaging may be helpful in guiding the ultrasound beam so that it is parallel with that of mitral inflow or pulmonary venous flow.

2. Sample volume size and location: To record peak mitral inflow velocities, the pulsed-wave Doppler technique is

Events of the Cardiac Cycle
(Left Heart)

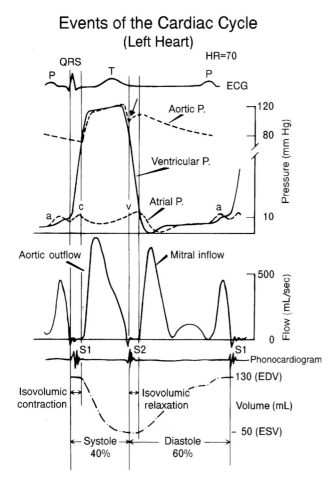

FIG. 5-1. Diagram of intracardiac pressures **(top)**, aortic outflow and mitral inflow **(middle)**, and volumetric changes in the left ventricle **(bottom)** to illustrate the hemodynamic events during the cardiac cycle. *ECG*, electrocardiogram; *EDV*, end-diastolic volume; *ESV*, end-systolic volume; *P*, pressure; *S1*, first heart sound; *S2*, second heart sound. (Courtesy of Dr. Yellin.)

TABLE 5-1. *Factors that influence LV diastolic chamber distensibility*

Factors extrinsic to the LV chamber
  Pericardial restraint
  Right ventricular loading
  Coronary vascular turgor (erectile effect)
  Extrinsic compression by tumor, pleural pressure, etc.
Factors intrinsic to LV chamber
  Passive elasticity of LV wall (stiffness or compliance when myocytes are completely relaxed)
    Thickness of LV wall
    Composition of LV wall (muscle, fibrosis, amyloid, hemosiderin), including both endocardium and myocardium
    Temperature, osmolality
  Active elasticity of LV wall due to residual cross-bridge activation (cycling and/or latch state) through part or all of diastole
    Slow relaxation affecting early diastole only
    Incomplete relaxation affecting early, mid-, and end-diastolic distensibility
    Diastolic tone, contracture, or rigor
  Elastic recoil (diastolic suction)
  Viscoelasticity (stress relaxation, creep)

LV, left ventricular.
From Grossman W. Evaluation of systolic and diastolic function of the myocardium. In: Grossman W, ed. *Cardiac catheterization and angiography*, 3rd ed. Philadelphia: Lea & Febiger, 1986:301–319, with permission.

used, with a sample volume size of 1 to 2 mm between the tips of the mitral leaflets during diastole (Fig. 5-4). The sample volume may be moved toward the mitral annulus to better record the duration of the A velocity.

For recording pulmonary venous flow velocity from an apical view, the sample volume size is usually larger (2 to 4 mm) and is placed 1 to 2 cm into the right upper pulmonary vein (Fig. 5-5 and 5-6).

To measure LV isovolumic relaxation time (IVRT), the interval from aortic valve closure to mitral valve opening, a 3- to 4-mm–size sample volume is placed in the area of the mitral leaflet tips. Next, the transducer beam is angulated toward the LV outflow tract until aortic valve closure appears above and below the baseline. An alternative technique is to use continuous-wave Doppler echocardiography to record simultaneously aortic and mitral flow.

Hepatic vein Doppler velocities are recorded with subcostal imaging, using a 2- to 3-mm pulsed-wave sample volume positioned 1 to 2 cm proximal to the junction with the inferior vena cava (IVC). Flow velocity in the superior vena cava (SVC) is obtained using a 2- to 3-mm pulsed-wave sample volume at a depth of 5 to 7 cm from the right supraclavicular area.

3. Velocity scale and filter: These should be adjusted according to the peak velocities of Doppler recording. Compared with mitral and tricuspid flow velocities (range, 0.5 to 1.5 m/sec), venous flow velocities are lower (range, 0.1 to 0.5 m/sec), and because of this, velocity scales should be expanded and the velocity filter should be low.

Mitral Flow Velocities

The initial classification of diastolic filling is usually attempted from peak mitral flow velocity of the early rapid filling wave (E), peak velocity of the late filling wave due to atrial contraction (A), and the E/A ratio (Fig. 5-7). To measure E and A velocities reliably, the Doppler velocity recording should be satisfactory. Tachycardia or first-degree atrioventricular block may result in fusion of the E and A velocities (Fig. 5-8). In fact, A velocity may be relatively increased if it starts before E velocity has reached zero. As a general rule, if E velocity is higher than 20 cm/sec at the beginning of A velocity (E at A), both the A velocity and E/A ratio are affected by the fusion of the two diastolic components (Fig. 5-9).

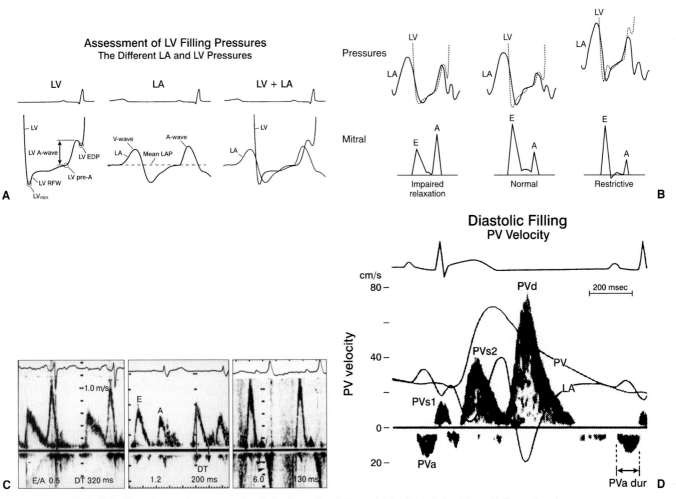

Assessment of LV Filling Pressures
The Different LA and LV Pressures

A: LV / LA / LV + LA

LV A-wave, LV EDP, LV pre-A, LV RFW, LV$_{min}$

V-wave, Mean LAP, A-wave

B: Pressures — LV, LA; Mitral — E, A
Impaired relaxation / Normal / Restrictive

Diastolic Filling
PV Velocity

PVd, PVs2, PVs1, PVa, PVa dur

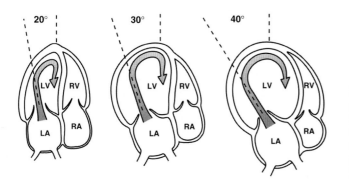

E/A 0.5   DT 320 ms   1.2   200 ms   6.0   130 ms

FIG. 5-2. Drawings of pressure tracings from the left ventricle (*LV*), left atrium (*LA*), and pulmonary vein (*PV*) and corresponding Doppler signals. **A:** Various phases of LV and LA pressure during diastole. LV pre-A indicates LV pressure just before atrial contraction; it correlates well with mean LA pressure (*LAP*). Pressure difference between LA and LV is reflected by mitral inflow velocities. *LV$_{min}$*, minimal LV pressure. *LV RFW*, LV rapid filling wave. *LV EDP*, LV end-diastolic pressure. **B:** LV and LA pressure relationship and corresponding mitral inflow velocities in three different diastolic filling patterns: impaired relaxation, normal, and restrictive. **C:** Actual Doppler recording of mitral inflow velocities, representing impaired relaxation **(left)**, normal **(center)**, and restrictive filling **(right)** patterns. *Arrowheads* indicate diastolic mitral regurgitation. *DT*, deceleration time. **D:** Pressure relationship between pulmonary vein (*PV*) and LA and the corresponding pulsed-wave Doppler recording from PV. *PVa, PVd, PVs1,* and *PVs2*, velocity components in PV (see text). *PVa dur*, PV atrial flow reversal duration. (**A** and **C** courtesy of Christopher P. Appleton, M.D.; **D** from ref. 9, with permission.)

20°   30°   40°

LV   RV   LA   RA

FIG. 5-3. Diagram of direction of mitral inflow in a normal and a diseased heart. In a normal heart, mitral inflow is directed toward the mid to distal portion of the posterolateral wall of the left ventricle (*LV*), which is approximately 20 degrees lateral to the apex. With dilatation of the LV, mitral inflow is directed more laterally and posteriorly. (From ref. 6, with permission.)

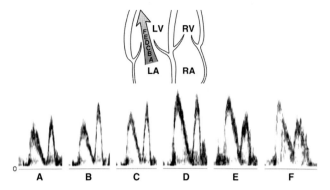

FIG. 5-4. Diagram of the heart **(top)** and pulsed-wave Doppler mitral recordings **(bottom)** illustrate typical changes in flow velocity profiles with different positions of the sample volume. Recordings are from the same person with the Doppler beam aligned parallel to flow and sample volume size (1.5 mm) and Doppler gain held constant. Recordings obtained from the mitral annulus **(A)** or between the body of the leaflets **(B,C)** have lower peak velocities and shorter mitral deceleration times than those obtained between mitral leaflet tips **(D)**, with the E wave decreasing proportionately more than the A wave. However, the spectral envelope remains relatively "sharp" at all locations. With the sample volume placed in the ventricle below the tips of the mitral leaflets **(E,F)**, lower peak velocity of both E and A waves is also seen, as compared with that between the tips of the mitral leaflets. More strikingly, the flow velocity envelope at ventricular locations also shows spectral broadening, with longer mitral deceleration time and longer A wave duration. These changes reflect greater diameter and less laminar flow in the midventricle compared with that between the mitral leaflets. (From ref. 6, with permission.)

The diastolic filling pattern is characterized further by measuring deceleration time (DT), the interval from the peak of the E velocity to its extrapolation to baseline. DT is prolonged in patients with a relaxation abnormality as the predominant diastolic dysfunction, because it takes longer for LA and LV pressures to be equilibrated with a slower and continued decrease in LV pressure until mid to late diastole. DT is shortened when there is rapid filling due to vigorous LV relaxation and elastic recoil, as in normal young subjects, or, conversely, if there is a decrease in LV compliance or marked increase in LA pressure. The IVRT is the interval from aortic valve closure to mitral valve opening. It generally parallels DT, becoming prolonged with abnormal relaxation and shorter with rapid relaxation or increasing filling pressure (or both). The duration of mitral flow with atrial contraction is a helpful means of estimating LV end-diastolic pressure (7,8).

Pulmonary Vein Flow Velocities

There are four distinct velocity components in pulmonary vein (PV) Doppler recordings (Fig. 5-10): two systolic velocities (PVs1 and PVs2), diastolic velocity (PVd), and atrial flow reversal (PVa). PVs1 occurs early in systole and

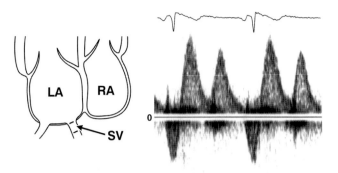

FIG. 5-5. Diagram of the heart and pulsed-wave pulmonary venous flow velocity recordings demonstrate the optimal location of sample volume placement (1 to 2 cm into the pulmonary vein). *SV*, sample volume. (From ref. 6, with permission.)

is related to atrial relaxation, which decreases LA pressure and fosters pulmonary venous flow into the LA. PVs2, the second systolic forward flow, occurs in mid to late systole and is produced by the increase in pulmonary venous pressure (5). At normal LA pressure, the late systolic increase in PV pressure is larger and more rapid than LA pressure. At elevated filling pressures, however, the late systolic pressure increase in the LA is equal to or more rapid than that in the PV, resulting in earlier peak of PVs2. The remaining PV flow velocity components (PVd, PVa, PVs1) follow phasic changes in LA pressure (9).

With normal atrioventricular conduction, the systolic components are closely connected and a distinct PVs1 peak velocity may not be seen in 70% of patients. During diastole, forward flow velocity (PVd) occurs after mitral valve opening and in conjunction with the decrease in LA pressure. With atrial contraction, the increase in LA pressure may result in flow reversal into the pulmonary vein, the extent and the duration of which are related to LV diastolic pressure, LA compliance, and heart rate. The diastolic phase of pulmonary venous flow resembles early mitral flow (E). The peak velocity and DT correlate well with those of mitral E velocity because the LA functions mainly as a passive conduit for flow during early diastole.

The analysis of pulmonary vein flow velocities complements the assessment of the mitral flow velocity pattern. This is especially true when there is fusion of mitral E and A waves. In this situation, the ratio between pulmonary vein systolic and diastolic flow velocities can be helpful in characterizing diastolic filling in patients with sinus rhythm (PVs2 >> PVd in impaired relaxation, and PVs2 << PVd in restrictive filling). In patients with atrial fibrillation, the PVs1 component is lost and PVs2 is usually smaller than that of PVd. Both peak velocity (PVa) and duration of pulmonary vein atrial flow reversal (PVa dur) are important measurements that increase with higher LV end-diastolic pressure (LVEDP) (8,9).

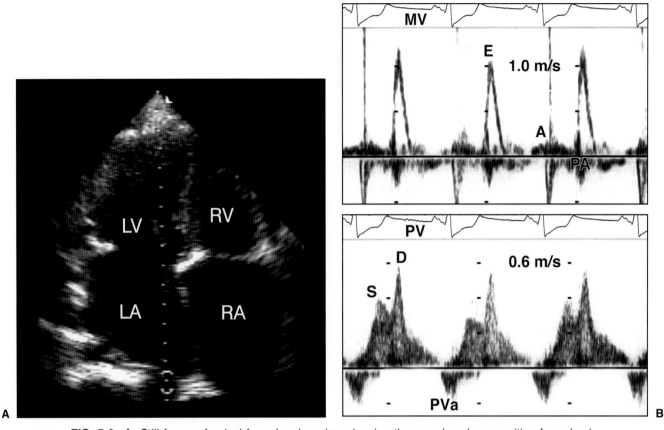

A

B

FIG. 5-6. A: Still frame of apical four-chamber view showing the sample volume position for pulsed-wave Doppler recording of right upper pulmonary vein flow in a patient with restrictive cardiomyopathy. Both atria are dilated. **B:** Mitral valve (*MV*) and pulmonary vein (*PV*) flow velocity recording from the same patient. Atrial flow reversal (*PVa*) and MV atrial velocity (*A*) are small, probably because of atrial failure. *S*, systolic flow; *D*, diastolic flow.

LV Diastolic Filling
Mitral Flow Velocity Variables

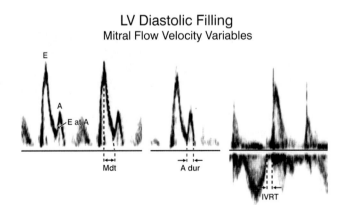

FIG. 5-7. Pulsed-wave Doppler recording of mitral flow velocity **(left** and **middle)** and left ventricle (*LV*) outflow tract velocity **(right)**. Deceleration time of mitral flow (*Mdt*) is the interval from the peak velocity of early filling velocity (*E*) to the time it reaches baseline. The descending slope of E velocity is usually extrapolated to baseline. Mitral inflow velocity has two components, E and A, in sinus rhythm. Duration of A wave (*A dur*) is important in determining LV diastolic pressure and is measured as the interval from the beginning to the end of the A wave. A dur is easier to measure when the sample volume is moved closer to the mitral annulus area **(middle)**. Isovolumic relaxation time (*IVRT*) is measured from the click of aortic valve closure to the beginning of mitral flow. (From ref. 4, with permission.)

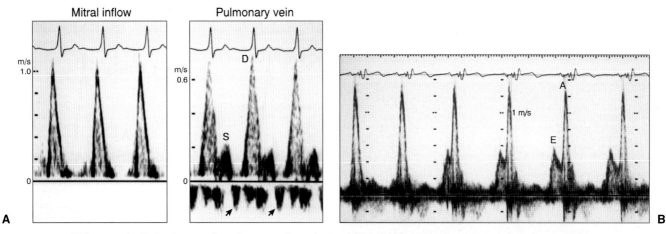

FIG. 5-8. A: Pulsed-wave Doppler recording of mitral flow **(left)** and pulmonary venous flow velocity pattern **(right)** in a patient with a very prolonged P wave to R wave (PR) interval. Mitral inflow velocity has only one velocity component, so that the diastolic filling pattern is difficult to assess. However, pulmonary venous flow velocity shows a predominant diastolic forward flow velocity and diminutive systolic forward flow velocity, consistent with restrictive filling. *Arrows,* pulmonary vein flow reversal before diastolic flow due to early atrial contraction; *D,* diastolic flow; *S,* systolic flow. **B:** Mitral flow velocity recording by pulsed-wave Doppler echocardiography. There is only one velocity component for the first two cardiac cycles, but with slight slowing of the heart rate induced by carotid sinus massage, the E velocity becomes separated from the A velocity in the third beat. Last velocity recording shows E at A velocity of 0.3 m/sec and E velocity of 0.6 m/sec and A velocity of 1.3 m/sec. Pulmonary venous flow velocity recording showed a characteristic impaired relaxation pattern. (From ref. 4, with permission.)

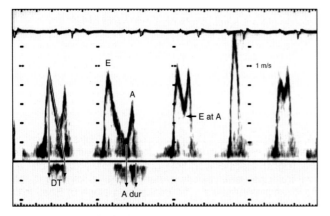

FIG. 5-9. Pulsed-wave Doppler recording of mitral inflow velocity in a patient with varying RR intervals. E at A velocity is greater than 20 cm/sec for all cycles except for the second signal. Increased E at A velocity is related to partial (first, third, and fifth signals) to complete (fourth signal) fusion of E and A, from short RR interval and prolonged pulmonary regurgitation interval. The second Doppler signal is optimal for characterizing diastolic filling. *DT,* deceleration time; *A dur,* duration of A wave.

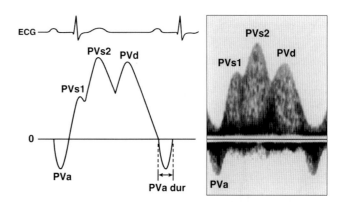

FIG. 5-10. Pulsed-wave Doppler recording of the pulmonary vein (PV) to demonstrate the four velocity components: *PVa, PVs1, PVs2,* and *PVd. PVa dur,* duration of PVa. See text for details.

Tricuspid Flow Velocities

Just as mitral flow velocity variables characterize the LV diastolic filling pattern, so tricuspid flow velocity recordings characterize the RV diastolic filling pattern, using the same criteria. Left and right diastolic filling patterns are not necessarily the same in a patient. The main difference between mitral and tricuspid velocities is a respiratory variation in tricuspid flow velocities in normal subjects; in mitral flow velocities, a respiratory variation is not usually seen.

Hepatic Vein Velocities

Hepatic vein velocities reflect changes in the pressure, volume, and compliance of the right atrium (RA). In normal subjects, hepatic vein flow velocities consist of four components (Fig. 5-11): systolic forward flow (S), diastolic forward flow (D), systolic flow reversal (SR), and diastolic flow reversal (DR). Under normal hemodynamic conditions, S is greater than D, and there are no prominent reversal velocities. Timing and respiratory changes in forward and reversal velocities of hepatic vein flow are important in the assessment of tricuspid regurgitation, constriction, tamponade, restriction, and pulmonary hypertension (10).

Superior Vena Cava Flow Velocities

SVC flow velocities are similar to hepatic vein flow velocities, but they are easier to record in subjects with normal hemodynamics on the right side of the heart. Flow reversal is less prominent in comparison with that of hepatic vein flow velocities. SVC flow velocities are useful in assessing the effect of increased respiratory effort on intrathoracic pressure (11).

DIASTOLIC FILLING PATTERNS

Normal Diastolic Filling Pattern

The rates of myocardial relaxation and compliance change with aging, so that different diastolic filling patterns are expected for different age groups (Fig. 5-12 and Table 5-2). In normal young subjects, LV elastic recoil is vigorous and myocardial relaxation is swift; therefore, most filling is completed during early diastole, with only a small contribution at atrial contraction (4,12).

With aging, there is a gradual decrease in the rate of myocardial relaxation as well as in elastic recoil, resulting in slow LV pressure declines and filling becomes slower. With normal LA pressure, the pressure crossover between the LV and LA (i.e., mitral valve opening) occurs later and the early transmitral pressure gradient is decreased. Hence, the IVRT becomes longer and the E velocity in normal subjects gradually decreases with increasing age. Decreased filling in early diastole retards the equilibration of pressure between the LV and LA, resulting in a longer DT. Because early LV filling is reduced, the contribution of atrial contraction to LV filling becomes more important. This results in *a gradual increase in A velocity with aging*. At the age of 65 years, E velocity approaches A velocity, and in persons older than 70 years, the E/A ratio is usually less than 1.0. Pulmonary venous flow velocities show similar changes with aging: diastolic forward flow velocity decreases as more filling of the LV occurs at atrial contraction and systolic forward flow velocity becomes more prominent. Normal values of various diastolic filling variables are listed for different age groups in Table 5-2 and in the Appendix (13).

Abnormal Patterns

Impaired Myocardial Relaxation Pattern

In nearly all types of cardiac disease, *the initial abnormality of diastolic filling is slowed or impaired myocardial*

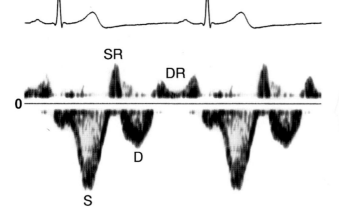

FIG. 5-11. Pulsed-wave Doppler recording of hepatic vein flow velocities in a normal subject. Systolic velocity (*S*) is usually greater than diastolic velocity (*D*) with no prominent reversal velocities (*SR* and *DR*). Both velocities are higher with inspiration than with expiration.

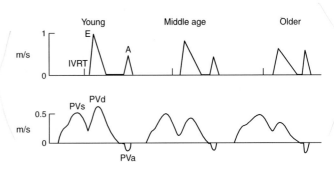

FIG. 5-12. Diagram of mitral inflow [*E, A,* isovolumic relaxation time (*IVRT*)] **(top)** and pulmonary venous flow velocities (*PVs, PVd,* and *PVa*) **(bottom)** in normal young, middle-aged, and older subjects, demonstrating gradual changes in the diastolic variables with aging. (From ref. 12, with permission.)

TABLE 5-2. *Normal values for diastolic variables[a]*

Variable	Age group (yr)			
	2–20 (n = 46)	21–40 (n = 51)	41–60 (n = 33)	>60 (n = 10)
Heart rate (beats/min)	78 ± 16	74 ± 11	73 ± 10	70 ± 14
Blood pressure (mm Hg)				
Systolic		111 ± 14	117 ± 14	121 ± 11
Diastolic		71 ± 10	73 ± 9	75 ± 12
IVRT (msec)	50 ± 9	67 ± 8	74 ± 7	87 ± 7
E (cm/sec)	88 ± 14	75 ± 13	71 ± 13	71 ± 11
A (cm/sec)	49 ± 12	51 ± 11	57 ± 13	75 ± 12
E/A	1.88 ± 0.45	1.53 ± 0.40	1.28 ± 0.25	0.96 ± 0.18
DT (msec)	142 ± 19	166 ± 14	181 ± 19	200 ± 29
A dur (msec)	113 ± 17	127 ± 13	133 ± 13	138 ± 19
PVs (cm/sec)	48 ± 10	44 ± 10	49 ± 8	52 ± 11
PVd (cm/sec)	60 ± 10	47 ± 11	41 ± 8	39 ± 11
PVa (cm/sec)	16 ± 10	21 ± 8	23 ± 3	25 ± 9
PVa dur (msec)	66 ± 39	96 ± 33	112 ± 15	113 ± 30
PVs/PVd	0.82 ± 0.18	0.98 ± 0.32	1.21 ± 0.20	1.39 ± 0.47

A, filling wave due to atrial contraction; A dur, duration of mitral flow with atrial contraction; BP, blood pressure; DT, deceleration time; E, early rapid filling wave: IVRT, isovolumic relaxation time; PVa, PVd, PVs, velocity components in pulmonary vein (see text).

[a] Normal values for mitral flow, pulmonary venous flow velocities, and other Doppler diastolic variables in different age groups. (Courtesy of Liv K. Hatle, M.D.)

relaxation (Fig. 5-13) that is more than that expected with aging (12). Typical examples of cardiac lesions that produce impaired relaxation include LV hypertrophy, hypertrophic cardiomyopathy, and myocardial ischemia/infarction. The IVRT is prolonged. *Mitral E velocity is decreased and A velocity is increased, producing an E/A ratio < 1, with prolonged DT.* Whenever the E/A ratio is below 1, impaired relaxation is usually present. (The reverse is not true.) PVd parallels mitral E velocity and is also decreased with compensatory increased flow in systole. The duration and velocity of PVa are usually normal, but they may be increased if LV end-diastolic pressure is high.

Restrictive Filling (or Decreased Compliance) Pattern

The term *restrictive diastolic filling,* or *restrictive physiology,* should be distinguished from *restrictive cardiomyopathy.* Restrictive physiology can be present in any cardiac abnormality or in a combination of abnormalities that produce decreased LV compliance and markedly increased LA pressure. Examples include patients with decompensated congestive heart failure, advanced restrictive cardiomyopathy, severe coronary artery disease, acute severe aortic regurgitation, and constrictive pericarditis. The increase in LA pressure results in earlier opening of the mitral valve, shortened IVRT, and a greater initial transmitral gradient (high E velocity). Early diastolic filling into a noncompliant LV causes a rapid increase in early LV diastolic pressure, with rapid equalization of LV and LA pressures producing a shortened DT. Atrial contraction increases LA pressure, but A velocity and duration are shortened because LV pressure increases even more rapidly. When LV diastolic pres-

sure is markedly increased, there may be diastolic mitral regurgitation during mid-diastole or with atrial relaxation. Therefore, *restrictive physiology is characterized by mitral flow velocities that show increased E velocity, decreased A velocity (<<E), and shortened DT (< 160 msec) and IVRT (< 70 msec).* Typically, the E/A ratio is greater than 2.0 and occasionally increases to 5 (e.g., E velocity of 1.5 m/sec and A velocity of 0.3 m/sec). It should be emphasized, however, that myocardial relaxation continues to be impaired in patients with restrictive filling, but it is masked by decreased LV compliance, with markedly increased LA pressure. Systolic forward flow velocity in the pulmonary vein is decreased because of increased LA pressure and decreased LA compliance. Pulmonary vein forward flow stops at mid to late diastole, reflecting the rapid increase in LV pressure; at atrial contraction, the increase in LA pressure can produce a prolonged PVa; however, PVa may not be seen if atrial contraction occurs when pulmonary vein flow velocity is relatively high because of tachycardia (Fig. 5-14).

Pseudonormalized Pattern

As diastolic function deteriorates, a transition from impaired relaxation to restrictive filling occurs. During this transition, mitral inflow pattern goes through a phase resembling a normal diastolic filling pattern, that is, E/A ratio of 1 to 1.5 and normal DT (160 to 200 ms). This is the result of a moderately increased LA pressure superimposed on a relaxation abnormality (14). This is referred to as the *pseudonormalized* filling pattern, and it represents a moderate stage of diastolic dysfunction. The pseudonormal pat-

Abnormal LV Filling Patterns

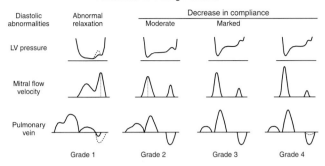

FIG. 5-13. Diagram of left ventricular (*LV*) pressure, mitral inflow velocity, and pulmonary vein Doppler signal in early-to-advanced diastolic dysfunction, with grading system. With worsening diastolic function, LV diastolic pressure is increased further, producing ↑ E, ↓ A, ↑ E/A, ↓ deceleration time (DT) in mitral inflow and ↓ S, ↑ D in pulmonary venous flow velocities. In grade 1 diastolic dysfunction, mean left atrial (LA) pressure and pre-A wave LV diastolic pressure are not elevated. However, LV end-diastolic pressure after atrial contraction may be elevated (*dotted line*). In that case, mitral A duration is usually shorter than PVa duration (*dotted lines*). In grade 2 diastolic dysfunction, mitral inflow velocity appears normal because of a moderately elevated filling pressure superimposed on an abnormal relaxation pattern. This can revert to grade 1 pattern with decreased filling pressure (Valsalva maneuver, nitroglycerin, or sitting position). With further increase in filling pressures, mitral E velocity becomes higher with shorter DT. When this restrictive filling pattern is reversed to grade 2 pattern by preload reduction (Nipride, diuresis, Valsalva maneuver), it is designated as grade 3 diastolic dysfunction. When restrictive filling pattern is irreversible, diastolic dysfunction becomes end-stage grade 4. As long as atrial contraction is preserved in grade 4 diastolic dysfunction, PVa is increased in velocity and duration. If the atrium fails, PVa is not prominent (*dotted line*). Prognosis of a patient with restrictive filling pattern depends on whether or not it can be reversed to a less restrictive filling pattern.

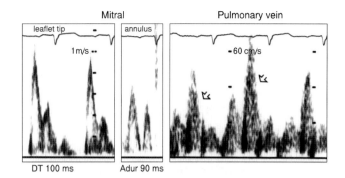

FIG. 5-14. Pulsed-wave Doppler recording of mitral inflow at the mitral leaflet tip **(left)** and at the annulus **(center)** and of the pulmonary vein flow velocities **(right)**. E velocity is 1 m/sec and A velocity is 0.4 m/sec, with an E/A ratio of 2.5, and deceleration time (*DT*) is shortened to 100 msec, consistent with restrictive filling. A duration (*Adur*) was obtained with the sample volume at the annulus and was measured as 90 msec. However, there was no pulmonary vein atrial flow reversal because the pulmonary venous flow velocity was relatively high at the time of atrial contraction (*arrows*). PVs1 occurs at the onset of QRS because of prolonged pulmonary regurgitation interval.

and flow propagation is slow, even when LA pressure and mitral E velocity are increased (Fig. 5-17).

The classification of diastolic filling patterns based on two-dimensional (2D) echocardiographic and Doppler variables is summarized in Table 5-3.

Variations in Mitral Inflow Patterns

Not all mitral flow velocity patterns fit nicely into one of these three patterns. The spectrum is wide as a result of different contributions and degrees of underlying disease, abnormal relaxation, changes in compliance, and volume status. The same degree of decrease in compliance or volume change will result in different mitral flow velocity curves, depending on whether there is abnormal relaxation. In the presence of significant LV hypertrophy, the DT still can be prolonged even with increased LA pressure, whereas a similar increase in pressure in other patients results in a shortened DT. In severe LV hypertrophy, a triphasic mitral flow pattern with prominent mid-diastolic flow can be seen as a result of markedly prolonged relaxation continuing into mid-diastole. Even if the initial slope gives a short DT, the continued filling indicates that abnormal relaxation, not a decrease in compliance, is the main problem. This may help explain why the use of mitral filling patterns in estimating filling pressures works less well in hypertrophic cardiomyopathy. An opposite example is constrictive pericarditis, in which normal relaxation and decreased compliance may result in markedly shortened mitral DTs without markedly increased filling pressures. These variations illustrate the importance of evaluating mitral flow velocity over the entire diastolic filling period, instead of relying on a single

tern can be distinguished from a true normal pattern by the following:

1. In patients with an LV of abnormal size or systolic dysfunction or with increased wall thickness, impaired relaxation is expected, and a normal E/A ratio suggests that increased LA pressure is masking the abnormal relaxation.

2. By demonstrating a shortening of mitral A duration in the absence of a short PR interval or by demonstrating prolonged PVa exceeding mitral A duration (Fig. 5-15).

3. A reduction in preload by sitting or by Valsalva maneuver or sublingual nitroglycerin may be able to unmask the underlying impaired relaxation of the LV (Fig. 5-16), decreasing the E/A ratio to less than 1.0 (15). In normal subjects, both the E and A velocities decrease more proportionally with a decrease in filling.

4. Color M-mode of mitral inflow can determine the rate of flow propagation in the LV (16,17). With worsening of diastolic function, myocardial relaxation is always impaired

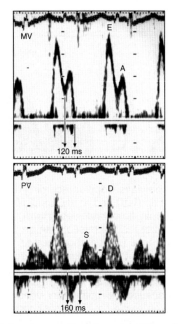

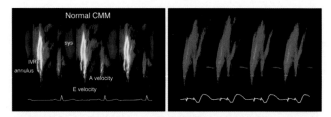

FIG. 5-17. Color M-mode (*CMM*) recordings of mitral inflow from two patients with normal-appearing pulsed-wave Doppler recordings of mitral inflow. In a patient with a pseudo-normalized mitral inflow, CMM shows slow flow propagation because of impaired myocardial relaxation **(right)**, whereas flow reaches the apex immediately in normal subjects with intact elastic recoil and suction **(left)**. *IVRT*, isovolumic relaxation time; *sys*, systolic. (Courtesy of Christopher P. Appleton, M.D. and Joan Jensen.)

FIG. 5-15. Pulsed-wave Doppler recording of mitral inflow (*MV*) **(top)** and pulmonary vein (*PV*) **(bottom)** flow velocities. E/A ratio is slightly < 2 and deceleration time is 180 msec. PV flow velocity shows predominant diastolic forward flow velocity, which indicates increased left atrial pressure. PV atrial flow reversal is also longer (160 msec) than the duration of the A wave (120 msec), indicating that MV is a "pseudonormalized" filling pattern. *D*, diastolic flow; *S*, systolic flow.

Valsalva Maneuver

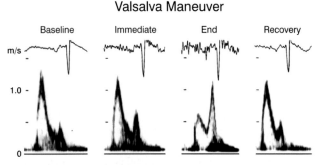

FIG. 5-16. Four separate recordings of mitral inflow velocity at baseline, immediately after the Valsalva maneuver, at the end of the Valsalva maneuver, and during the recovery phase. With reduction of preload by the Valsalva maneuver, the underlying impaired relaxation of the left ventricle was unmasked **(End)**, with a decrease in E velocity and an increase in A velocity.

TABLE 5-3. *Classification of diastolic filling*

Normal filling
    DT 160–240 msec (but can be lower, especially in young persons)
    IVRT 70–90 msec; E/A 1–2
    Mitral A duration ≥ PVa duration
    PV_{S2} ≥ PVd (PV_{S2} can be smaller than PVd in young persons)
    No anatomic abnormalities
Impaired (or abnormal) relaxation
    DT > 240 msec
    IVRT > 90 msec
    E/A < 1.0
    PV_{S2} >> PVd
    Mitral A duration ≥ or < PVa duration (depending on LVEDP)
Pseudonormal pattern
    DT 160–200 msec
    IVRT < 90 msec; E/A 1–1.5
    PV_{S2} < PVd
    Mitral A duration < PVa duration
    PVa velocity ↑ (> 35 cm/sec)
    2D echocardiographic evidence of structural heart disease (↓ EF, ↑ LA, LVH)
    Reversal of E/A ratio (to < 1.0) with preload reduction (e.g., Valsalva maneuver)
Restrictive filling
    DT < 160 msec
    IVRT < 70 ms; E/A > 1.5
    PV_{S2} << PVd
    Mitral A duration < PVa duration
    PVa velocity ↑ (≥ 35 cm/sec, usually but not always)
    2D echocardiographic evidence of structural heart disease
    Decreased E/A ratio with preload reduction (e.g., Valsalva)

A, filling wave due to atrial contraction; DT, deceleration time; E, early rapid filling wave; EF, ejection fraction; IVRT, isovolumic relaxation time; LA, left atrial; LVEDP, LV end-diastolic pressure; LVH, left ventricular hypertrophy; PVa, PVd, PV_{S2}, velocity components in pulmonary vein (see text); 2D, two dimensional.

variable for characterization. This approach helps avoid interpretive errors made by trying to fit all patients into rigid diagnostic algorithms. In these cases, 2D echocardiography is also often helpful by demonstrating the presence and absence of structural heart disease.

Mitral Annulus Velocity by Doppler Tissue Imaging

Doppler tissue imaging (DTI), or tissue Doppler, has been applied to evaluate diastolic function by measuring mitral annulus velocity during diastole. The mitral annulus velocity profile during diastole reflects the rate of changes in the long-axis dimension and in LV volume. When myocardial relaxation is abnormal, the ratio of mitral annulus motion during atrial systole to the total diastolic annular motion is increased. Sohn et al. (18) demonstrated that mitral annulus velocity determined by DTI is relatively preload-independent and is useful in differentiating pseudonormal (grade 2 diastolic dysfunction) from normal mitral inflow velocity pattern. Various patterns of mitral inflow and mitral annulus velocity are shown in Fig. 5-18 (18). Mitral annulus velocities are markedly decreased in patients with restrictive cardiomyopathy, which is clinically useful in distinguishing it from constrictive pericarditis, which has a preserved mitral annulus velocity (20). Using the early diastolic velocity of the mitral annulus (E′) as a preindependent index of LV relaxation, E/E′ has been found to

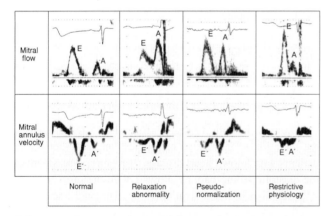

FIG. 5-18. Patterns of mitral inflow and mitral annulus velocity from normal to restrictive physiology. The mitral annulus velocity was obtained from the septal side of the mitral annulus using Doppler tissue imaging. Each calibration mark in the recording of mitral annulus velocity respresents 5 cm/sec. Early diastolic annulus velocity (E′) is greater than late diastolic annulus velocity (A′) in a normal pattern. In all other patterns, E′ is not greater than A′. In relaxation abnormality, E′ and A′ parallel E and A velocities of mitral inflow. However, when filling pressure is increased (pseudonormalization and restrictive physiology), E′ remains decreased (i.e., persistent underlying relaxation abnormality) while mitral inflow E velocity increases. Hence, E/E′ may be useful in estimating LV filling pressure (19). (From ref. 18, with permission.)

correlate well with mean pulmonary capillary wedge pressure (19). This finding needs further clinical validation.

Diastolic Filling Pattern in Atrial Fibrillation

The usual criteria for classifying diastolic filling patterns cannot be applied to patients with atrial fibrillation. There is no A wave in mitral inflow, and systolic forward flow in the pulmonary vein is almost always diminished. Peak velocity and DT of mitral E vary with length of the cardiac cycle. Peak acceleration rate of E velocity was found to correlate well with LV filling pressure (21), but it is difficult to measure. It appears from clinical observations that DT becomes shortened with increased LV filling pressure, as in patients with sinus rhythm, especially when LV systolic function is decreased (22,23); however, DT should be measured only when E velocity ends before the onset of QRS (Fig. 5-19A). When the diastolic filling period is too short, E velocity is terminated prematurely with a shorter DT (Fig. 5-19B). Diastolic flow is a predominant pulmonary vein forward flow in patients with atrial fibrillation. Duration and the initial deceleration slope time of pulmonary vein diastolic flow may be useful in determining LV filling pressure (24). Further clinical studies are needed to understand the diastolic filling pattern in patients with atrial fibrillation.

Index of Myocardial Performance

An index of myocardial performance (IMP) has been devised to incorporate both systolic and diastolic time intervals in expressing global ventricular performance (25). Systolic dysfunction results in a prolongation of the preejection (isovolumic contraction time; ICT) and a shortening of the ejection time (ET). Both systolic and diastolic dysfunction result in abnormality in myocardial relaxation, which prolongs the relaxation period (isovolumic relaxation time; IRT).

$$IMP = \frac{ICT + IRT}{ET}$$

The time intervals necessary for calculating IMP are easily obtained with Doppler echocardiography (Fig. 5-20). It was measured in normal subjects and patients with dilated cardiomyopathy. The normal value was 0.39 ± 0.05, and it was increased to 0.59 ± 0.10 in those with dilated cardiomyopathy. IMP was evaluated for the RV, especially in patients with pulmonary hypertension (26). This index was the single most powerful variable for discriminating patients with primary pulmonary hypertension from normal subjects (0.93 ± 0.34 vs 0.28 ± 0.04). It may have an important role in assessing RV function. Further clinical studies are needed to assess the incremental role of IMP in the evaluation of ventricular function.

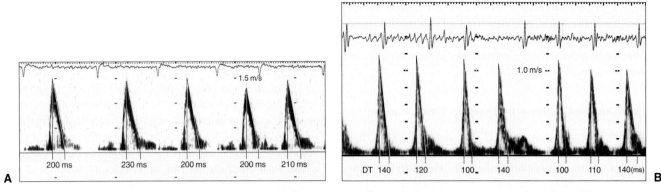

FIG. 5-19. A: Pulsed-wave Doppler recording of mitral inflow velocity in an asymptomatic patient with atrial fibrillation after aortic replacement. All E velocities were completed before the onset of QRS, and their deceleration time ranges from 200 to 230 msec. **B:** Pulsed-wave Doppler recording of mitral inflow from an elderly woman with congestive heart failure in the setting of atrial fibrillation. Peak E velocity and deceleration time (*DT*) vary depending on cardiac cycle length. When E velocity is terminated before the onset of QRS (third, fifth, and sixth signals), DT is shorter (100–110 msec) than that (120–140 msec) of mitral inflow velocity, which were completed before the QRS (first, second, fourth, and seventh signals).

Grading of Diastolic Dysfunction

In most (if not all) cardiac diseases, the initial diastolic dysfunction is impaired relaxation. With further progression of disease and a mild-to-moderate increase in LA pressure, the mitral inflow velocity pattern appears similar to a normal filling pattern (pseudonormalized). With further decrease in LV compliance and increase in LA pressure, di-

astolic filling becomes restrictive. Most patients with restrictive filling are symptomatic and have a poor prognosis unless the restrictive filling can be reversed by treatment (22,27). However, restrictive filling may be irreversible and represent the end stage of diastolic heart failure. Therefore, diastolic dysfunction can be graded as follows according to the diastolic filling pattern (4,28):

Grade 1 = impaired relaxation
Grade 2 = pseudonormalized pattern
Grade 3 = reversible restrictive pattern
Grade 4 = irreversible restrictive pattern (see Fig. 5-13)

Clinical Applications of Diastolic Function Assessment

Although diastolic filling is affected by various factors, the direction of its change or progression is predictable in patients with known heart disease. Therefore, assessment of the diastolic filling pattern allows LV filling pressures and LV compliance and relaxation to be estimated and understood so that optimal treatment strategies can be offered to symptomatic patients with diastolic dysfunction. The estimation of LV filling pressure by diastolic filling variables is discussed in Chapter 6. Another important application is to provide prognosis in various cardiac diseases. A restrictive filling pattern indicates a poor prognosis and treatments aimed at making diastolic filling less restrictive improve the clinical outcome of patients. The Doppler echocardiographic evaluation of the diastolic filling pattern may be helpful in assessing the response to treatment of patients with heart failure.

Evaluation of the diastolic filling pattern is extremely valuable in differentiating constrictive pericarditis from restrictive cardiomyopathy; this is discussed in Chapter 14.

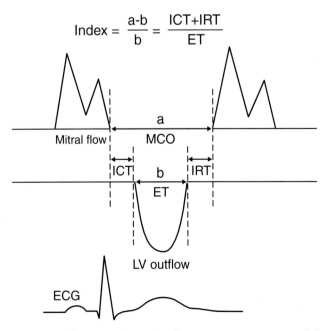

$$\text{Index} = \frac{a-b}{b} = \frac{ICT+IRT}{ET}$$

FIG. 5-20. Diagram illustrating how to measure myocardial performance index. *ECG*, electrocardiogram; *ET*, ejection time; *ICT*, isovolumic contraction time; *IRT*, isovolumic relaxation time; *MCO*, mitral valve closure to opening.

REFERENCES

1. Kitabatake A, Inoue M, Asao M, et al. Transmitral blood flow reflecting diastolic behavior of the left ventricle in health and disease—a study by pulsed Doppler technique. *Jpn Circ J* 1982;46:92–102.

2. Appleton CP, Hatle LK, Popp RL. Relation of transmitral flow velocity patterns to left ventricular diastolic function: new insights from a combined hemodynamic and Doppler echocardiographic study. *J Am Coll Cardiol* 1988;12:426–440.

3. Nishimura RA, Abel MD, Hatle LK, Tajik AJ. Assessment of diastolic function of the heart: Background and current applications of Doppler echocardiography. Part II. Clinical studies. *Mayo Clin Proc* 1989;64:181–204.

4. Oh JK, Appleton CP, Hatle LK, Nishimura RA, Seward JB, Tajik AJ. The noninvasive assessment of left ventricular diastolic function with two-dimensional and Doppler echocardiography. *J Am Soc Echocardiogr* 1997;10:246–270.

5. Jensen JL, Williams FE, Beilby BJ, et al. Feasibility of obtaining pulmonary venous flow velocity in cardiac patients using transthoracic pulsed wave Doppler technique. *J Am Soc Echocardiogr* 1997;10:60–66.

6. Appleton CP, Jensen JL, Hatle LK, Oh JK. Doppler evaluation of left and right ventricular diastolic function: a technical guide for obtaining optimal flow velocity recordings. *J Am Soc Echocardiogr* 1997;10:271–292.

7. Rossvoll O, Hatle LK. Pulmonary venous flow velocities recorded by transthoracic Doppler ultrasound: relation to left ventricular diastolic pressures. *J Am Coll Cardiol* 1993;21:1687–1696.

8. Yamamoto K, Nishimura RA, Burnett JC Jr, Redfield MM. Assessment of left ventricular end-diastolic pressure by Doppler echocardiography: contribution of duration of pulmonary venous versus mitral flow velocity curves at atrial contraction. *J Am Soc Echocardiogr* 1997;10:52–59.

9. Appleton CP. Hemodynamic determinants of Doppler pulmonary venous flow velocity components: new insights from studies in lightly sedated normal dogs. *J Am Coll Cardiol* 1997;30:1562–1574.

10. Oh JK, Hatle LK, Seward JB, et al. Diagnostic role of Doppler echocardiography in constrictive pericarditis. *J Am Coll Cardiol* 1994;23:154–162.

11. Boonyaratavej S, Olson LJ, Beck KC, Swee CM, Oh JK, Seward JB. Respiratory variation of superior vena cava Doppler in patients with severe emphysema: correlation with intrapleural and intraabdominal pressure. *J Am Coll Cardiol* 1996;27:212A(abst).

12. Appleton CP, Hatle LK. The natural history of left ventricular filling abnormalities: assessment by two-dimensional and Doppler echocardiography. *Echocardiography* 1992;9:437–457.

13. Klein AL, Burstow DJ, Tajik AJ, Zachariah PK, Bailey KR, Seward JB. Effects of age on left ventricular dimensions and filling dynamics in 117 normal persons. *Mayo Clin Proc* 1994;69:212–224.

14. Nishimura RA, Schwartz RS, Holmes DR Jr, Tajik AJ. Failure of calcium channel blockers to improve ventricular relaxation in humans. *J Am Coll Cardiol* 1993;21:182–188.

15. Dumesnil JG, Gaudreault G, Honos GN, Kingma JG Jr. Use of Valsalva maneuver to unmask left ventricular diastolic function abnormalities by Doppler echocardiography in patients with coronary artery disease or systemic hypertension. *Am J Cardiol* 1991;68:515–519.

16. Takatsuji H, Mikami T, Urasawa K, et al. A new approach for evaluation of left ventricular diastolic function: spatial and temporal analysis of left ventricular filling flow propagation by color M-mode Doppler echocardiography. *J Am Coll Cardiol* 1996;27:365–371.

17. Stugaard M, Steen T, Lundervold A, Smiseth OA, Ihlen H. Visual assessment of intraventricular flow from colour M-mode Doppler images. *Int J Card Imaging* 1994;10:279–287.

18. Sohn DW, Chai IH, Lee DJ, et al. Assessment of mitral annulus velocity by Doppler tissue imaging in the evaluation of left ventricular diastolic function. *J Am Coll Cardiol* 1997;30:474–480.

19. Nagueh SF, Middleton KJ, Kopelen HA, Zoghbi WA, Quiñones MA. Doppler tissue imaging: a noninvasive technique for evaluation of left ventricular relaxation and estimation of filling pressures. *J Am Coll Cardiol* 1997;30:1527–1533.

20. Garcia MJ, Rodriguez L, Ares M, Griffin BP, Thomas JD, Klein AL. Differentiation of constrictive pericarditis from restrictive cardiomyopathy: assessment of left ventricular diastolic velocities in longitudinal axis by Doppler tissue imaging. *J Am Coll Cardiol* 1996;27:108–114.

21. Nagueh SF, Kopelen HA, Quinones MA. Assessment of left ventricular filling pressures by Doppler in the presence of atrial fibrillation. *Circulation* 1996;94:2138–2145.

22. Lee DC, Oh JK, Osborn SL, Mahoney DW, Seward JB. Repeat evaluation of diastolic filling pattern after treatment of congestive heart failure in patients with restrictive diastolic filling: Implication for long-term prognosis. *J Am Soc Echocardiogr* 1997;10:431(abst).

23. Hurrell DG, Oh JK, Mahoney DW, Miller FA Jr, Seward JB. Short deceleration time of mitral inflow E velocity: prognostic implication with atrial fibrillation versus sinus rhythm. *J Am Soc Echocardiogr* 1998;11:450–457.

24. Chirillo F, Brunazzi MC, Barbiero M, et al. Estimating mean pulmonary wedge pressure in patients with chronic atrial fibrillation from transthoracic Doppler indexes of mitral and pulmonary venous flow velocity. *J Am Coll Cardiol* 1997;30:19–26.

25. Tei C, Ling LH, Hodge DO, et al. New index of combined systolic and diastolic myocardial performance: a simple and reproducible measure of cardiac function—a study in normals and dilated cardiomyopathy. *J Cardiol* 1995;26:357–366.

26. Tei C, Dujardin KS, Hodge DO, et al. Doppler echocardiographic index for assessment of global right ventricular function. *J Am Soc Echocardiogr* 1996;9:838–847.

27. Pinamonti B, Zecchin M, Di Lenarda A, Gregori D, Sinagra G, Camerini F. Persistence of restrictive left ventricular filling pattern in dilated cardiomyopathy: an ominous prognostic sign. *J Am Coll Cardiol* 1997;29:604–612.

28. Nishimura RA, Tajik AJ. Evaluation of diastolic filling of left ventricle in health and disease: Doppler echocardiography is the clinician's Rosetta Stone. *J Am Coll Cardiol* 1997;30:8–18.

CHAPTER 6

Hemodynamic Assessment

Before the application of Doppler echocardiography, cardiac hemodynamics were obtained by invasive cardiac catheterization. Now, echocardiography is the preferred method for determining various hemodynamic data noninvasively. These are listed in Table 6-1.

M-mode and two-dimensional (2D) echocardiography alone can provide only indirect evidence of hemodynamic abnormalities, but this evidence may be the initial clue to such problems. Table 6-2 and Figs. 6-1 through 6-4 demonstrate various M-mode and 2D echocardiographic signs of hemodynamic derangements; however, these signs are qualitative at best. Intracardiac hemodynamic assessment requires Doppler echocardiography, and the accuracy of Doppler-derived hemodynamic measurements has been validated by comparison with simultaneously derived catheterization data (1–4).

STROKE VOLUME AND CARDIAC OUTPUT

Flow across a fixed orifice is equal to the product of the cross-sectional area (CSA) of the orifice and flow velocity (Fig. 6-5).

$$Flow\ rate\ =\ CSA\ \times\ Flow\ velocity$$

Because flow velocity varies during ejection in a pulsatile system, such as the cardiovascular system, individual velocities of the Doppler spectrum need to be summed (i.e., integrated) to measure the total volume of flow during a given ejection period. The sum of velocities is called the *time velocity integral* (TVI), or *velocity time integral* (VTI), and is equal to the area enclosed by the baseline and Doppler spectrum. It is also equal to stroke distance (i.e., the distance blood travels with each beat of the heart). TVI can be measured readily with the built-in calculation package in the ultrasound unit by tracing the Doppler velocity signal. After TVI is determined, stroke volume (SV) is calculated by multiplying TVI by CSA.

$$SV\ =\ CSA\ \times\ TVI$$

The location most frequently used to determine stroke volume is the LV outflow tract (LVOT) (5). Figure 6-6 demonstrates how to calculate stroke volume from the LVOT. Flow across the other cardiac orifices can be calculated by using the same formula. The CSA of orifices in the heart is usually assumed to be a circle, and it is determined from measurement of the orifice diameter (D):

$$CSA\ =\ \left(\frac{D}{2}\right)^2\ \times\ \pi\ =\ D^2\ \times\ 0.785$$

hence,

$$SV\ =\ D^2\ \times\ 0.785\ \times\ TVI$$

Table 6-3 lists orifice areas according to measured diameters.

Cardiac output (CO) is obtained by multiplying stroke volume by heart rate and cardiac index (CI) by dividing CO by body surface area (BSA).

$$CO\ =\ SV\ \times\ Heart\ rate$$

$$CI\ =\ CO/BSA$$

TABLE 6-1. *Hemodynamic data that can be obtained with two-dimensional Doppler echocardiography*

Volumetric measurements
  Stroke volume and cardiac output
  Regurgitant volume and fraction
  Pulmonary-systemic flow ratio (Qp/Qs)
Pressure gradients
  Maximal instantaneous gradient
  Mean gradient
Valve area
  Stenotic valve area
  Regurgitant orifice area
Intracardiac pressures
  Pulmonary artery pressures
  Left atrial pressure
  Left ventricular end-diastolic pressure

TABLE 6-2. *M-mode/two-dimensional (2D) echocardiographic signs of hemodynamic abnormalities*

M-mode/2D findings	Hemodynamic abnormality
Fluttering of mitral valve	Aortic regurgitation
Midsystolic aortic valve closure	Dynamic obstruction of LVOT
Systolic anterior motion of mitral valve	Dynamic obstruction of LVOT
Midsystolic pulmonary valve closure	Pulmonary hypertension
Dilated RV + D-shaped LV	Increased RV systolic pressure
Dilated IVC with lack of inspiratory collapse	Increased RA pressure
Persistent bowing of atrial septum	
To RA	Increased LA pressure
To LA	Increased RA pressure
Diastolic RA and RV wall inversion or collapse	Cardiac tamponade
Abnormal ventricular septal motion	Constrictive pericarditis

IVC, inferior vena cava; LVOT, left ventricular outflow tract; RV, right ventricle; LV, left ventricle; RA, right atrium; LA, left atrium; 2D, two dimensional.

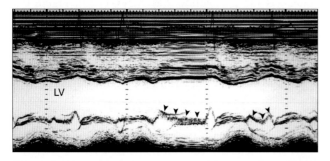

FIG. 6-1. M-mode echocardiogram of the mitral valve, with fluttering (*arrowheads*) from aortic regurgitation. However, this M-mode sign may not be present if the aortic regurgitation jet is eccentric toward the ventricular septum rather than toward the mitral valve. Left ventricle (*LV*) is enlarged and systolic function is reduced.

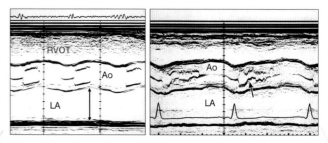

FIG. 6-2. M-mode echocardiograms of the aortic valve and the aorta (*Ao*). **Left:** Normal aortic valve, with the same amount of opening throughout systole. **Right:** Midsystolic closure (*arrow*) due to dynamic obstruction of the left ventricular outflow tract. *RVOT,* RV outflow tract.

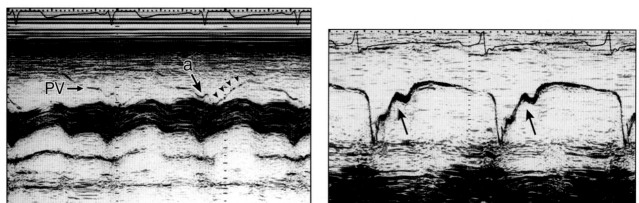

FIG. 6-3. M-mode echocardiograms of the pulmonary valve (*PV*). **A:** Normal PV with prominent "a" wave (*a*). The valve closure is smooth (*arrowheads*). **B:** Midsystolic closure (*arrows*) of PV, producing a W shape in pulmonary hypertension. There is no "a" wave.

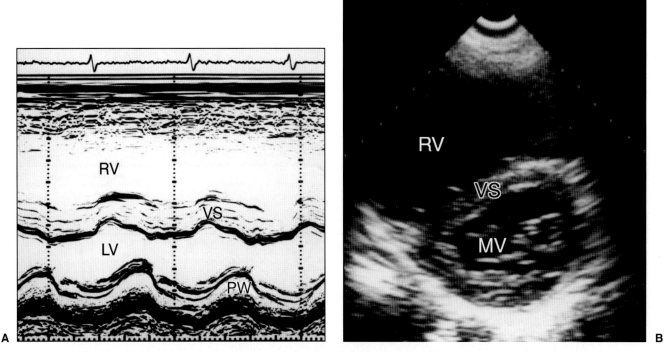

FIG. 6-4. A: M-mode echocardiogram of the dilated right ventricle (*RV*), flattened ventricular septum (*VS*) with abnormal motion, and small left ventricular (*LV*) cavity. This is typical of RV systolic pressure overload. **B:** Two-dimensional echocardiogram of the dilated RV, flattened VS, and D-shaped LV typically seen in patients with pulmonary hypertension. *MV*, mitral valve; *PW*, posterior wall.

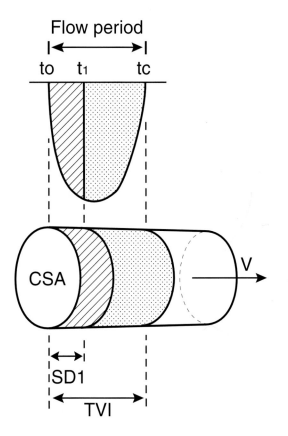

FIG. 6-5. A schematic example of a Doppler spectrum of the left ventricular outflow tract. The amount of blood flow going through a fixed orifice is directly proportional to the product of the orifice cross-sectional area (*CSA*) and flow velocity (flow = CSA × velocity). Flow velocities vary during the ejection or filling period (from "*to*" to "*tc*") and provide a distinct Doppler profile for a given orifice in the pulsatile cardiovascular system. The area enclosed by the velocity curve is equivalent to the distance blood flow travels with one stroke [stroke distance (SD)]; that is, the area of the velocity curve indicated by diagonal lines is equal to the distance blood travels (*SD1*) from the time of valve opening (*to*) to time 1 (*t₁*). The entire area under the velocity curve represents the total distance the blood travels with each stroke and is the same as integration of the entire velocity spectrum (*TVI*). *V,* velocity.

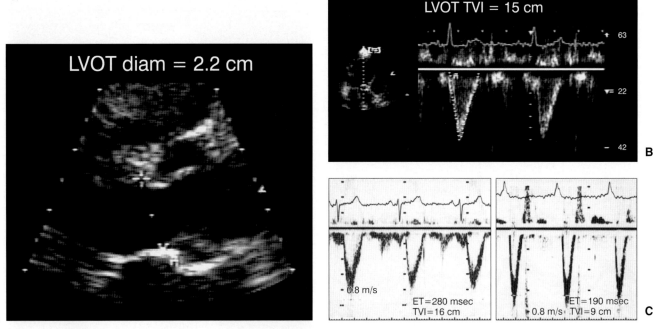

FIG. 6-6. How to calculate stroke volume from the left ventricle outflow tract (*LVOT*).
Step 1: **A:** Measurement of LVOT diameter (D) from the expanded (zoom) parasternal long-axis view. The diameter is measured at the level of the aortic annulus during systole. The line is drawn from where the anterior aortic cusp meets the ventricular septum to where the posterior aortic cusp meets the anterior mitral leaflet and perpendicular to the anterior aortic wall. D = 2.2 cm.
Step 2: Calculation of LVOT area. Assuming a circular shape of LVOT,

$$\text{LVOT area (cm}^2) = \left(\frac{D}{2}\right)^2 \times \pi$$
$$= D^2 \times 0.785$$

Table 6-3 lists area in square centimeters according to the measured diameters. LVOT area = 3.8 cm^2 when D = 2.2 cm.
Step 3: **B:** Measurement of LVOT velocity and time velocity integral (*TVI*) from the apical long-axis view. Pulsed-wave sample volume is placed at the center of the aortic annulus or 0.5 cm proximal to it (in a patient with aortic stenosis). TVI (cm) is the area under the velocity curve and is equal to the sum of velocities (cm/sec) during the ejection time (sec). TVI was measured to be 15 cm.
Step 4: Calculation of stroke volume (*SV*) across the LVOT.

$$SV \text{ (mL)} = \text{Area (cm}^2) \times TVI$$
$$= D^2 \times 0.785 \times TVI$$
$$SV = 3.8 \text{ cm}^2 \times 15 \text{ cm} = 57 \text{ mL}.$$

C: Two different LVOT velocity Doppler signals. Despite similar peak velocities, the TVI is different because of a difference in ejection time (*ET*).

Regurgitant Volume and Regurgitant Fraction

Regurgitant volume can be estimated two different ways with echocardiography: by the *volumetric method,* and the *proximal isovelocity surface area* (PISA) *method.* The hydraulic orifice formula given above is used in both methods:

$$Flow = CSA \times Velocity$$
$$or$$
$$Volume = CSA \times TVI$$

Volumetric Method

Total forward volume across a regurgitant valve (Q total) is the sum of systemic stroke volume (Qs) and regurgitant volume. Hence, regurgitant volume (Fig. 6-7) can be obtained by calculating the difference between the total forward stroke volume and systemic stroke volume.

$$Regurgitant \ volume + Qs = Q \ total$$

$$Regurgitant \ volume = Q \ total - Qs$$

TABLE 6-3. *Area calculation from diameter (D): area = D²*
× 0.785

Diameter (cm)	Area (cm²)	Diameter (cm)	Area (cm²)	Diameter (cm)	Area (cm²)
1.5	1.77	2.7	5.72	3.9	11.94
1.6	2.01	2.8	6.15	4.0	12.56
1.7	2.27	2.9	6.60	4.1	13.20
1.8	2.54	3.0	7.06	4.2	13.85
1.9[a]	2.83	3.1	7.54	4.3	14.51
2.0	3.14	3.2	8.04	4.4	15.20
2.1[b]	3.46	3.3	8.55	4.5	15.90
2.2	3.80	3.4	9.07	4.6	16.61
2.3	4.15	3.5	9.62	4.7	17.34
2.4	4.52	3.6	10.17	4.8	18.09
2.5	4.90	3.7	10.75	4.9	18.73
2.6	5.31	3.8	11.34	5.0	19.63

[a] Mean diameter of left ventricular outflow tract for adult woman.

[b] Mean diameter of left ventricular outflow tract for adult man.

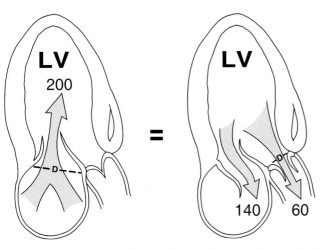

FIG. 6-7. Estimation of regurgitant volume and regurgitant fraction using mitral regurgitation as an example. Assume that regurgitation is present only in the mitral valve. Therefore, diastolic forward flow across the mitral valve (200 mL; **left**) is the sum of systolic flow across the left ventricular (*LV*) outflow tract (60 mL) and mitral regurgitant volume (140 mL); what goes into the LV during diastole (mitral inflow) must come out of the LV during systole [left ventricular outflow tract (LVOT)] flow + mitral regurgitant flow). The diagram shows a flail posterior mitral leaflet. Mitral inflow volume is the product of mitral annulus area and mitral flow TVI (flow = area × TVI). For this volumetric calculation, the sample volume is placed at the level of the mitral annulus.

Mitral regurgitant volume = Mitral inflow − LVOT flow

= (D² × 0.785 × TVI) MV − (D² × 0.785 × TVI) LVOT

Regurgitant fraction (%)

$$= \frac{\text{Mitral regurgitant volume}}{\text{Mitral inflow volume}} \times 100 \ (\%)$$

$$= \frac{140 \text{ mL}}{200 \text{ mL}} \times 100\% = 70\%$$

D, diameter; TVI, time velocity integral.

In mitral regurgitation, the Q total is the mitral inflow volume, calculated as a product of mitral valve annulus area and mitral inflow TVI. Mitral inflow TVI is obtained by placing a sample volume at the center of the mitral annulus. Systemic stroke volume (Qs) is obtained from multiplying the LVOT area by LVOT TVI. Mitral valve regurgitant volume is estimated as the mitral inflow volume minus the LVOT stroke volume (6). This calculation is not accurate (i.e., regurgitant volume is underestimated) if there is significant aortic regurgitation. In aortic regurgitation, the aortic valve regurgitant volume is obtained by subtracting the mitral inflow stroke volume (Qs) from the LVOT forward stroke volume (Q total).

The *regurgitant fraction* is simply the percentage of regurgitant volume compared with the total flow across the regurgitant valve.

Regurgitant fraction = (Regurgitant volume/Q total)

× 100%

Proximal Isovelocity Surface Area (PISA) Method

If the regurgitant orifice area is known, the regurgitant volume can be estimated as the product of effective regurgitant orifice area (ERO) and regurgitant velocity TVI.

Regurgitant volume = ERO × Regurgitant TVI

The regurgitant orifice area can be estimated using the concept of PISA. As blood flow converges toward the regurgitant orifice, blood flow velocity increases, with the formation of multiple shells of isovelocity of hemispheric shape. The flow rate at the surface of a hemispheric shell with the same flow velocity (isovelocity) should be equal to the flow rate across the regurgitant orifice (conservation of flow). By adjusting the Nyquist limit of the color-flow map, the flow velocity at a hemispheric surface proximal to the regurgitant orifice can be determined. In mitral valve regurgitation (MR), regurgitant flow travels away from the position of the apical transducer and toward the mitral regurgitation orifice. Hence, the blood flow converging toward the mitral regurgitant orifice in the LV is color-coded blue until the velocity reaches the negative aliasing velocity of the selected color-flow map, at which time the flow is color-coded light orange-red. If the negative aliasing velocity is reduced, the transition from blue to red-orange will occur farther from the regurgitant orifice, providing a larger hemispheric shell radius (r) (Fig. 6-8). After a hemisphere of blood flow with known velocity (equal to negative aliasing velocity) is identified, the rate of flow through a hemispheric shell is equal to the area of the hemisphere multiplied by the flow velocity (which is the aliasing velocity). The area of hemisphere is calculated as $2\pi \times r^2$. Hence,

Flow rate = 6.28 × r² × Aliasing velocity

This flow rate across the proximal isovelocity surface

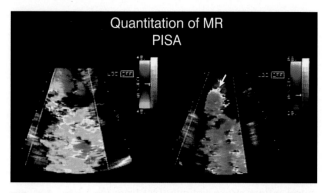

FIG. 6-8. Color-flow imaging of mitral regurgitation (*MR*) and proximal isovelocity surface area (*PISA*) at baseline without shift in aliasing velocity **(left)** and after baseline shift **(right)** to reduce the negative aliasing velocity from 48 cm/sec to 29 cm/sec. With the reduced aliasing velocity, PISA is larger (*arrow*).

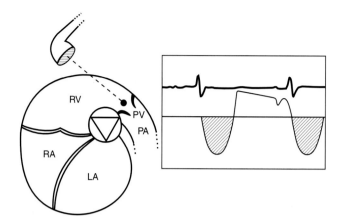

FIG. 6-9. Diagram of parasternal short-axis view to illustrate how to obtain right ventricular outflow tract (RVOT) velocity. The sample volume is located at the level of the pulmonary valve annulus, then

$$Qp = RVOT\ diameter^2 \times 0.785 \times TVI$$

Systemic flow is estimated from the LV outflow tract (LVOT) as in Fig. 6-6 unless there is significant aortic regurgitation. *LA*, left atrium; *RA*, right atrium; *RV*, right ventricle; *PA*, pulmonary artery; *PV*, pulmonary valve; *Qp*, blood flow through the pulmonary circulation.

area is equal to the flow rate across the ERO:

$$Flow\ rate = ERO \times Regurgitant\ velocity$$

Therefore, ERO can be obtained by dividing the flow rate by peak MR velocity across the regurgitant orifice.

$$ERO = \frac{Flow\ rate}{Peak\ MR\ velocity}$$

$$= 6.28 \times r^2 \times \frac{Aliasing\ velocity}{MR\ velocity}$$

Regurgitant volume is equal to regurgitant orifice area multiplied by the mitral regurgitation TVI.

$$Regurgitant\ volume = ERO \times MR\ TVI$$

$$= 6.28 \times r^2 \times \frac{Aliasing\ velocity}{MR\ velocity} \times MR\ TVI$$

Pulmonary–Systemic Flow Ratio (Qp/Qs)

In the presence of an intracardiac shunt, the flow ratio between the pulmonary and the systemic circulations usually indicates the magnitude of shunt. Pulmonary flow (Qp) is calculated from the RV outflow tract (RVOT) and systemic flow (Qs) from the LVOT.

$$Qp = RVOT\ CSA \times RVOT\ TVI$$

$$Qs = LVOT\ CSA \times LVOT\ TVI$$

Hence,

$$\frac{Qp}{Qs} = \frac{RVOT\ CSA \times RVOT\ TVI}{LVOT\ CSA \times LVOT\ TVI}$$

Figure 6-9 demonstrates the calculation of RVOT flow from the parasternal or subcostal short-axis view.

Transvalvular Gradients

Based on the Doppler shift (see Chapter 2), Doppler echocardiography measures blood-flow velocities in the cardiac chambers as well as in the great vessels (7,8). Blood-flow velocities can be converted to pressure gradients [in millimeters of mercury (mm Hg)] according to the Bernoulli equation (Fig. 6-10).

In most clinical situations, flow acceleration and viscous friction terms can be ignored. Furthermore, flow velocity proximal to a fixed orifice (v_1) is much lower than the peak flow velocity (v_2); hence, v_1 also can frequently be ignored. Therefore, pressure gradient (or pressure drop) across a fixed orifice can be calculated with the *simplified Bernoulli equation:*

$$Pressure\ gradient\ (\Delta P) = 4 \times (v_2)^2\ or\ (2\ v_2)^2$$

Blood-flow velocity measured with Doppler echocardiography is an *instantaneous event,* and the pressure gradients derived from Doppler velocities are *instantaneous gradients.* When maximal Doppler velocity is converted to pressure gradient using the simplified Bernoulli equation, it represents *maximal instantaneous gradient.* It should be noted that the maximal instantaneous gradient by Doppler will always be higher than the customary peak-to-peak gradient measured in the catheterization laboratory (Fig. 6-11). *Peak-to-peak gradient* in aortic stenosis is the pressure difference between the peak LV and peak aortic pressures, which do not occur simultaneously and, hence, is a nonphysiologic measurement. *Mean gradient* is an average of pressure gradients during the entire flow period, and mean gradient by

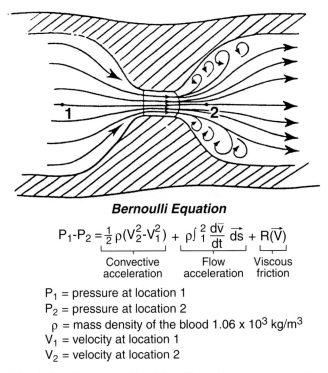

Bernoulli Equation

$$P_1-P_2 = \underbrace{\frac{1}{2}\rho(V_2^2-V_1^2)}_{\substack{\text{Convective}\\\text{acceleration}}} + \underbrace{\rho\int_1^2 \frac{d\vec{v}}{dt}\,\vec{ds}}_{\substack{\text{Flow}\\\text{acceleration}}} + \underbrace{R(\vec{V})}_{\substack{\text{Viscous}\\\text{friction}}}$$

P_1 = pressure at location 1
P_2 = pressure at location 2
ρ = mass density of the blood 1.06×10^3 kg/m^3
V_1 = velocity at location 1
V_2 = velocity at location 2

FIG. 6-10. Diagram of blood flow through a narrowed orifice to illustrate the *Bernoulli equation*, which measures pressure gradient across the orifice using blood-flow velocities. The Bernoulli equation has three components: convective acceleration, flow acceleration, and viscous friction. Because the velocity profile in the center of the lumen is usually flat, the viscous friction factor can be ignored in the clinical setting. The flow acceleration term causes a delay between the pressure drop curve and the velocity curve but provides a reasonably accurate estimation of pressure gradient, and this flow acceleration factor is ignored. Therefore, in a clinical situation, the flow gradient across a narrowed orifice can be derived from the convective acceleration term alone. (From ref. 7, with permission.)

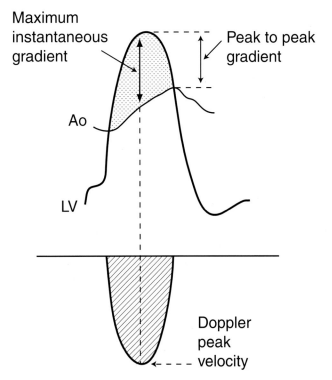

FIG. 6-11. Diagram of pressure tracings of left ventricle (*LV*) and aorta (*Ao*) in aortic stenosis along with the corresponding Doppler velocity spectrum. It is important to understand how different pressure gradients are derived. The average of pressure differences between LV and Ao (*stippled area*) represents the mean gradient (see text).

Doppler has been shown to correlate well with one simultaneously measured by cardiac catheterization. From the Doppler tracing, mean gradient can be derived by the built-in calculation package. Doppler velocity signals are traced manually, but recently they have been traced by automated border detection to provide peak velocity, maximal instantaneous gradient, and mean gradient (Fig. 6-12). Several studies have validated that Doppler-derived pressure gradients are highly accurate, with an excellent correlation with catheter-derived pressure gradients across LV or RVOT obstruction, mitral stenosis, pulmonary artery band, and various prosthetic valves (1–4,9–11) (Fig. 6-13).

Transmitral (normal, stenotic, native, or prosthetic valve) pressure gradient may be overestimated by cardiac catheterization if pulmonary capillary wedge pressure is used (instead of direct LA pressure) to calculate the pressure gradient (12). Doppler velocity recording is the optimal way to determine transmitral pressure gradient.

Valve Area (Stenotic or Regurgitant)

Continuity Equation

The *continuity equation* (Fig. 6-14) is the Gorlin formula of echocardiography and is used to calculate the area of a stenotic or regurgitant valve (13). It uses the concept of conservation of flow, namely, ''what comes in must go out.''

Because flow rate (or volume) is the product of the area and velocity (or TVI) of flow, a stenotic or regurgitant orifice area can be calculated from measurement of flow and flow velocity. Flow across a stenotic or regurgitant orifice is the same as a proximal (or upstream) flow across a known area and velocity. Hence,

$$A_1 \times TVI_1 = A_2 \times TVI_2$$

where A_1 is a known area at a location proximal to the unknown area, A_2. TVI is measured with pulsed- or continuous-wave Doppler.

$$A_2 = A_1 \times \left(\frac{TVI_1}{TVI_2}\right)$$

In aortic stenosis, flow across the aortic valve area (A_2) is the same as flow across the LVOT (A_1). In mitral re-

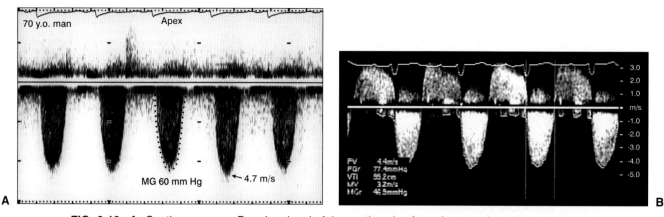

FIG. 6-12. A: Continuous-wave Doppler signal of the aortic valve from the apex in a 70-year-old man with severe aortic stenosis. Peak velocity is 4.7 m/sec, and tracing of the velocity yields a mean gradient (*MG*) of 60 mm Hg. **B:** Automated border detection of Doppler signals. Doppler velocity obtained from the apex is automatically traced to provide peak velocity (*PV*), maximal or peak gradient (*PGr*), time velocity integral (*VTI*), mean velocity (*MV*), and mean gradient (*MGr*) instantly. The two *lines* that are perpendicular to the baseline define the Doppler signal being interrogated.

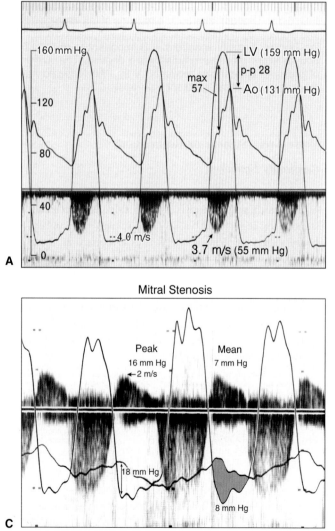

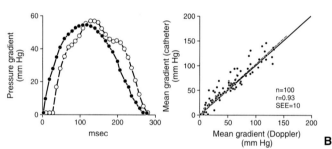

FIG. 6-13. A: Simultaneous Doppler and cardiac pressure recordings show an excellent correlation between Doppler-derived and catheter-derived pressure gradients in aortic stenosis. Peak Doppler velocity (3.7 m/sec) from the third cardiac cycle is converted to a maximal instantaneous gradient (*max*) of 55 mm Hg, which corresponds well to the maximal gradient determined by catheter (57 mm Hg) but not to the peak-to-peak (*p-p*) gradient of 28 mm Hg. *Ao*, aorta. **B:** Digitization of Doppler spectral velocity envelope and (LV-Ao) pressure waveforms of the third beat in panel A. The phase delay of the catheter gradient (*closed circles*) compared with the Doppler-derived gradient (*open circles*) is related to the fluid-filled catheter system **(left)**. Plot of mean gradients by Doppler echocardiography and catheterization showing a good correlation in 100 patients with aortic stenosis **(right)**. *r*, correlation coefficient; *SEE*, standard error of estimate. **C:** Simultaneous left ventricular and left atrial pressure measurements and Doppler velocity recording of the mitral valve in mitral stenosis. Peak instantaneous and mean gradients correlate well. (**B** from Currie PJ, Seward JB, Reeder GS, et al. Continuous-wave Doppler echocardiographic assessment of severity of calcific aortic stenosis: a simultaneous Doppler-catheter correlative study in 100 adult patients. *Circulation* 1985;71:1162–1169, with permission.)

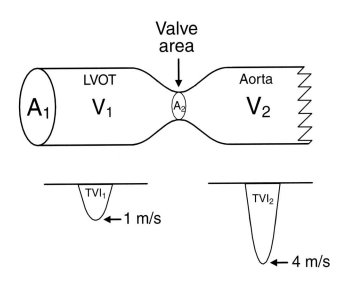

FIG. 6-14. Diagram to illustrate the continuity equation. Area₁ is the known cross-sectional area. Area₂ is the unknown cross-sectional area to be calculated.

$$(Stroke\ volume)_2 = (Stroke\ Volume)_1$$

$$A_2 \times TVI_2 = A_1 \times TVI_1$$

$$A_2 = A_1 \times TVI_1/TVI_2$$

LVOT, LV outflow tract; *TVI*, time velocity integral.

gurgitation, flow across the regurgitant mitral valve orifice (A_2) is the same as flow at a proximal isovelocity surface area (A_1). It should be noted that the ratio of the areas is inversely proportional to their TVI ratio.

$$\frac{A_2}{A_1} = \frac{TVI_1}{TVI_2}$$

Pressure Half-Time

Pressure half-time (PHT) (Fig. 6-15) is the time interval for the peak pressure gradient to reach its half level (14) and is the same as the interval for the peak a velocity to decline to a velocity equal to the peak velocity divided by $\sqrt{2}$ ($=1.4$) (15,16). It is always proportionally related to deceleration time (DT).

$$PHT = 0.29 \times DT$$

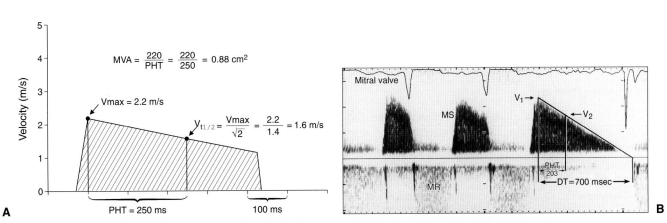

A

B

FIG. 6-15. A: Diagram to illustrate the calculation of pressure half-time. Pressure half-time (*PHT*) is the time interval required for maximal pressure gradient (*Pmax*) to reach its half level (P½). Hence,

$$P\tfrac{1}{2} = \tfrac{1}{2}Pmax$$

$$4 \times (V_{t1/2})^2 = \tfrac{1}{2}(4 \times Vmax^2)$$

$$V_{t1/2} = \frac{Vmax}{\sqrt{2}} = Vmax/1.4$$

where *V* is velocity. In this example, *Vmax* = 2.2 m/sec; hence, $V_{t1/2}$ = 2.2/1.4 = 1.6 m/sec. The time interval from the Vmax (2.2 m/sec) to V (1.6 m/sec) is the pressure half-time (PHT = 250 msec). In patients with native mitral valvular stenosis, mitral valve area (*MVA*) is estimated by dividing the constant, 220, by PHT. $V_{t1/2}$ = velocity at PHT. **B:** Continuous-wave Doppler velocity recording from the apex of the mitral valve in a 45-year-old woman with mitral stenosis (MS) and atrial fibrillation. V_2 is the velocity at which the pressure gradient is a half of the peak gradient at V_1.

$$V_2 = V_1/1.4$$

Deceleration time (*DT*) is the time interval from the peak velocity to when it reaches zero baseline. PHT is always 29% of DT. *MR*, mitral regurgitation.

Pressure half-time is used to estimate stenotic native mitral valve area (MVA) with the empiric formula:

$$MVA = \frac{220}{PHT}$$

It overestimates the area of normal prosthetic mitral valves, however. Another important clinical application of PHT is to assess the severity of aortic regurgitation. The PHT of aortic regurgitation Doppler velocity becomes significantly shorter (< 250 msec) with severe aortic regurgitation, because of a rapid increase in LV diastolic pressure and decrease in aortic pressure (17,18).

PISA Method

The concept of PISA, as discussed above for determining regurgitant orifice and volume, can be applied for calculating the area of a stenotic orifice. This method has been validated for mitral valve area in patients with mitral stenosis; however, it should be considered that PISA proximal to a stenotic mitral orifice may not be a complete hemisphere but rather a portion of a hemisphere because of the geometry of mitral leaflets on the atrial side. Therefore, an angle correction factor may be necessary (but not in all cases):

$$MVA = 6.28 \times r^2 \times \frac{Aliasing\ velocity}{Peak\ mitral\ stenosis\ velocity} \times \frac{\alpha^\circ}{180^\circ}$$

where α is the angle between two mitral leaflets on the atrial side (see Chapter 9).

Intracardiac Pressures

The velocity of a regurgitant valve is directly related to the pressure drop across that valve and therefore is used to determine intracardiac pressure (Table 6-4).

Tricuspid regurgitation (TR) velocity reflects the systolic pressure difference between the RV and the RA (2) (see also Chapter 17). Therefore, RV systolic pressure can be obtained by adding the estimated RA pressure to the TR velocity^2 × 4 (19,20). For example, if TR velocity is 3.8 m/sec, the pressure drop across the tricuspid valve during systole is 58 mm Hg (= 3.8^2 × 4) (Fig. 6-15). If the RA pressure is 10 mm Hg, the RV systolic pressure is 58 + 10 = 68 mm Hg. In the absence of RVOT obstruction, the pulmonary artery systolic pressure will be the same as the calculated RV systolic pressure. RVOT and pulmonary valve flow velocities should be measured in all patients with increased TR velocity to ensure that there is no RVOT obstruction.

Pulmonary regurgitation (PR) velocity represents the diastolic pressure difference between the pulmonary artery and the RV. Hence, pulmonary artery end-diastolic pressure (PAEDP) can be obtained by adding RV end-diastolic pressure (RVEDP) (which is equal to RA pressure) to (PR end-diastolic velocity)^2 × 4. The pulmonary artery mean pressure correlates well with the early diastolic pressure difference between the pulmonary artery and RV; hence, (PR peak velocity)^2 × 4. For example, PR end-diastolic velocity is about 1.0 m/sec when the pulmonary artery pressure is normal; PAEDP − RVEDP = 1.0^2 × 4 = 4 mm Hg. PAEDP = RA pressure + 4 = 14 mm Hg, if RA pressure is assumed to be 10 mm Hg. When pulmonary artery pressure is elevated, PR end-diastolic velocity is increased. If PR end-diastolic velocity is 2.3 m/sec (Fig. 6-16), PAEDP − RVEDP = 2.3^2 × 4 = 21 mm Hg. Therefore, PAEDP is equal to 21 + RA pressure. RA pressure is roughly estimated by inspecting at the bedside the jugular venous pressure, or an empiric value of 10 or 14 mm Hg can be used (i.e., PAEDP = 21 + 14 = 35).

Mitral regurgitation velocity (MRV) represents the systolic pressure difference between the LV and the LA. In patients without LV outflow obstruction, systolic blood

TABLE 6-4. *Doppler estimation of intracardiac pressures*

Peak TR velocity→	RV systolic pressure
	PA systolic pressure
Peak PR velocity→	Mean PA pressure
End-diastolic PR velocity→	PA end-diastolic pressure
Peak MR velocity→	LA pressure
End-diastolic AR velocity→	LV end-diastolic pressure
Diastolic filling pattern→	LA pressure
Mitral inflow	LV end-diastolic pressure
Pulmonary vein	
PFO velocity→	LA pressure

AR, aortic regurgitation; LA, left atrium; LV, left ventricle; MR, mitral regurgitation; PA, pulmonary artery; PFO, patent foramen ovale; PR, pulmonary regurgitation; RV, right ventricle; TR, tricuspid regurgitation.

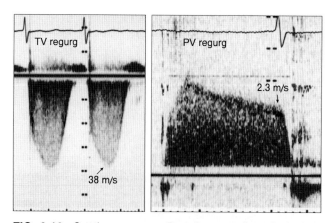

FIG. 6-16. Continuous-wave Doppler recording of tricuspid valve regurgitation (*TV regurg*) and pulmonary valve regurgitation (*PV regurg*) in a patient with pulmonary hypertension. Systolic and end-diastolic pulmonary artery pressures are derived from peak tricuspid regurgitation velocity and end-diastolic pulmonary regurgitation velocity, respectively.

pressure is practically the same as LV systolic pressure; hence,

$$LA\ pressure = SBP - 4 \times MRV^2$$

where *SBP* is the systolic blood pressure.

Aortic regurgitation (AR) velocity reflects the diastolic pressure difference between the aorta and the LV. Hence,

$$LVEDP = DBP - (AR\ EDV)^2 \times 4$$

where DBP is the diastolic blood pressure and EDV = end-diastolic velocity.

This is illustrated in Fig. 6-17. LVEDP and LA pressure can also be estimated by various diastolic filling variables from mitral inflow and pulmonary venous flow velocities (Fig. 6-18). As LA pressure increases, the mitral valve opens earlier, the initial transmitral gradient is higher, and the LV diastolic pressure increases faster. Therefore, the mitral inflow velocity pattern shows shortened IVRT, increased E velocity, reduced A velocity with increased E/A ratio, and shortened DT (21,22). Pulmonary venous velocity has a predominant diastolic forward-flow velocity (23,24). When LVEDP is increased, the velocity and duration of mitral inflow during atrial contraction are decreased, whereas pulmonary vein atrial flow reversal velocity (PVa) and duration increase. The difference between the duration of PVa and the duration of mitral inflow velocity with atrial systole is a reliable value for estimating LVEDP (25,26). The duration of mitral inflow is usually longer than that of PVa, with normal LVEDP. With increased LVEDP, the duration of PVa becomes longer than

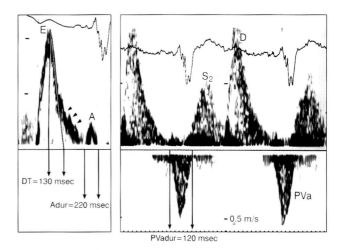

FIG. 6-18. Mitral inflow **(left)** and pulmonary venous flow **(right)** pulsed-wave Doppler velocity in a patient with elevated left atrial pressure (see text). Mitral A duration (120 msec) is much shorter than the duration of pulmonary vein atrial flow reversal (220 msec) because of increased left ventricular (*LV*) end-diastolic pressure. *Arrowheads* indicate flow from LA to LV caused by delayed relaxation. *DT*, deceleration time; *Pva*, pulmonary vein atrial flow reversal; *E*, early filling wave, *A*, late filling wave due to atrial contraction; *D*, diastolic pulmonary vein flow; *S₂*, systolic pulmonary vein flow.

that of mitral atrial flow. A difference of 50 msec or greater is quite specific for LVEDP greater than 20 mm Hg. Other mitral inflow velocity measures have been found to indicate increased LA pressure and include shortened DT of mitral E velocity, shortened DT of mitral A velocity, and reduced ratio of mitral atrial flow duration and PVa duration (22).

Therefore, LA pressure and LVEDP should be estimated collectively using various measures of mitral valve and pulmonary vein flow velocities. Most of these measurements have been validated best in patients with dilated cardiomyopathy or in patients after myocardial infarction. In patients with marked LV hypertrophy, as in hypertension or hypertrophic cardiomyopathy, as well as in those with normal LV function, these variables may not be as accurate as in patients with dilated cardiomyopathy (27,28). In patients with atrial fibrillation, varying RR intervals and the absence of mitral A velocity make the use of mitral flow velocity difficult for estimating mean LA pressure or LVEDP. It appears, however, that the shortened DT (≤130 msec) of mitral E flow velocity (averaged over five cardiac cycles) indicates increased LV filling pressure. In these patients, pulmonary venous forward flow velocity has a predominantly diastolic component and systolic flow velocity is decreased even without increased LA pressure. The correlation between the duration of the diastolic pulmonary venous flow, its initial deceleration slope time, and the mean pulmonary wedge pressure is good (29). Additional hemodynamic correlation studies are required to estimate LV filling pressure better in patients with atrial fibrillation.

LA pressure also can be estimated from velocity of flow

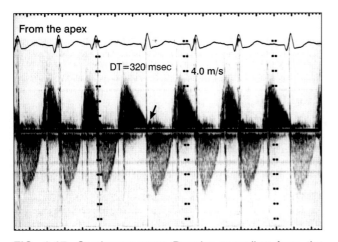

FIG. 6-17. Continuous-wave Doppler recording from the apex of severe aortic regurgitation with increased left ventricular end-diastolic pressure (LVEDP). Deceleration time (*DT*) of aortic regurgitation velocity is only 320 msec; hence, the pressure half-time is 93 msec (pressure half-time < 250 msec indicates severe aortic regurgitation). End-diastolic aortic regurgitation velocity (*arrow*) is 0 m/sec, and LVEDP is equal to diastolic blood pressure. Blood pressure in this patient was 84/40 mm Hg. Hence, LVEDP is about 40 mm Hg.

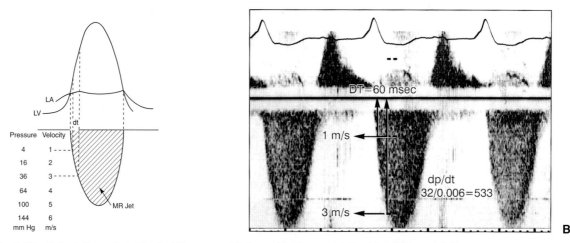

FIG. 6-19. Calculation of dp/dt. **A:** Diagram of left ventricular and left atrial (*LV* and *LA*) pressure tracings along with continuous-wave Doppler velocity spectrum of mitral regurgitation (*MR*). The rate of pressure rise in the LV is estimated from the time interval (*dt*) required to achieve MR velocity from 1 to 3 m/sec assuming no significant change in LA pressure during that period.

$$dp/dt = (4 \times 3^2 - 4 \times 1^2) \text{ mm Hg} \times 1,000/dt \text{ (in ms)}$$

$$= 32,000/dt \text{ (mm Hg/sec)}$$

Normal LV dp/dt is >1,000 mm Hg/s. **B:** Continuous-wave Doppler spectrum of MR in a patient with severe LV systolic dysfunction. To measure dt accurately, it is better to record the signal at 100 mm/sec. The velocity scale is expanded so that only a jet up to 3 m/sec is recorded. It should also be noted that the peak velocity of MR in this patient is 3.5 m/sec corresponding to only a 49-mm Hg gradient across the mitral valve during systole. Pulmonary capillary wedge pressure in this patient was 50 mm Hg and the systolic blood pressure was 96 mm Hg. The depressed systolic function is also reflected in a decreased dp/dt to 533 mm Hg/sec. *DT*, deceleration time.

across the patent foramen ovale (PFO) or atrial septal defect.

$$LA \text{ } pressure = (PFO \text{ } velocity)^2 \times 4 + RA \text{ } pressure$$

dp/dt

The rate of LV pressure change during the isovolumic contraction period, dp/dt, is another index of LV contractility. From a continuous-wave Doppler of mitral regurgitation jet, the rate of the LV pressure increase (dp/dt) can be estimated. During the isovolumic contraction, there is no significant change in LA pressure. Therefore, MR velocity changes during this period reflect dp/dt. Usually, the time interval between 1 m/sec and 3 m/sec on the mitral regurgitation velocity spectrum is measured (Fig. 6-19). Using the Bernoulli equation, the pressure change from 1 m/sec to 3 m/sec is 32 mm Hg ($4 \times 3^2 - 4 \times 1^2$). The dp/dt (in mm Hg/sec) is calculated from the following formula: dp/dt = 32 mm Hg/time (seconds). Several studies have demonstrated a good correlation between the noninvasive Doppler-derived and catheter-derived dp/dt (30,31). The actual measurement of dp/dt is illustrated in Fig. 6-19B. Normal dp/dt is 1,200 mm Hg/sec or greater. The rate of pressure change in the RV is derived similarly from the tricuspid regurgitation jet as in the LV, using the mitral regurgitation jet except that the time interval between 1

m/sec and 2 m/sec is used for the right side. Therefore, for the RV, dp/dt = ($4 \times 2^2 - 4 \times 1^2$)/time = 12 mm Hg/time (in seconds).

Also, dp/dt may be useful in predicting postoperative systolic function in patients with severe mitral valve regurgitation (32), but more clinical applications of dp/dt require further investigation.

REFERENCES

1. Callahan MJ, Tajik AJ, Su-Fan Q, Bove AA. Validation of instantaneous pressure gradients measured by continuous-wave Doppler in experimentally induced aortic stenosis. *Am J Cardiol* 1985;56:989–993.
2. Currie PJ, Seward JB, Chan KL. Continuous wave Doppler determination of right ventricular pressure: a simultaneous Doppler-catheterization study in 127 patients. *J Am Coll Cardiol* 1985;6:750–756.
3. Currie PJ, Hagler DJ, Seward JB, et al. Instantaneous pressure gradient: a simultaneous Doppler and dual catheter correlative study. *J Am Coll Cardiol* 1986;7:800–806.
4. Burstow DJ, Nishimura RA, Bailey KR, et al. Continuous wave Doppler echocardiographic measurement of prosthetic valve gradients: a simultaneous Doppler-catheter correlative study. *Circulation* 1989;80:504–514.
5. Zoghbi WA, Quinones MA. Determination of cardiac output by Doppler echocardiography: a critical appraisal. *Herz* 1986;11:258–268.
6. Rokey R, Sterling LL, Zoghbi WA, et al. Determination of regurgitant fraction in isolated mitral or aortic regurgitation by pulsed Doppler two-dimensional echocardiography. *J Am Coll Cardiol* 1986;7:1273–1278.

7. Hatle L, Angelsen B. *Doppler ultrasound in cardiology: physical principles and clinical applications*, 2nd ed. Philadelphia: Lea & Febiger, 1985.

8. Nishimura RA, Miller FA Jr, Callahan MJ, Benassi RC, Seward JB, Tajik AJ. Doppler echocardiography: theory, instrumentation, technique, and application. *Mayo Clin Proc* 1985;60:321–343.

9. Hatle L, Brubakk A, Tromsdal A, Angelsen B. Noninvasive assessment of pressure drop in mitral stenosis by Doppler ultrasound. *Br Heart J* 1978;40:131–140.

10. Teirstein PS, Yock PG, Popp RL. The accuracy of Doppler ultrasound measurement of pressure gradients across irregular, dual, and tunnel-like obstructions to blood flow. *Circulation* 1985;72:577–584.

11. Fyfe DA, Currie PJ, Seward JB, et al. Continuous-wave Doppler determination of the pressure gradient across pulmonary artery bands: Hemodynamic correlation in 20 patients. *Mayo Clin Proc* 1984;59: 744–750.

12. Nishimura RA, Rihal CS, Tajik AJ, Holmes DR Jr. Accurate measurement of the transmitral gradient in patients with mitral stenosis: a simultaneous catheterization and Doppler echocardiographic study. *J Am Coll Cardiol* 1994;24:152–158.

13. Skjaerpe T, Hegrenaes L, Hatle L. Noninvasive estimation of valve area in patients with aortic stenosis by Doppler ultrasound and two-dimensional echocardiography. *Circulation* 1985;72:810–818.

14. Libanoff AJ, Rodbard S. Atrioventricular pressure half-time: measurement of mitral valve orifice area. *Circulation* 1968;38:144–150.

15. Hatle L, Angelsen B, Tromsdal A. Noninvasive assessment of atrioventricular pressure half-time by Doppler ultrasound. *Circulation* 1979;60:1096–1104.

16. Thomas JD, Weyman AE. Doppler mitral pressure half-time: a clinical tool in search of theoretical justification. *J Am Coll Cardiol* 1987;10:923–929.

17. Samstad SO, Hegrenaes L, Skjaerpe T, Hatle L. Half time of the diastolic aortoventricular pressure difference by continuous wave Doppler ultrasound: a measure of the severity of aortic regurgitation? *Br Heart J* 1989;61:336–343.

18. Grayburn PA, Handshoe R, Smith MD, Harrison MR, DeMaria AN. Quantitative assessment of the hemodynamic consequences of aortic regurgitation by means of continuous wave Doppler recordings. *J Am Coll Cardiol* 1987;10:135–141.

19. Yock PG, Popp RL. Noninvasive estimation of right ventricular systolic pressure by Doppler ultrasound in patients with tricuspid regurgitation. *Circulation* 1984;70:657–662.

20. Chan KL, Currie PJ, Seward JB, Hagler DJ, Mair DD, Tajik AJ. Comparison of three Doppler ultrasound methods in the prediction of pulmonary artery pressure. *J Am Coll Cardiol* 1987;9:549–554.

21. Giannuzzi P, Imparato A, Temporelli PL, et al. Doppler-derived mitral deceleration time of early filling as a strong predictor of pulmonary capillary wedge pressure in postinfarction patients with left ventricular systolic dysfunction. *J Am Coll Cardiol* 1994;23:1630–1637.

22. Cecconi M, Manfrin M, Zanoli R, et al. Doppler echocardiographic evaluation of left ventricular end-diastolic pressure in patients with coronary artery disease. *J Am Soc Echocardiogr* 1996;9:241–250.

23. Kuecherer HF, Muhiudeen IA, Kusumoto FM, et al. Estimation of mean left atrial pressure from transesophageal pulsed Doppler echocardiography of pulmonary venous flow. *Circulation* 1990;82:1127–1139.

24. Nishimura RA, Abel MD, Hatle LK, Tajik AJ. Relation of pulmonary vein to mitral flow velocities by transesophageal Doppler echocardiography: effect of different loading conditions. *Circulation* 1990;81: 1488–1497.

25. Rossvoll O, Hatle LK. Pulmonary venous flow velocities recorded by transthoracic Doppler ultrasound: relation to left ventricular diastolic pressures. *J Am Coll Cardiol* 1993;21:1687–1696.

26. Chen C, Rodriguez L, Levine RA, Weyman AE, Thomas JD. Non-invasive measurement of the time constant of left ventricular relaxation using the continuous-wave Doppler velocity profile of mitral regurgitation. *Circulation* 1992;86:272–278.

27. Nishimura RA, Schwartz RS, Tajik AJ, Holmes DR Jr. Noninvasive measurement of rate of left ventricular relaxation by Doppler echocardiography: validation with simultaneous cardiac catheterization. *Circulation* 1993;88:146–155.

28. Symanski JD, Nishimura RA, Hurrell DG. Doppler parameters of left ventricular filling are poor predictors of diastolic performance in patients with hypertrophic cardiomyopathy. *Circulation* 1995;92(Suppl): 1:I–269(abst).

29. Chirillo F, Brunazzi MC, Barbiero M, et al. Estimating mean pulmonary wedge pressure in patients with chronic atrial fibrillation from transthoracic Doppler indexes of mitral and pulmonary venous flow velocity. *J Am Coll Cardiol* 1997;30:19–26.

30. Bargiggia GS, Bertucci C, Recusani F, et al. A new method for estimating left ventricular dP/dt by continuous wave Doppler-echocardiography: validation studies at cardiac catheterization. *Circulation* 1989;80:1287–1292.

31. Chung NS, Nishimura RA, Holmes DR Jr, Tajik AJ. Measurement of left ventricular dp/dt by simultaneous Doppler echocardiography and cardiac catheterization. *J Am Soc Echocardiogr* 1992;5:147–152.

32. Leung DY, Griffin BP, Stewart WJ, Cosgrove DM III, Thomas JD, Marwick TH. Left ventricular function after valve repair for chronic mitral regurgitation: predictive value of preoperative assessment of contractile reserve by exercise echocardiography. *J Am Coll Cardiol* 1996:28:1198–1205.

CHAPTER 7

Coronary Artery Disease

Coronary artery disease is the most commonly encountered problem in adult cardiology practice in the United States. Annually, acute myocardial infarction occurs in 1.2 million Americans, and more than half a million deaths are related to coronary artery disease. Knowledge of global and regional systolic function and global assessment of diastolic function is helpful in establishing the diagnosis, management strategy, and prognosis of patients with coronary artery disease. Myocardial contraction becomes abnormal immediately after the onset of ischemia, and the resulting regional wall motion abnormality (RWMA) is detected readily by echocardiography, even before other ischemic manifestations. The treatment of acute myocardial infarction with thrombolysis or coronary angioplasty (or both) has changed the outcome and the natural history of acute myocardial infarction (1,2). Systolic and diastolic ventricular function may change in the acute setting and require repeat assessment to determine the beneficial effects of acute reperfusion therapy. Without prompt diagnosis and early surgical intervention, mechanical complications of acute myocardial infarction are often fatal. Echocardiography, including transesophageal echocardiography (TEE), should be able to identify most, if not all, mechanical complications of myocardial infarction (3). Exercise or pharmacologic stress echocardiography is valuable in predicting myocardial viability and prognosis as well as detecting coronary artery disease (4,5). In this clinical context, echocardiography has an important role (Fig. 7-1), from the diagnosis of coronary artery disease, early detection of acute myocardial infarction (even in the absence of typical electrocardiographic evidence), evaluation of RWMAs after reperfusion therapy, detection of postinfarction mechanical and functional complications, assessment of myocardial viability, to prognostic risk stratification.

This chapter discusses all these applications, except stress echocardiography. Chapter 8 is concerned with stress echocardiography.

REGIONAL WALL MOTION ANALYSIS— CORRELATION WITH PERFUSION DEFECT AND PATHOLOGY

The immediate manifestation of myocardial ischemia is a decrease in or cessation of myocardial contractility (*systolic thickening*), even before the occurrence of ST-segment changes or the development of symptoms. Ischemic myocardium may continue to demonstrate some degree of passive forward motion because of the pulling action of adjacent nonischemic muscle, but the contractility (systolic thickening) of the ischemic myocardial segments is decreased (*hypokinesis*) or absent (*akinesis*). Normally, LV free wall thickness increases more than 40% during systole. In normal subjects, the percent of thickening of the ventricular septum is somewhat less than that of the free wall of the LV. *Hypokinesis* is defined as systolic wall thickening of less than 30%, and *akinesis* is defined as less than 10%. *Dyskinesis* is defined as a myocardial segment moving outward during systole, usually in association with systolic wall thinning.

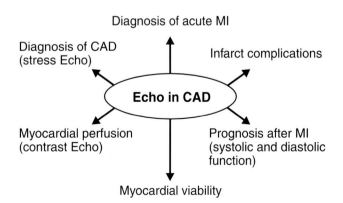

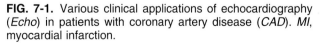

FIG. 7-1. Various clinical applications of echocardiography (*Echo*) in patients with coronary artery disease (*CAD*). *MI,* myocardial infarction.

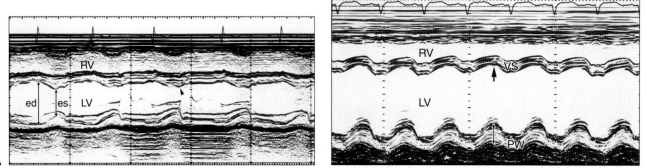

FIG. 7-2. M-mode echocardiogram of normal **(A)** and abnormal **(B)** ventricular wall thickening. **A:** Normally, wall thickness at end systole (*es*) is more than 5 mm greater than that at end diastole (*ed*). *Arrowhead* indicates maximal systolic thickening. **B:** The ventricular septum is thinned and dyskinetic (*arrow*), moving toward the right ventricle (*RV*) during end systole. The thickening of the posterior wall is normal. This M-mode echocardiogram was obtained from a patient with anterior wall myocardial infarction. *LV*, left ventricle.

M-mode echocardiography is useful in recording the temporal changes in wall thickness (Fig. 7-2) and can be obtained by two-dimensional (2D) image guidance. With multiple tomographic imaging planes, 2D echocardiography allows visualization of all left ventricular (LV) wall segments. For purposes of regional wall motion analysis, the LV is divided into several segments. The American Society of Echocardiography has recommended a 16-segment model (6) (Fig. 7-3). Each segment is assigned a score based on its contractility as assessed visually: normal, 1; hypokinesis, 2; akinesis, 3; dyskinesis, 4; and aneurysm, 5. On the basis of this wall motion analysis scheme, a *wall motion score index* (WMSI) is calculated to semiquantitate the extent of regional wall motion abnormalities.

$$WMSI = \frac{Sum\ of\ wall\ motion\ scores}{Number\ of\ segments\ visualized}$$

A normally contracting LV has a WMSI of 1 (each of the 16 segments receives a wall motion score of 1; hence, the total score is 16 and WMSI is 16/16 = 1). The WMSI is higher with larger infarcts because wall motion abnormalities become more severe.

What does the WMSI indicate? Because the echocardiographic analysis of wall motion abnormality is subjective and the reduction of systolic myocardial thickening is not proportional to the incremental amount of infarcted or ischemic myocardial tissue (Fig. 7-4) (7), the correlation of the WMSI with the actual size of the myocardial infarct or

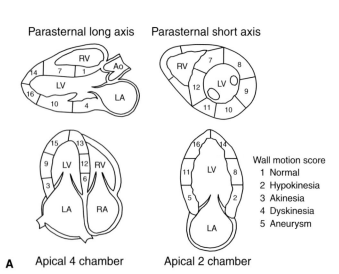

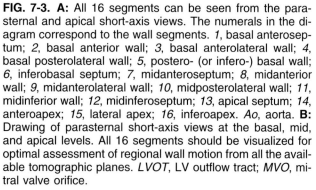

FIG. 7-3. A: All 16 segments can be seen from the parasternal and apical short-axis views. The numerals in the diagram correspond to the wall segments. *1*, basal anteroseptum; *2*, basal anterior wall; *3*, basal anterolateral wall; *4*, basal postero- (or infero-) basal wall; *5*, postero- (or infero-) basal wall; *6*, inferobasal septum; *7*, midanteroseptum; *8*, midanterior wall; *9*, midanterolateral wall; *10*, midposterolateral wall; *11*, midinferior wall; *12*, midinferoseptum; *13*, apical septum; *14*, anteroapex; *15*, lateral apex; *16*, inferoapex. *Ao*, aorta. **B:** Drawing of parasternal short-axis views at the basal, mid, and apical levels. All 16 segments should be visualized for optimal assessment of regional wall motion from all the available tomographic planes. *LVOT*, LV outflow tract; *MVO*, mitral valve orifice.

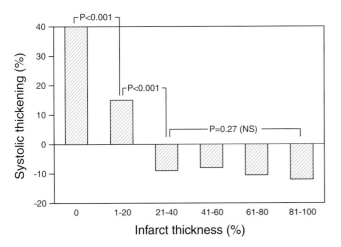

FIG. 7-4. A plot of percent systolic thickening versus percent of wall thickness involved with ischemia or infarction. Wall thickening stops (i.e., akinesis) when 25% or more of wall thickness is affected. Therefore, akinesis shown on echocardiography does not always indicate transmural involvement with ischemia or infarction. There may be significant viability in akinetic myocardium. (From ref. 7, with permission.)

the perfusion defect may not be good in the setting of acute myocardial infarction. A clinicopathologic study of 30 patients who had a 2D echocardiographic examination within 7 days before death demonstrated a reasonable quantitative relationship between the WMSI and segmental infarct size (8). The mean segmental infarct sizes were 9% ± 4%, 17% ± 17%, 30% ± 27%, and 44% ± 29% for regional wall motion scores of 1, 2, 3, and 4, respectively. When a 2D echocardiographic examination was performed simultaneously with an injection of sestamibi in patients with acute transmural myocardial infarction [with ST-segment elevation on the electrocardiogram (ECG)], the overall correlation between the WMSI and the perfusion defect was good (9). Patients with a WMSI greater than 1.7 had a perfusion defect greater than 20% (Fig. 7-5). The correlation was better in patients with an anterior wall myocardial infarction than in those with an inferior or lateral wall myocardial infarction with a smaller infarct size.

TECHNICAL CAVEATS

A comprehensive regional wall motion analysis is among the most challenging tasks in echocardiography. All available windows and tomographic planes should be used to visualize all the LV segments. Apical short- and long-axis views are especially useful in evaluating the apical third of

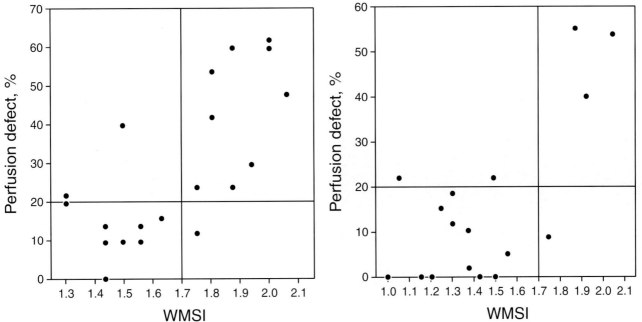

A   **B**

FIG. 7-5. Plot of perfusion defect detected by sestamibi imaging versus wall motion score index (*WMSI*) by two-dimensional echocardiography in patients with acute myocardial infarction at baseline **(A)** and several days after reperfusion therapy by thrombolysis or angioplasty **(B)**. There is a reasonable correlation between perfusion defect and WMSI at baseline. After reperfusion therapy, both the perfusion defect and WMSI decrease. Some patients, however, still had wall motion abnormalities (WMSI ≥1.0) when there was no perfusion defect (0% perfusion defect). This is thought to represent stunned myocardium; recovery of wall motion abnormalities generally occur after successful reperfusion therapy. (From ref. 9, with permission.)

the LV. Continuous scanning from the apical four-chamber to the apical long-axis to the apical two-chamber view allows complete visualization of all LV segments. In patients who have chronic obstructive pulmonary disease or are obese, a lower frequency (2.0 to 2.5 MHz) transducer should be used to optimize the definition of the endocardium, and the subcostal window may provide adequate visualization of the LV segments. A new imaging method that uses the principle of harmonic resonance (native harmonic imaging) can improve visualization of the endocardium (Fig. 7-6). In patients with a good apical window, the use of higher frequency transducers, with adjustment of the focal zone to the near region, may enhance the definition of the apical endocardium, help delineate apical wall motion abnormalities, and differentiate thrombus from apical trabeculation.

The assessment of regional wall motion on echocardiography is limited when visualization of the LV endocardium is inadequate. Several new modalities may enhance our ability to analyze regional wall motion. Intravenous administration of contrast agent may enhance endocardial definition; preliminary studies suggest that this increases the sensitivity of detecting wall motion abnormality during stress echocardiography, but additional clinical confirmation is required concerning its reliability, practicality, choice of contrast agent, and cost-effectiveness. Colorization of 2D echocardiographic images may improve visualization of the endocardial border. Newer ultrasound units hold promise in this regard, with more advanced technology to enhance visualization of the endocardium. Second harmonic imaging or frequency conversion technology, initially created for contrast echocardiography, is a new development that will improve visualization of cardiac structures as well as endocardial definition. More experience is needed with Doppler tissue imaging and color ki-

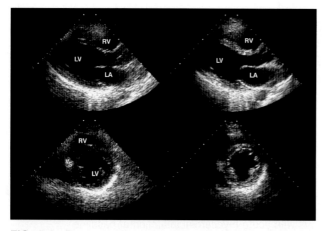

FIG. 7-6. Demonstration of better visualization of the left ventricular (*LV*) endocardial border by native harmonic imaging. Parasternal long-axis views (*upper panels*) and short-axis views (*lower panels*) were scanned by fundamental imaging (2.5 MHz; *left panels*) and by native harmonic imaging (*right panels*) for comparison. *VS*, ventricular septum.

nesis before they can be incorporated into routine regional wall motion analysis (10–12).

ACUTE MYOCARDIAL INFARCTION

The role of echocardiography in acute myocardial infarction has evolved as the management strategy of acute myocardial infarction has changed. Its current role can be classified as follows: (a) diagnosis and exclusion of acute myocardial infarction in patients with prolonged chest pain and nondiagnostic electrocardiographic (ECG) findings, (b) estimation of the amount of myocardium at risk and final infarct size after reperfusion therapy, (c) detection of infarct complications, (d) evaluation of myocardial viability, and (e) risk stratification. Therefore, at various stages of acute myocardial infarction, echocardiography is important in providing anatomic, functional, and hemodynamic information.

EVALUATION OF CHEST PAIN SYNDROME

Not all patients with prolonged chest pain resulting from myocardial ischemia or infarction present with typical ECG changes. More than 50% of patients with myocardial infarction show nonspecific findings on the initial ECG. In most patients admitted to the hospital because of chest pain syndrome, the chance of detecting a myocardial infarction is less than 30%. Rapid assay of subforms of creatine kinase (muscle-brain subunits) (CK-MB) is reliable in detecting myocardial infarction within the first 6 hours after the onset of chest pain (13); however, the sensitivity of CK-MB subform assays may not be satisfactory if the assay is obtained within 4 hours after the onset of chest pain. Troponin T and troponin I are being investigated as sensitive markers of necrotic myocardial tissue (14). The sensitivity and specificity of perfusion imaging technique used in the emergency room to detect a perfusion defect in patients with chest pain are good, but this technique requires a 2- to 3-hour delay in detecting a perfusion defect. The main advantage of echocardiography is that the examination can be performed in the emergency room and the findings are immediately available.

As mentioned, myocardial contractility diminishes or ceases immediately after ischemia or infarction and is manifested as an RWMA that is readily identified in most patients by 2D echocardiography. Therefore, the use of RWMAs as a marker of myocardial infarction in patients with prolonged chest pain and nondiagnostic ECG findings is attractive. Several studies have confirmed the usefulness of echocardiography in this setting. The absence of LV wall motion abnormalities usually excludes detecting myocardial infarction subsequently, and the presence of RWMAs has a high sensitivity for detecting myocardial infarction; however, the positive predictive value is about 30%, because RWMAs are not specific for myocardial infarction and some patients have unstable angina without myocardial damage (15). Echocardiography may not be helpful or cost-effective in patients with a low to intermediate risk of acute myocardial infarction, however. Occasionally, echocardiography may be useful in detecting not an ischemic but a potentially fatal cause of chest pain syndrome, such as pulmonary embolism, aortic dissection, or pericardial disease. The incidence of these findings is small, but use of anti-coagulation or thrombolytic therapy in a subset of these patients may result in a disastrous clinical outcome. The approach outlined here requires that the echocardiographic examination and interpretation in the emergency room be prompt. Recently, digitized real-time echocardiographic images have been transmitted over existing telephone lines to a laptop computer (16). This approach will improve the use of echocardiography, providing that the transmission can be prompt and without significant deterioration in image quality.

Two-dimensional echocardiographic analysis of RWMAs is important diagnostically and clinically even in patients with classic chest pain and ST-segment elevation on the ECG. The amount of myocardium at risk can be estimated by calculating the WMSI. A WMSI greater than 1.7 usually suggests a perfusion defect greater than 20% (Fig. 7-5) (9) and increased complications unless the wall motion abnormalities are reversed with reperfusion therapy. Regional wall motion analysis can be performed several days after reperfusion therapy to identify recovery of RWMAs (17,18).

The amount of myocardium at risk from the affected artery also may determine who will receive the greatest benefit from acute interventional therapy. Patients with a large amount of myocardium at risk will derive more benefit from reperfusion therapy than those with a small amount of myocardium at risk. When a patient presents with transmural acute myocardial infarction (ST-segment elevation in the ECG), the affected myocardium on the echocardiogram is akinetic or dyskinetic. After the myocardium has been reperfused successfully within an appropriate time frame (usually within 4 hours), it becomes more contractile on subsequent 2D echocardiographic studies. Serial echocardiographic studies have demonstrated that the improvement in regional myocardial contractility is evident within 24 to 48 hours and that the improvement continues for several days to months. Therefore, follow-up 2D echocardiographic imaging is useful in detecting reperfused myocardial segments or infarct expansion, especially using digital echocardiography, by which serial images of the same tomographic planes can be compared side by side.

Persistent akinesis does not always indicate failed reperfusion. Unless reperfusion therapy achieves recovery of more than 75% of the transmural thickness involved with infarction, the myocardium may remain akinetic, although the more myocardium is reperfused, the less tendency there is for infarct expansion to develop. When the myocardium remains akinetic while being viable, low-dose dobutamine or contrast echocardiography may be helpful to demonstrate

its viability (discussed in Chapter 8). LV enlargement, one of the strongest predictors of a cardiac event after myocardial infarction, is readily assessed with serial 2D echocardiography (see Risk Stratification).

DETECTION OF MECHANICAL COMPLICATIONS

According to a community-based study, the incidence and mortality of cardiogenic shock after acute myocardial infarction remained unchanged at 7.5% and 80%, respectively, from 1975 to 1988 (19). The incidence of shock in patients who had thrombolytic therapy was 5.7%. Because patients who have cardiogenic shock after myocardial infarction have a poor prognosis unless the cause is reversible, it is of paramount clinical importance to identify promptly the underlying cause so that proper treatment can be given. In a study of an international registry from 19 medical centers, the cause of cardiogenic shock in 251 patients after myocardial infarction was severe LV failure in 85%, mechanical complications in 8%, right ventricular (RV) infarct in 2%, and other comorbid conditions in 5% (20). Two-dimensional and Doppler echocardiography with color-flow imaging are useful in promptly identifying the cause in these patients, especially in looking for mechanical complications. In addition, TEE should be used promptly in patients in whom precordial echocardiography may not be possible or if images obtained in the intensive care unit are suboptimal (21). The presence of normal systolic function in a critically ill patient should immediately lead to a suspicion of a mechanical complication. Acute and chronic complications of myocardial infarction are listed in Table 7-1.

TABLE 7-1. *Complications of myocardial infarction*

Acute phase
  LV systolic dysfunction
  Rupture
    Free wall rupture
    Ventricular septal defect
    Papillary muscle rupture
    Subepicardial aneurysm
  Mitral regurgitation
    LV dilatation
    Papillary muscle dysfunction
    Papillary muscle rupture
  LV thrombus
  Pericardial effusion/tamponade
  RV infarct
  LV outflow tract obstruction
Chronic phase
  Infarct expansion
  Ventricular aneurysm
    True aneurysm
    Pseudoaneurysm
  LV thrombus

LV, left ventricle; RV, right ventricle.

FREE WALL RUPTURE

Cardiac free wall rupture usually is a fatal complication of acute myocardial infarction (Fig. 7-7A) that occurs in about 1% of all patients with myocardial infarction. It accounts for up to 7% of all infarct-related deaths. Typically, it produces a sudden hemodynamic collapse due to cardiac tamponade and electromechanical dissociation. Most ruptures occur within the first week after the infarction (median time, 4 days), and this problem is more common in women and elderly patients. Patients with rupture have less severe coronary artery disease and usually have a small myocardial infarction. Another clinical situation that potentially enhances cardiac rupture is the use of thrombolytic therapy (usually more than 10 hours after the onset of chest pain), presumably because of a hemorrhagic infarct.

Although patients with infarct expansion are at higher risk for cardiac rupture, no specific echocardiographic features have been found to predict this almost always fatal complication. Echocardiographic diagnosis of cardiac rupture depends on a high degree of clinical acumen, because a subset of patients may present subacutely with hypotension, recurrent chest pain, or emesis (or some combination of these) (22). A meticulous search by the echocardiographer for the site of rupture is mandatory if a region of thin myocardium or a small amount of pericardial effusion is present, particularly if a loculated effusion or clot is detected (Fig. 7-7B). Detection of a free wall rupture in these patients allows surgical repair, with a survival rate greater than 50%.

Although transthoracic 2D echocardiography may not be able to show the site of rupture, it can demonstrate a pericardial effusion with or without 2D and Doppler characteristics of pericardial tamponade. The presence of pericardial effusion alone is not sufficient to diagnose a subacute free wall rupture, because it is relatively common after acute myocardial infarction. In some cases, a pseudoaneurysm forms after a free wall rupture is contained within a limited portion of the pericardial space (most frequently in the inferolateral wall) (Fig. 7-8A). A pseudoaneurysm is usually characterized by a small neck communication (Fig. 7-8B) between the LV and the aneurysmal cavity (the ratio of the diameter of entry and the maximal diameter of the pseudoaneurysm is <0.5). Some pseudoaneurysms may have a wide neck communication (Fig. 7-9). There is always to-and-fro blood flow through the rupture site that can be documented by Doppler and color-flow imaging. The clinical features of chronic pseudoaneurysm are nonspecific, and its detection is frequently incidental. Although there is concern that pseudoaneurysms have a high incidence of rupture compared with true aneurysms, death due to cardiac rupture is infrequent in patients with chronic pseudoaneurysm who do not undergo surgical repair (23).

Occasionally, a free wall rupture does not extend through the entire thickness of the wall and is contained by the epicardial layer (''subepicardial aneurysm'') (24). This can create an intramyocardial cavity or an aneurysmal sac similar to a pseudoaneurysm (Fig. 7-9 and 7-10). This condition should be treated surgically.

VENTRICULAR SEPTAL RUPTURE

Postinfarct ventricular septal rupture occurs in 1% to 3% of all patients with infarcts, and it occurs during the early phase of acute infarction (within the first week). As in free wall rupture, ventricular septal rupture is more common in elderly women who have not had a previous myocardial infarction. Nearly half of the patients in whom infarct-related ventricular septal rupture develops have single-vessel

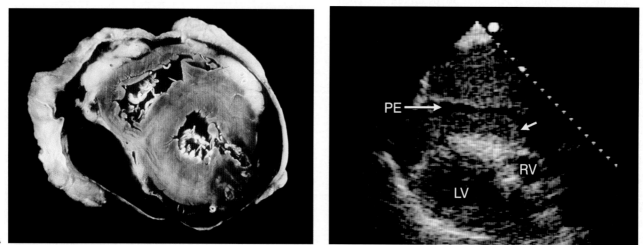

FIG. 7-7. A: Cross section of a heart with a lateral wall rupture that resulted in fatal hemopericardium. **B:** Transthoracic subcostal view demonstrating hemopericardium with gelatinous echo-dense material (*small arrow*) in the pericardium in a hypotensive patient with a recent myocardial infarction. The pericardial effusion (*PE*) was drained urgently, and the myocardial rupture was repaired.

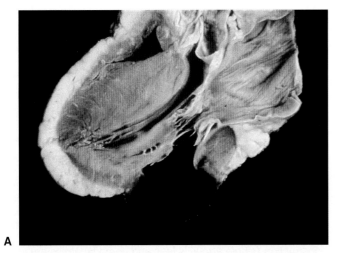

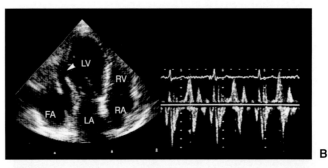

FIG. 7-8. A: Gross pathologic specimen showing a pseudoaneurysm at the level of the midinferolateral segment. B: Two-dimensional imaging (left) of a free wall rupture (*arrowhead*) resulting in a false aneurysm (*FA*). The pulsed-wave Doppler (right) shows to and fro blood flow velocities.

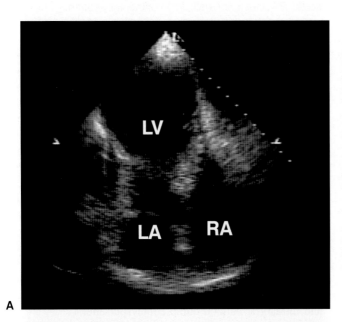

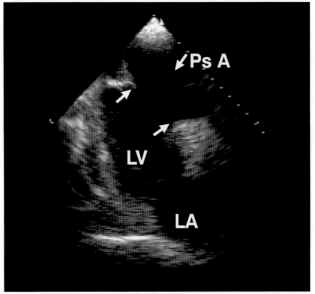

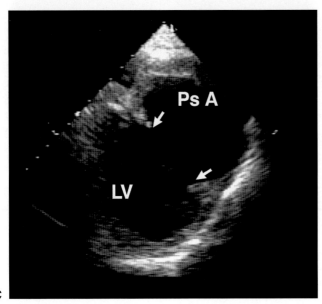

FIG. 7-9. Echocardiographic examination in a 54-year-old man who had a myocardial infarction 5 months earlier caused by complete occlusion of the diagonal artery. The patient had a syncopal spell 3 weeks after the acute myocardial infarction, and echocardiography showed a small amount of pericardial effusion. The patient came to the Mayo Clinic for further cardiac evaluation, and because chest radiography showed an abnormal cardiac contour, echocardiography was performed. A: Apical four-chamber view showed apical dilatation consistent with an aneurysm cavity. In this view, the aneurysm appears to be a true aneurysm, with a relatively large neck. B: An apical two-chamber view showed an abrupt discontinuity of the anterior wall (*arrows*) communicating with a large cavity that appeared to be a pseudoaneurysm (*Ps A*). The aneurysm cavity was pulsatile during systole in real-time imaging. C: Parasternal short-axis view also showing the tear or rupture of the anterolateral wall of the left ventricle (*LV*) communicating with a PsA cavity. *Arrows*: The mouth of the aneurysm cavity, which is relatively large. The patient underwent surgical repair of the myocardial rupture. The rupture turned out to be contained by the epicardial layer of the LV and pericardium. This entity has been termed *subepicardial aneurysm*.

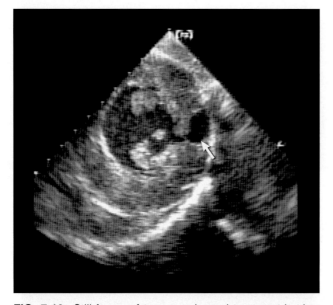

FIG. 7-10. Still-frame of transesophageal transgastric view of the left ventricle in a 61-year-old patient who had acute inferolateral myocardial infarction and persistent back pain. The patient was thought to have aortic dissection; however, transesophageal echocardiography showed incomplete rupture of the myocardium, resulting in a subepicardial aneurysm (*arrow*). The cavity was contained by the epicardial layer. On the basis of these transesophageal echocardiographic findings, the patient underwent resection of the infarcted area and aneurysm.

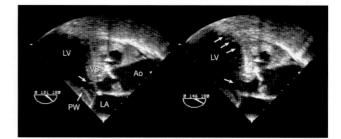

FIG. 7-11. Transesophageal systolic frame of long-axis view in a 72-year-old woman with chest pain, hypotension, and systolic murmur. **Left:** Note large apical aneurysm, hyperdynamic inferobasal area (*upward arrow*) resulting in systolic anterior motion of the mitral valve (*downward arrow*), and dynamic left ventricular (*LV*) outflow tract obstruction. **Right:** With infusion of phenylephrine (α-agonist), LV outflow tract obstruction (*single arrow*) is less and hemodynamics are improved. Apical aneurysm (*three arrows*) is not improved. *Ao,* aorta; *PW,* posterior wall; *VS,* ventricular septum.

coronary artery disease. The typical clinical presentation is a new systolic murmur, with abrupt and progressive hemodynamic deterioration.

The differential diagnosis of a new systolic murmur in patients with acute myocardial infarction includes infarct-related ventricular septal rupture, papillary muscle dysfunction or rupture, pericardial rub, acute LV outflow tract (LVOT) obstruction (Fig. 7-11), and free wall rupture (Table 7-2). After physical examination, echocardiography is the next logical noninvasive diagnostic procedure for all patients with a new murmur, especially for those who are hemodynamically unstable. Infarct-related ventricular septal defect is diagnosed by demonstration of a disrupted ventricular septum with a left-to-right shunt (Fig. 7-12). The defect is always located in the region of the thinned myocardium with dyskinetic motion. The diagnosis can be

established in 90% of cases with a transthoracic 2D echocardiographic examination (3). Transesophageal echocardiography (TEE) may be necessary in a small subgroup of patients with a suboptimal precordial study (Fig. 7-12). Peak flow velocity across the rupture measured by continuous-wave Doppler can be used to estimate RV systolic pressure (Fig. 7-12E). When it is located at the inferoseptum, the RV usually is involved with myocardial infarction, which portends a poor prognosis. An inferoseptal ventricular septal rupture can have a serpiginous septal tear, and an anteroapical septal ventricular septal rupture may be extended to an LV free wall rupture.

Currently, the therapeutic approach for infarct-related ventricular septal rupture is urgent surgical intervention (25). Until the time of surgery, the patient's condition should be stabilized by afterload reduction (nitroprusside) and intraaortic balloon pump counterpulsation.

PAPILLARY MUSCLE RUPTURE

Mitral regurgitation is common after acute myocardial infarction. Among 206 patients entering the Thrombolysis in Myocardial Infarction (TIMI) Phase I trial, mitral regurgitation was present in 13% (26). The incidence may be more common (up to 50% to 60%) if transient mitral regurgitation is included. In the TIMI-I trial, the presence of

TABLE 7-2. *Differential diagnosis of a new murmur in patients with acute myocardial infarction*

	Ventricular septal rupture	Papillary muscle rupture	LVOT obstruction
Location	Anterior/inferior	Inferior > anterior	Usually anterior
Signs	Low output	Pulmonary edema	Hypotension
Hemodynamics	O_2 sat. stepup (RA → PA) > 10%	V wave on PCWP tracing	Dynamic LVOT gradient
Treatment	Operation	Operation	Fluids, β-blocker, α-agonist

LVOT, LV outflow tract; PA, pulmonary artery; PCWP, pulmonary capillary wedge pressure; RA, right atrium; sat., saturation.

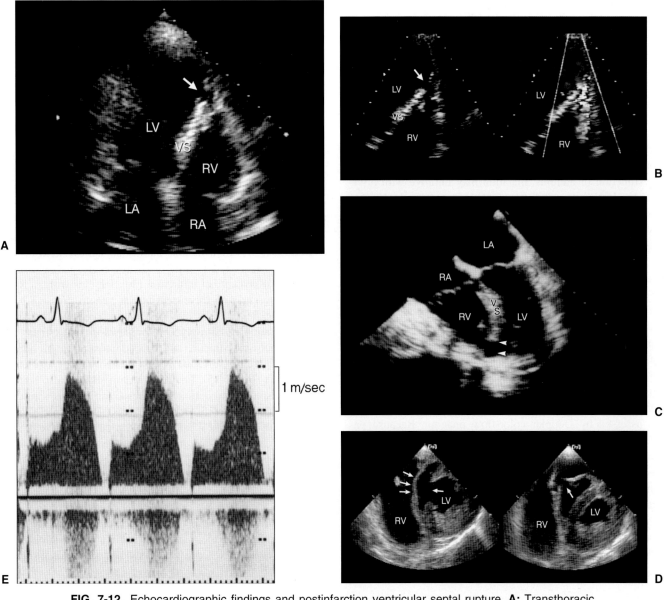

FIG. 7-12. Echocardiographic findings and postinfarction ventricular septal rupture. **A:** Transthoracic apical four-chamber view demonstrating ventricular septal (*VS*) rupture (*arrow*) in a patient with antero-apical myocardial infarction. **B:** Zoomed ventricular septal rupture (*arrow*) and color-flow imaging demonstrating a shunt from left ventricle (*LV*) to right ventricle (*RV*). **C:** Transesophageal transverse view with the transducer in the midesophagus position demonstrating an apical anteroseptal ventricular septal rupture (*arrowheads*). This ventricular septal rupture was the first to be detected with transesophageal echocardiography at the Mayo Clinic; the patient was an 81-year-old woman with an anterior wall infarct and new systolic murmur. **D:** Transesophageal transgastric view of the LV demonstrating a serpiginous tear of the ventricular septum. **Left image:** The tear in the left side of the ventricular septum (*single arrow* in LV), with the dissection into the myocardial cavity at that level; the right side of the septum was intact (*three arrows*). **Right image:** A tear in the right side of the ventricular septum, more toward the apical level (*arrow*). **E:** Continuous-wave Doppler recording from the parasternal position of an infarct-related ventricular septal defect. The peak systolic flow velocity is 3 m/sec, corresponding to a 36-mm Hg pressure gradient between the LV and RV. Systolic blood pressure was 90 mm Hg; hence, RV systolic pressure = 90 − 36 = 54 mm Hg. There is a continuous shunt through the ventricular septal defect except during early diastole.

early mitral regurgitation independently predicted 1-year cardiovascular mortality, but a murmur of mitral regurgitation was heard in fewer than 10% of the patients.

There are three separate pathophysiologic mechanisms of acute mitral regurgitation after myocardial infarction: (a) LV cavity and mitral annulus dilatation, (b) papillary muscle dysfunction, and (c) papillary muscle rupture. Therapeutically, it is important to recognize the exact underlying cause of ischemic mitral regurgitation, because papillary muscle rupture mandates urgent mitral valve replacement or repair, but mitral regurgitation due to papillary muscle dysfunction or annulus dilatation may improve with afterload reduction or coronary revascularization (or both). According to a large clinical study, however, acute reperfusion with thrombolysis or coronary angioplasty did not reliably reverse severe mitral regurgitation (27).

Hemodynamically, papillary muscle rupture is the most serious complication involving the mitral valve. The patients usually have a small infarct in the distribution of the right or circumflex coronary artery. Because the posteromedial papillary muscle is supplied by a single coronary artery (as opposed to the dual supply of the anterolateral papillary muscle), rupture of the posteromedial papillary muscle is six to ten times more frequent. Echocardiography is the best way to diagnose papillary muscle dysfunction and rupture (Fig. 7-13). The severity of mitral regurgitation is assessed by Doppler color-flow imaging. Because patients with severe mitral regurgitation usually present with hemodynamic decompensation, TEE may be necessary to establish clearly the diagnosis and to assess the severity of mitral regurgitation (Fig. 7-14) (28). After papillary muscle rupture has been diagnosed, urgent mitral valve replacement with or without coronary revascularization is necessary for survival. The long-term survival rate is excellent after successful surgery (29).

PERICARDIAL EFFUSION AND TAMPONADE

Hemodynamically insignificant pericardial effusion is common after myocardial infarction, especially a large transmural anterior infarct. It is treated symptomatically [e.g., indomethacin (Indocin) therapy for pericarditic chest pain]; however, cardiac rupture may present as cardiac tamponade. In this situation, the pericardial sac may be filled with a gelatinous-appearing clot (Fig. 7-7B). If so, urgent cardiac surgery is needed, and emergency pericardiocentesis may be required to stabilize the patient's condition until surgery.

RIGHT VENTRICULAR INFARCT

The RV frequently is involved in acute myocardial infarction; however, a hemodynamically significant RV infarct is infrequent and almost always associated with inferior wall myocardial infarction (30). Patients with an RV infarct present with increased jugular venous pressure but clear lung fields. They may become hypotensive after the administration of nitroglycerin or develop shock that requires inotropic support and the administration of fluid. Echocardiographically, the RV is dilated and hypokinetic to akinetic (Fig. 7-15). The right atrium (RA) is also large, and tricuspid regurgitation becomes significant as a result of tricuspid annulus dilatation. Because RV systolic pressure is not increased, peak tricuspid regurgitation velocity is not high, usually lower than 2 m/sec. In patients with a patent foramen ovale (PFO), an RV infarct creates an optimal clinical setting for significant right-to-left shunt through the PFO because of abnormal RV compliance and markedly increased RA pressure. If a patient presents with hypoxemia after inferior wall myocardial infarction, RV infarct and right-to-left shunt through a PFO should be strongly considered (31). This diagnosis can be confirmed

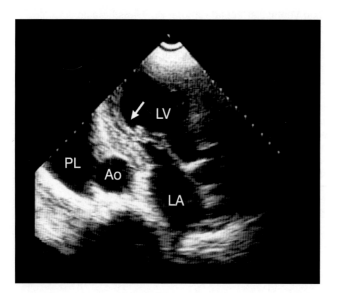

FIG. 7-13. Apical long-axis view on transthoracic examination demonstrating a partial rupture of the papillary muscle (*arrow*). Incidentally, a large amount of pleural effusion (*PL*) is noted. In real time, the inferolateral wall was akinetic and the anteroseptum was hyperdynamic. *Ao*, aorta.

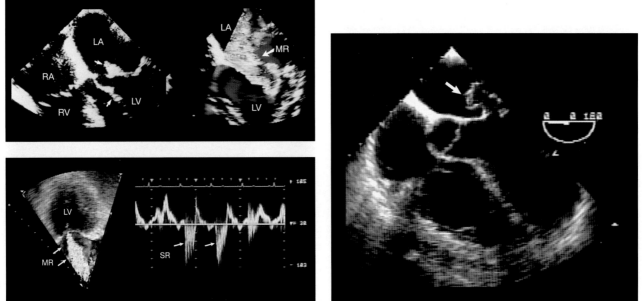

FIG. 7-14. Transesophageal echocardiographic (TEE) images demonstrating rupture and dysfunction of papillary muscle, with severe mitral valve regurgitation. **A:** This was the first TEE diagnosis at the Mayo Clinic of complete rupture of papillary muscle. Transverse view (using monoplane) demonstrating a ruptured papillary muscle prolapsing into the left atrium (*LA*) during diastole attached to the posterior mitral leaflet (*arrow* in LA); *arrow* in left ventricle (*LV*) indicates anterior mitral leaflet. Color-flow imaging shows severe mitral regurgitation with broad mitral regurgitation (*MR*) jet. **B:** Multiplane TEE image with the transducer at zero degree. This demonstrates a ruptured papillary muscle (*arrow*) that is still attached to both mitral leaflets. **C:** It was difficult to assess the severity of MR with surface echocardiography in an elderly woman with her first inferolateral acute myocardial infarction and cardiogenic shock but global systolic function was normal. TEE showed severe MR caused by papillary muscle dysfunction and an akinetic inferolateral wall. Pulsed-wave Doppler echocardiography **(right)** of the pulmonary vein shows systolic flow reversal (*SR*), indicating severe mitral regurgitation. Coronary angiography showed complete occlusion of the left circumflex coronary artery. The patient underwent urgent mitral valve repair and recovered satisfactorily. (**A:** from Patel AM, Miller FA Jr, Khandheria BK, Mullany CJ, Seward JB. Role of transesophageal echocardiography in the diagnosis of papillary muscle rupture secondary to myocardial infarction. *Am Heart J* 1989;118:1330–1333, with permission.)

with contrast echocardiography (peripheral venous injection of agitated saline). Following opacification of the RA, the contrast medium enters the LA via the PFO. This situation is best assessed by TEE (Fig. 7-15). The PFO and the shunt in this clinical setting can be closed temporarily by inflation of a balloon catheter into the LA. Placement of the balloon catheter across the PFO and sufficient inflation of the balloon to obliterate the right-to-left shunt can be guided by TEE. Surgical or device closure of the PFO may be indicated in certain cases.

TRUE VENTRICULAR ANEURYSM AND THROMBUS

A ventricular aneurysm is characterized by myocardial thinning and bulging motion during systole (Fig. 7-16). Aneurysm formation is related to transmural myocardial infarction and is found most frequently at the apex, followed by the inferobasal area. The apical view is the best window

to visualize an apical aneurysm. An inferobasal aneurysm is visualized best from a parasternal long or apical two-chamber view. A ventricular aneurysm is the consequence of infarct expansion, which indicates a poor prognosis. Ventricular aneurysms frequently harbor a thrombus and can be the focus of malignant ventricular arrhythmias. Because of concern about a potential embolic event, patients with a large apical infarct or a ventricular aneurysm are given anticoagulation therapy for at least 6 months after an infarct, at which time the chance for systemic embolism diminishes. The frequency of apical thrombus has decreased with thrombolytic therapy and therapeutic heparinization during hospitalization. Unless apical wall motion improves with reperfusion therapy, patients with an apical infarct remain at higher risk for developing thrombus after anticoagulation therapy is stopped. Two-dimensional echocardiography has become the most practical and reliable imaging modality for detecting LV thrombus. It is important to differentiate thrombus from chordae or artifacts fre-

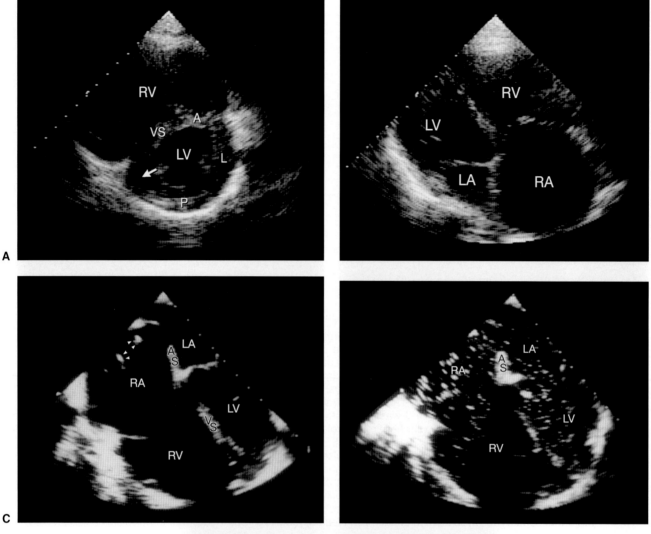

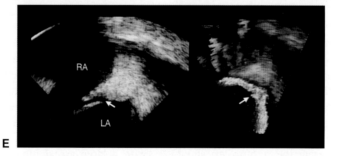

FIG. 7-15. Transthoracic parasternal short-axis **(A)** and apical four-chamber **(B)** views showing a dilated right ventricle (*RV*) and right atrium (*RA*) in a patient with an RV infarct associated with inferior wall myocardial infarction, indicated by an *arrow* pointing to thinned akinetic inferior and inferoseptal segments. *A,* anterior wall; *L,* lateral wall; *P,* posterior wall; *VS,* ventricular septum. **C:** Transesophageal four-chamber view demonstrating RV infarct. The chambers on the right side are markedly dilated, and the atrial septum (*AS*) is deviated toward the left atrium (*LA*) because of increased RA pressure. A Swan-Ganz catheter and temporary pacemaker leads (*arrowheads*) are seen in the RA. **D:** Injection of contrast agent into a vein in the right arm opacifies the left-sided cardiac chambers immediately after opacification of the RA. **E:** Long-axis view of a transesophageal examination **(left)** showing the atrial septum and patent foramen ovale (*arrow*) in a patient with RV infarct and hypoxemia. Color-flow imaging **(right)** showing continuous right-to-left shunt (*arrow*) via a patent foramen ovale that was responsible for the patient's hypoxemia in the setting of RV infarct.

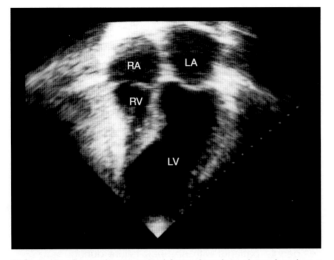

FIG. 7-16. Apex-down, apical four-chamber view showing a large apical aneurysm. The apex is thinned and dilated, with dyskinetic motion in real time.

quently seen at the apex (Fig. 7-17). Characteristically, a thrombus has a nonhomogeneous echo density with a margin distinct from the underlying wall, which is akinetic to dyskinetic. With these criteria, 2D echocardiography has a sensitivity of 95% and a specificity of 86% in detecting thrombus, as compared with a pathologic study (32). A pedunculated thrombus has a greater chance of embolization than a sessile or a laminated thrombus.

DIASTOLIC FUNCTION

Myocardial ischemia alters diastolic function of the LV. The most prominent initial diastolic abnormality due to ischemia is prolonged and delayed myocardial relaxation. Re-

laxation becomes slower, resulting in prolongation of the isovolumic relaxation time (IVRT) as well as in a lower transmitral pressure gradient at the time of mitral valve opening, which decreases early rapid filling (E) of the LV. The deceleration time (DT) of the E velocity is prolonged because of continued slow relaxation with an incompletely emptied LA, resulting in augmented LA contraction (increased A velocity), which augments LV filling.

The typical mitral flow pattern of a relaxation abnormality ($\downarrow$E, $\uparrow$DT, $\uparrow$A, $\downarrow$E/A) is seen during transient myocardial ischemia and in patients with coronary artery disease (33). When a patient has a myocardial infarction, the mitral flow velocity pattern depends on the interaction of various factors: relaxation abnormalities, ventricular compliance, LA pressure, loading conditions, heart rate, medications, and pericardial compliance in the setting of acute cardiac dilatation. Therefore, no particular mitral inflow pattern is seen consistently in patients with myocardial infarction. Although numerous factors influence transmitral Doppler velocities, increased LA pressure is one of the most important determinants and produces a restrictive diastolic filling pattern ($\uparrow$E, $\downarrow$DT, $\downarrow$A, $\uparrow$E/A). Patients with acute myocardial infarction who demonstrate a restrictive filling pattern on transmitral Doppler echocardiography are more likely to experience heart failure (Fig. 7-18) from severe LV systolic dysfunction or severe underlying coronary artery disease (or both) (33).

RISK STRATIFICATION

The most powerful prognostic indicators after myocardial infarction are the degree of systolic dysfunction, the extent of coronary artery disease, and the presence of heart failure. Therefore, it is reasonable to predict that patients with a

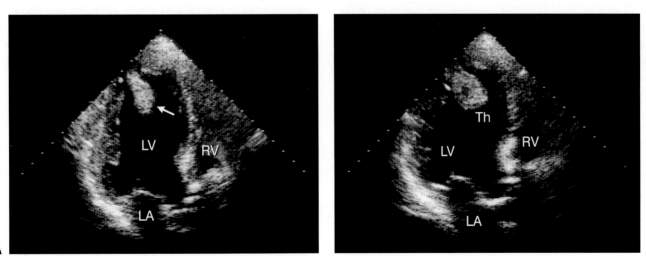

A   B

FIG. 7-17. A, B: Example of a pedunculated mobile apical thrombus (*arrow* in **A** and *Th* in **B**) in a patient with an anteroapical infarct. The mobile nature of the thrombus can be appreciated by varying shapes of the thrombus in two separate frames. This appearance suggests a high probability of embolization.

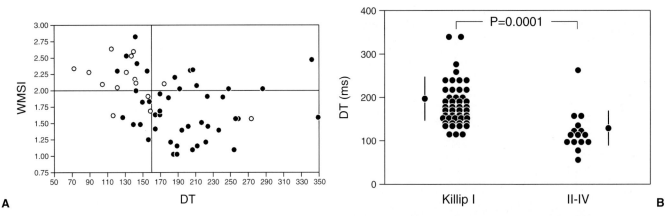

FIG. 7-18. A: Plot of wall motion score index (*WMSI*) and deceleration time (*DT*) from mitral inflow velocity in patients with acute myocardial infarction. *Open circles* denote patients who had heart failure at admission or during hospitalization. *Darkened circles* denote patients with no heart failure during hospitalization. Note that many patients with a high wall motion index score (>2.0) are not in heart failure despite a large myocardial infarction. Most patients with a deceleration time <160 ms were in heart failure at admission or heart failure developed during hospitalization. **B:** Patients in Killip class II–IV had a much shorter deceleration time than those in Killip class I. (From ref. 33, with permission.)

high WMSI have a greater chance of subsequently developing cardiac events. Nishimura and associates (34) demonstrated that patients with postmyocardial infarction complications had a higher WMSI than those without complications (2.4 versus 1.7, using a 14-segment model). Furthermore, among patients with no heart failure (Killip class I) at admission, a subgroup of patients with a WMSI greater than 2.0 were more likely to develop heart failure during hospitalization. Myocardial RWMAs can return to normal contractility after successful reperfusion therapy, however, and in this situation the high WMSI on the initial echocardiogram may not necessarily predict in-hospital complications. Our more recent study using the American Society of Echocardiography-recommended 16-segment wall motion analysis model demonstrated that most of the patients with Killip class II–IV heart failure after an acute myocardial infarction had a WMSI of 1.7 or higher, but many patients with this score did not develop any complications (33). Evaluation of diastolic filling as well as systolic function was more discriminative in risk stratification.

In addition to the WMSI, restrictive Doppler filling variables derived from mitral inflow velocities correlate well with the incidence of postinfarct heart failure and LV filling pressures (33,35). Stress echocardiography is sensitive in detecting residual ischemia, myocardial viability, and multivessel disease soon after myocardial infarction occurs. Usually, however, patients are unable to exercise adequately soon after an acute myocardial infarction. Many studies have demonstrated that stress echocardiography using dobutamine can be performed safely soon after an acute myocardial infarction (3 to 5 days) and can provide predictable stress to the heart (36–38). Carlos and colleagues (37) demonstrated that the following information on do-

butamine stress echocardiography was predictive of future adverse outcome (Fig. 7-19): (a) lack of myocardial viability (i.e., no increase in wall motion of the infarcted segment with a low dose of dobutamine) and (b) involvement of four or more segments with acute myocardial infarction (i.e., ≥25% of the LV). Enlargement of the LV after myocardial infarction is associated with adverse cardiac events. Attenuation of LV enlargement with captopril treatment was demonstrated by 2D echocardiography in the Survival and Ventricular Enlargement (SAVE) trial (39). This was associated with fewer cardiac events.

In summary, patients at increased risk for future cardiac events after acute myocardial infarction can be identified by (a) systolic dysfunction (ejection fraction <40%), (b) extensive infarction (WMSI ≥1.7), (c) restrictive diastolic filling, (d) LV enlargement, and (e) abnormal stress test findings on echocardiography. Multivessel coronary artery disease (i.e., ischemia of noninfarcted segments with a high

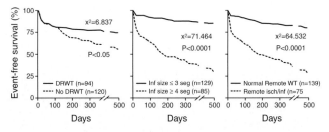

FIG. 7-19. Kaplan-Meier life table curves to show dobutamine stress echocardiography variables for predicting future outcome in patients with acute myocardial infarction. *DRWT*, dobutamine-responsive wall thickening at low dose; *Inf*, infarction; *Isch*, ischemia; *WT*, wall thickening. (From ref. 37, with permission.)

dose of dobutamine) detected on dobutamine stress echocardiography was more predictive of an adverse event than the anatomic detection of multivessel coronary disease on angiography (37).

VISUALIZATION OF THE CORONARY ARTERIES

Visualization of the coronary arteries has been one of the most challenging tasks for echocardiography. Since Weyman and coauthors (40) first described the feasibility of visualizing the left main coronary artery with transthoracic echocardiography, numerous attempts have been made to improve its sensitivity and specificity. It became clear, however, that the transthoracic approach could not visualize the coronary arteries adequately, reliably, and consistently, although it was demonstrated that high-frequency (7.5 MHz) transthoracic imaging could visualize the distal left anterior descending coronary artery in 85% of patients studied (41).

The advent of TEE renewed enthusiasm for echocardiographic visualization of the coronary arteries. The left main and proximal portions of the left coronary arterial tree are located within the domain of the basal short-axis view (see Fig. 3-16). The ostium and proximal portions of the right coronary artery are seen best from the long-axis view of the heart with multiplane imaging (~135 degrees). Anomalous coronary arteries, coronary aneurysm (Kawasaki disease), and coronary fistula can be identified on TEE (Fig. 7-20 and 7-21) (42). Coronary-flow reserve can be assessed by recording coronary-flow velocities before and after the administration of a vasodilator (adenosine), but its clinical role is limited. Contrast echocardiography using second-harmonic imaging has identified intramural coronary arteries and has been able to demonstrate flow reserve (43). This interesting observation needs to be investigated further for clinical application.

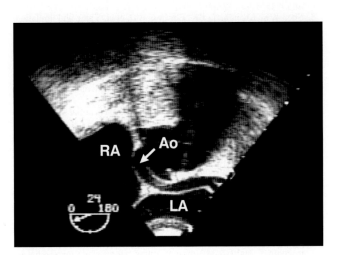

FIG. 7-20. Multiplane transesophageal image (transducer at 29 degrees) of anomalous left circumflex artery (*arrow*), which originates from the right coronary cusp. *Ao*, aorta.

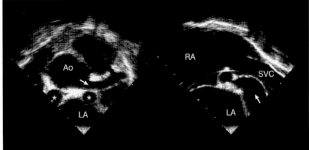

FIG. 7-21. Transesophageal images of coronary artery fistula. **Left:** Transverse view showing dilated coronary arteries. *Arrow*, Left anterior descending coronary artery; *, cross sections of other segments of the enlarged coronary artery. Ao = aorta. **Right:** Longitudinal view showing a dilated coronary artery (*arrow*) draining to the right atrium (*RA*). *SVC*, superior vena cava.

INTRAVASCULAR ULTRASONOGRAPHY

Miniaturized high-frequency (20 to 40 MHz) ultrasound crystals have been incorporated into the tip of a catheter to image the structure and lumen size of coronary arteries. A small (3F to 5F) ultrasound imaging catheter can be manipulated into the coronary arteries. The catheter system allows circumferential tomographic imaging of the artery. Normally, the wall of a coronary artery has three layers: the intima, media, and adventitia. Intravascular ultrasonography shows that the thickness of the inner layer is increased in atherosclerotic arteries. The composition of the atherosclerotic plaque can be characterized by its ultrasonographic appearance. Hence, intravascular ultrasonography provides better definition of the thickness and morphology of an atherosclerotic plaque, characterization of tissue, and measurement of the vascular lumen (44). This system has been used in conjunction with peripheral vascular imaging, evaluation of the left main coronary artery (45), percutaneous transluminal coronary angioplasty, and coronary stenting. In patients undergoing a coronary stent procedure, intracoronary ultrasonography guides the optimal expansion and application of the stent device, which helps to minimize restenosis and avoid unnecessary anticoagulation (46). Another exciting area is intracoronary Doppler echocardiography, which can measure increased flow velocity caused by coronary stenosis and can assess coronary flow reserve (Fig. 7-22).

SUMMARY AND CLINICAL IMPACT

Echocardiography has become an essential part of the evaluation of patients who have various manifestations of ischemic heart disease (see Fig. 7-1). No other imaging technique can provide readily, noninvasively, and relatively inexpensively such a wealth of information at the patient's bedside. Most of adult cardiology practice is concerned with coronary artery disease: chest pain, stress testing, my-

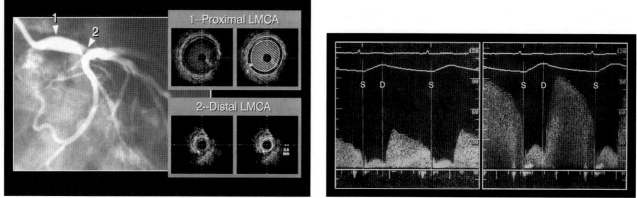

FIG. 7-22. A: Coronary angiogram and left main coronary artery (*LMCA*) intravascular sonograms. **Left:** Right anterior oblique view of an indeterminate lesion (*2*) in the distal LMCA. **Right:** Intravascular ultrasonographic images from the proximal (*1*) and distal (*2*) LMCA. The distal LMCA has an 80% area stenosis. *Hatched area* denotes the luminal area. The internal and external elastic membranes are outlined. *A*, adventitia; *M*, media. (From ref. 45, with permission.) **B:** Intracoronary Doppler study showing measurement of coronary flow reserve. Tracings are from the left anterior descending coronary artery before **(left)** and after **(right)** 18 μg of adenosine was delivered by intracoronary administration. *D*, onset of diastole; *S*, onset of systole. (From Higawo ST, Nishimura RA. Coronary circulation. B. Intravascular ultrasonography. In: Giuliani ER, Gersh BJ, McGoon MD, Hayes DL, Schaff HV, eds. *Mayo Clinic practice of cardiology,* 3rd ed. St. Louis: Mosby, 1996:1049–1055, with permission.)

ocardial infarction, postinfarction complications, risk stratification, and preoperative cardiac evaluation. Echocardiography helps to evaluate every aspect of coronary artery disease short of visualization of the entire coronary arterial tree and evaluation of arrhythmias. Serial regional wall motion analysis using digital echocardiography is an excellent way of evaluating the beneficial effects of thrombolytic therapy on regional myocardial function and should become a routine part of managing acute myocardial infarction. When a complication develops after myocardial infarction, echocardiography should be the first diagnostic procedure used so that potentially fatal complications can be diagnosed and intervention can be started expeditiously to improve the chance of survival. In patients with uncomplicated myocardial infarction, systolic and diastolic filling variables at rest or with stress (exercise or pharmacologic stress) determined by 2D Doppler echocardiography provide prognostic information and guide optimal management strategies.

REFERENCES

1. The GUSTO Investigators. An international randomized trial comparing four thrombolytic strategies for acute myocardial infarction. *N Engl J Med* 1993;329:673–682.
2. Every NR, Parsons LS, Hlatky M, Martin JS, Weaver WD, for the Myocardial Infarction Triage and Intervention Investigators. A comparison of thrombolytic therapy with primary coronary angioplasty for acute myocardial infarction. *N Engl J Med* 1996;335:1253–1260.
3. Kishon Y, Iqbal A, Oh JK, et al. Evolution of echocardiographic modalities in detection of postmyocardial infarction ventricular septal defect and papillary muscle rupture: study of 62 patients. *Am Heart J* 1993;126:667–675.
4. Meluzin J, Cigarroa CG, Brickner ME, et al. Dobutamine echocardiography in predicting improvement in global left ventricular systolic function after coronary bypass or angioplasty in patients with healed myocardial infarcts. *Am J Cardiol* 1995;76:877–880.
5. Picano E, Pingitore A, Sicari R, et al. on behalf of the Echo Persantine International Cooperative (EPIC) Study Group. Stress echocardiographic results predict risk of reinfarction early after uncomplicated acute myocardial infarction: large-scale multicenter study. *J Am Coll Cardiol* 1995;26:908–913.
6. Schiller NB, Shah PM, Crawford M, et al. for the American Society of Echocardiography Committee on Standards, Subcommittee on Quantitation of Two-Dimensional Echocardiograms. Recommendations for quantitation of the left ventricle by two-dimensional echocardiography. *J Am Soc Echocardiogr* 1989;2:358–367.
7. Lieberman AN, Weiss JL, Jugdutt BI, et al. Two-dimensional echocardiography and infarct size: relationship of regional wall motion and thickening to the extent of myocardial infarction in the dog. *Circulation* 1981;63:739–746.
8. Shen WK, Khandheria BK, Edwards WD, et al. Value and limitations of two-dimensional echocardiography in predicting myocardial infarct size. *Am J Cardiol* 1991;68:1143–1149.
9. Oh JK, Gibbons RJ, Christian TF, et al. Correlation of regional wall motion abnormalities detected by two-dimensional echocardiography with perfusion defect determined by technetium 99m sestamibi imaging in patients treated with reperfusion therapy during acute myocardial infarction. *Am Heart J* 1996;131:32–37.
10. Uematsu M, Miyatake K, Tanaka N, et al. Myocardial velocity gradient as a new indicator of regional left ventricular contraction: detection by a two-dimensional tissue Doppler imaging technique. *J Am Coll Cardiol* 1995;26:217–223.
11. McDicken WN, Sutherland GR, Moran CM, Gordon LN. Colour Doppler velocity imaging of the myocardium. *Ultrasound Med Biol* 1992;18:651–654.
12. Mor-Avi V, Vignon P, Koch R, et al. Segmental analysis of color kinesis images: New method for quantification of the magnitude and timing of endocardial motion during left ventricular systole and diastole. *Circulation* 1997;95:2082–2097.
13. de Winter RJ, Koster RW, Sturk A, Sanders GT. Value of myoglobin, troponin T, and CK-MB mass in ruling out an acute myocardial infarction in the emergency room. *Circulation* 1995;92:3401–3407.
14. Hamm CW, Goldmann BU, Heeschen C, Kreymann G, Berger J, Meinertz T. Emergency room triage of patients with acute chest pain by

means of rapid testing for cardiac Troponin T or Troponin I. *N Engl J Med* 1997;337:1648–1653.

15. Sabia P, Afrookteh A, Touchstone DA, Keller MW, Esquivel L, Kaul S. Value of regional wall motion abnormality in the emergency room diagnosis of acute myocardial infarction. A prospective study using two-dimensional echocardiography. *Circulation* 1991;84(Suppl 1): I85–I92.

16. Trippi JA, Lee KS, Kopp G, Nelson DR, Yee KG, Cordell WH. Dobutamine stress tele-echocardiography for evaluation of emergency department patients with chest pain. *J Am Coll Cardiol* 1997;30:627–632.

17. Oh JK, Gersh BJ, Nassef LA Jr, et al. Effects of acute reperfusion on regional myocardial function: serial two-dimensional echocardiography assessment. *Int J Cardiol* 1989;22:161–168.

18. Broderick TM, Bourdillon PD, Ryan T, Feigenbaum H, Dillon JC, Armstrong WF. Comparison of regional and global left ventricular function by serial echocardiograms after reperfusion in acute myocardial infarction. *J Am Soc Echocardiogr* 1989;2:315–323.

19. Goldberg RJ, Gore JM, Alpert JS, et al. Cardiogenic shock after acute myocardial infarction: incidence and mortality from a community-wide perspective, 1975 to 1988. *N Engl J Med* 1991;325:1117–1122.

20. Hochman JS, Boland J, Sleeper LA, et al. and the SHOCK Registry Investigators. Current spectrum of cardiogenic shock and effect of early revascularization on mortality: results of an International Registry. *Circulation* 1995;91:873–881.

21. Sohn DW, Shin GJ, Oh JK, et al. Role of transesophageal echocardiography in hemodynamically unstable patients. *Mayo Clin Proc* 1995;70:925–931.

22. Oliva PB, Hammill SC, Edwards WD. Cardiac rupture, a clinically predictable complication of acute myocardial infarction: report of 70 cases with clinicopathologic correlations. *J Am Coll Cardiol* 1993;22: 720–726.

23. Yeo TC, Malouf JF, Reeder GS, Oh JK. Post infarction pseudoaneurysm: clinical and echocardiographic features in 22 cases. *J Am Soc Echocardiogr* 1997;10:432(abst).

24. Yamaura Y, Yoshikawa J, Yoshida K, Akasaka T. Echocardiographic findings of subepicardial aneurysm of the left ventricle. *Am Heart J* 1994;127:211–214.

25. Reeder GS. Identification and treatment of complications of myocardial infarction. *Mayo Clin Proc* 1995;70:880–884.

26. Lehmann KG, Francis CK, Dodge HT, and the TIMI Study Group. Mitral regurgitation in early myocardial infarction: incidence, clinical detection, and prognostic implications. *Ann Intern Med* 1992;117:10–17.

27. Tcheng JE, Jackman JD Jr, Nelson CL, et al. Outcome of patients sustaining acute ischemic mitral regurgitation during myocardial infarction. *Ann Intern Med* 1992;117:18–24.

28. Oh JK, Seward JB, Khandheria BK, et al. Transesophageal echocardiography in critically ill patients. *Am J Cardiol* 1990;66:1492–1495.

29. Kishon Y, Oh JK, Schaff HV, Mullany CJ, Tajik AJ, Gersh BJ. Mitral valve operation in postinfarction rupture of a papillary muscle: immediate results and long-term follow-up of 22 patients. *Mayo Clin Proc* 1992;67:1023–1030.

30. Kinch JW, Ryan TJ. Right ventricular infarction. *N Engl J Med* 1994;330:1211–1217.

31. Lin SS, Oh JK, Tajik AJ, Gay PC, Kishon Y, Seward JB. Right-to-left shunts in patients with severe hypoxemia: transesophageal contrast echocardiography study. *J Am Coll Cardiol* 1995;Special Issue: 17A(abst).

32. DeMaria AN, Bommer W, Neumann A, et al. Left ventricular thrombi identified by cross-sectional echocardiography. *Ann Intern Med* 1979;90:14–18.

33. Oh JK, Ding ZP, Gersh BJ, Bailey KR, Tajik AJ. Restrictive left ventricular diastolic filling identifies patients with heart failure after acute myocardial infarction. *J Am Soc Echocardiogr* 1992;5:497–503.

34. Nishimura RA, Tajik AJ, Shub C, Miller FA Jr, Ilstrup DM, Harrison CE. Role of two-dimensional echocardiography in the prediction of in-hospital complications after acute myocardial infarction. *J Am Coll Cardiol* 1984;4:1080–1087.

35. Giannuzzi P, Imparato A, Temporelli PL, et al. Doppler-derived mitral deceleration time of early filling as a strong predictor of pulmonary capillary wedge pressure in postinfarction patients with left ventricular systolic dysfunction. *J Am Coll Cardiol* 1994;23:1630–1637.

36. Bolognese L, Antoniucci D, Rovai D, et al. Myocardial contrast echocardiography versus dobutamine echocardiography for predicting functional recovery after acute myocardial infarction treated with primary coronary angioplasty. *J Am Coll Cardiol* 1996;28:1677–1683.

37. Carlos ME, Smart SC, Wynsen JC, Sagar KB. Dobutamine stress echocardiography for risk stratification after myocardial infarction. *Circulation* 1997;95:1402–1410.

38. Smart SC, Knickelbine T, Stoiber TR, Carlos M, Wynsen JC, Sagar KB. Safety and accuracy of dobutamine-atropine stress echocardiography for the detection of residual stenosis of the infarct-related artery and multivessel disease during the first week after acute myocardial infarction. *Circulation* 1997;95:1394–1401.

39. St. John Sutton M, Pfeffer MA, Plappert T, et al. for the SAVE Investigators. Quantitative two-dimensional echocardiographic measurements are major predictors of adverse cardiovascular events after acute myocardial infarction: the protective effects of captopril. *Circulation* 1994;89:68–75.

40. Weyman AE, Feigenbaum H, Dillon JC, Johnston KW, Eggleton RC. Noninvasive visualization of the left main coronary artery by cross-sectional echocardiography. *Circulation* 1976;54:169–174.

41. Ross JJ Jr, Mintz GS, Chandrasekaran K. Transthoracic two-dimensional high frequency (7.5 MHz) ultrasonic visualization of the distal left anterior descending coronary artery. *J Am Coll Cardiol* 1990;15: 373–377.

42. Fernandes F, Alam M, Smith S, Khaja F. The role of transesophageal echocardiography in identifying anomalous coronary arteries. *Circulation* 1993;88:2532–2540.

43. Mulvagh SL, Foley DA, Aeschbacher BC, Klarich KK, Seward JB. Second harmonic imaging of an intravenously administered echocardiographic contrast agent: visualization of coronary arteries and measurement of coronary blood flow. *J Am Coll Cardiol* 1996;27:1519–1525.

44. Higano ST, Nishimura RA. Intravascular ultrasonography. *Curr Probl Cardiol* 1994;19:1–55.

45. Nishimura RA, Higano ST, Holmes DR Jr. Use of intracoronary ultrasound imaging for assessing left main coronary artery disease. *Mayo Clin Proc* 1993;68:134–140.

46. Colombo A, Hall P, Nakamura S, et al. Intracoronary stenting without anticoagulation accomplished with intravascular ultrasound guidance. *Circulation* 1995;91:1676—1688.

CHAPTER 8

Stress Echocardiography

Stress testing is a common diagnostic procedure, and many different types of stress tests are available, including treadmill exercise with electrocardiographic (ECG) monitoring, stress echocardiography, myocardial perfusion imaging, radionuclide angiography, positron emission tomography (PET), and cardiopulmonary exercise testing. Pharmacologic as well as exercise stress has been used in conjunction with an imaging technique.

Common indications for a stress test are the diagnosis of myocardial ischemia, identification of severe coronary artery disease, prognostication, risk stratification after acute myocardial infarction, and a preoperative evaluation for a major noncardiac surgical procedure. The choice of an optimal stress modality depends on local expertise, the patient's ability to exercise, body weight, resting ECG, and clinical questions to be answered. The Mayo Clinic Cardiovascular Working Group on Stress Testing has published a guideline for selecting a stress test for individual patients (Fig. 8-1) (1).

Myocardial ischemia has various manifestations, including ST-segment depression on ECG, perfusion defect on nuclear imaging or contrast echocardiography, metabolic abnormalities on PET, and abnormal contractility on radionuclide angiography or echocardiography (Fig. 8-2). Stress echocardiography is based on the concept that new or worsening regional myocardial contractility induced by ischemia is reliably detected by echocardiographic wall motion analysis. Comparison of left ventricular (LV) segmental wall motion during or soon after stress with resting wall motion is accomplished with side-by-side review of digitized cine-loop images of all 16 segments of the LV.

This chapter discusses the concept and application of digitized echocardiography and stress echocardiography.

DIGITIZED ECHOCARDIOGRAPHY

Echocardiographic data can be digitized for easier and more convenient storage and for display, retrieval, and comparison of serial studies (Fig. 8-3) (2). Digital echo-cardiography allows on-line grabbing, or capturing, of an entire cardiac cycle(s) or a portion of a representative cardiac cycle using a continuous cine-loop. Initiation of capturing is triggered by the QRS complex and the programmed length of initial delay. If the initial delay is set at 0 msec, the first image will be grabbed at the onset of the QRS complex. Subsequent images are digitized at a preset interval delay, usually 50 msec. When only the systolic period needs to be digitized, eight sequential images (seven intervals) with 50 msec between each image provide 350 msec of the cardiac cycle, which is enough to acquire the entire systolic phase at various heart rates. The interval delay may be shortened to 33 msec when heart rate is fast. Alternatively, one or more consecutive cardiac cycles can be captured to minimize sampling errors, and the best image can be selected for storage and review. It also is possible to digitize color-flow imaging and Doppler velocity recordings as well as several cycles continuously. The captured images are stored on a floppy, hard, or optic disk for archiving, retrieval, and display. The continuous cine-loop can be displayed in a split-screen or a quad-screen format for showing multiple views simultaneously or multiple studies of the same view for purposes of comparison. One quad-screen systolic cine-loop takes 1 megabyte (MB) of memory. Digitized images are essential in performing stress echocardiography, which requires simultaneous comparison of rest and exercise wall motion abnormalities, and in transmitting images over a telephone line and a modem (3). The transmission of digitized images over telephone lines allows immediate expert echocardiographic interpretation at a distance, which is especially helpful in the interpretation of off-hour emergency or out-reach echocardiographic studies.

Currently, interpretation of an echocardiographic study is based on review of 10 to 15 minutes of videotape recording. This is time-consuming, and review at a later time requires a lengthy search for a desired study. With the current videotape storage system, it is almost impossible for nonechocardiographer physicians to have access to tapes to review

91

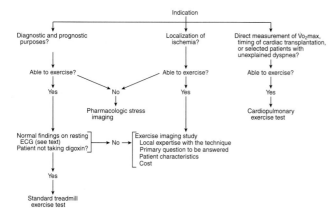

FIG. 8-1. Algorithm proposed by the Mayo Clinic Cardiovascular Working Group on Stress Testing for choosing the most appropriate stress test modality. *ECG*, electrocardiography; *VO₂max*, maximal oxygen consumption. (From ref. 1, with permission.)

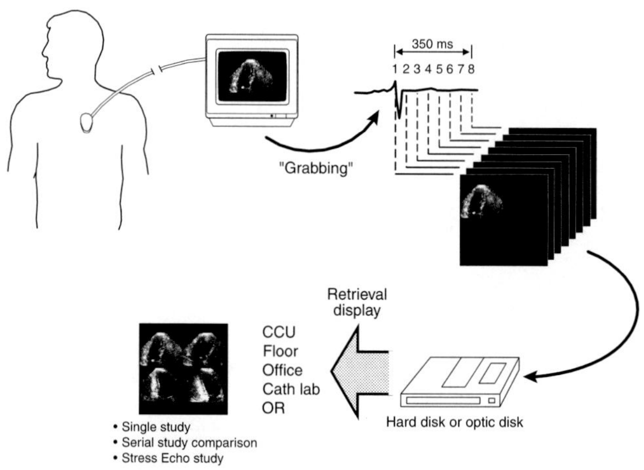

studies performed on their patients; thus, they rely on the report of the study for further evaluation and management of the patient. Digitization of echocardiographic images and their storage in a central area by a network allow easy access and retrieval of image data.

TYPES OF STRESS ECHOCARDIOGRAPHY

Stress echocardiography is performed with exercise, administration of a pharmacologic agent, or transesophageal atrial pacing. The exercise protocol includes a standard treadmill exercise test, with immediate postexercise echocardiographic images obtained within 1.5 minutes (3) or upright or supine bicycle echocardiographic images ob-

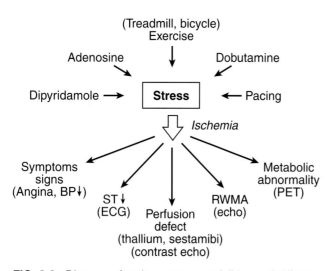

FIG. 8-2. Diagram of various stress modalities and different manifestations of myocardial ischemia and techniques to detect those ischemic markers. *BP*, blood pressure; *ECG*, electrocardiogram; *echo*, echocardiography; *PET*, positron emission tomography; *RWMA*, regional wall motion abnormality.

FIG. 8-3. Diagram of digitized echocardiography and concept of network using digitized echocardiography. Echocardiographic information (two-dimensional, Doppler, or color-flow imaging) can be digitized. A segment of the cardiac cycle, the entire cardiac cycle, or several cardiac cycles can be digitized according to clinical needs. The digitized images are stored in a server; they can be retrieved from multiple terminals. This is essential for comparing studies and for easy retrieval of echocardiographic images without having to always review videotape. *CCU*, cardiac care unit; *OR*, operating room.

tained at peak exercise (4). Because exercise-induced regional wall motion abnormalities usually last for a few minutes after termination of exercise, immediate postexercise images can be compared with the baseline preexercise images to detect exercise-induced regional wall motion abnormalities. Therefore, treadmill exercise with echocardiographic images obtained immediately after termination of exercise is the most frequently used form of exercise echocardiography. By allowing several successive cardiac cycles to be captured and stored in memory, digitized echocardiography enhances the capability of acquiring satisfactory comparative postexercise images. The most satisfactory postexercise image is selected and compared with the baseline image by side-by-side quad-screen display (see Fig. 8-3). The typical exercise echocardiography protocol used at the Mayo Clinic is shown in Table 8-1 and Fig. 8-4A.

When a patient cannot exercise, stress is induced pharmacologically with dobutamine, dipyridamole, or adenosine (Table 8-2) (5,6). Dobutamine is the agent used most commonly in stress echocardiography and is the one used most commonly at the Mayo Clinic (7). Albutamine is another pharmacologic agent with more chronotropic and less inotropic properties than dobutamine. A flowchart for dobutamine stress echocardiography is shown in Fig. 8-4B. Atrial pacing with a transesophageal lead is another option for inducing stress in patients who cannot exercise or when no exercise stress equipment is available. When the surface echocardiographic image is inadequate, transesophageal

TABLE 8-1. *Exercise echocardiography protocol*

Baseline blood pressure, heart rate, and electrocardiogram.
Baseline echocardiography; resting images are digitized and stored.
Exercise test according to the needs of the patient and clinician.
  Treadmill exercise, then immediate postexercise echocardiogram, preferably within 1 min.
  Bicycle or arm ergometer; images are obtained at low and peak levels of exercise; these images are digitized and stored.
Display of baseline and peak exercise (in case of bicycle), or postexercise images (in case of treadmill) side by side using continuous cine-loop.
Review of echocardiographic images (first, digitized images for comparison of rest and postexercise, then selected videotaped images if necessary).
Interpretation of study incorporating other clinical variables (workload, electrocardiographic changes, heart rate and blood pressure response).
End points.
  Severe symptoms (chest pain, dyspnea).
  Severe ischemia (ST ↓ ≥5 mm).
  Complex ectopy or ventricular tachycardia.
  Hypertensive blood pressure response (>220 mm Hg systolic, >110 mm Hg diastolic).
  Hypotension (>20 mm Hg ↓, compared with previous stage).
  Target heart rate.

TABLE 8-2. *Dobutamine echocardiography protocol.*

Baseline heart rate, blood pressure, and electrocardiogram.
Baseline echocardiogram; resting images are digitized and stored.
Begin dobutamine infusion at 5 μg/kg per min.
Increase dobutamine infusion every 3 minutes to 10, 20, 30, and 40 μg/kg per min or until patient develops symptoms, side effects, or new regional wall motion abnormalities.
In patients taking β-blocker, the heart rate response to dobutamine may not be satisfactory. If the heart rate is not within 10% of the target rate with 40 μg/kg per min of dobutamine, atropine (0.2–1.0 mg i.v.) is given to increase heart rate.
Digitize and store echocardiographic images during a low dose (5 or 10 μg/kg per min), prepeak, and peak (or after atropine). Compare images in a quad-screen format. Wall motion is compared with that of preceding level as well as baseline wall motion.
If a patient develops symptoms or persistent tachycardia after termination of dobutamine, esmolol (0.5–1.0 mg/kg i.v.) usually terminates the side effects of dobutamine.
End points.
  Target heart rate (85% of age-predicted maximal heart rate or, if soon after myocardial infarction, 70% of age-predicted maximal heart rate.
  Development of new regional wall motion abnormalities of at least moderate severity.
  Peak dose.
  Ventricular tachycardia or sustained supraventricular tachycardia.
  Severe hypertension (systolic blood pressure >220 mm Hg or diastolic blood pressure >110 mm Hg.
  Substantial decrease in systolic blood pressure (a decrease of 20 mm Hg from previous level of infusion may be used as a guideline for terminating the test, but amount depends on baseline blood pressure and judgment of person monitoring the test).
Intolerable symptoms.

End points from ref. 7, with permission.

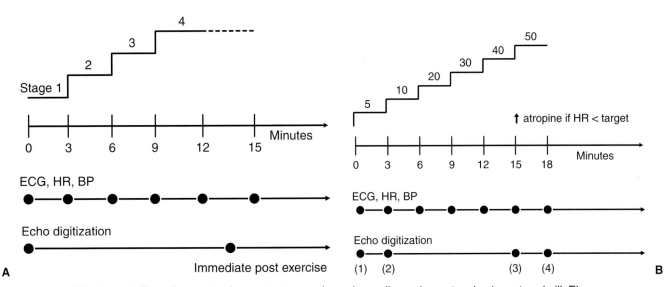

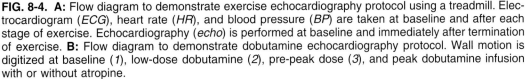

FIG. 8-4. **A:** Flow diagram to demonstrate exercise echocardiography protocol using a treadmill. Electrocardiogram (*ECG*), heart rate (*HR*), and blood pressure (*BP*) are taken at baseline and after each stage of exercise. Echocardiography (*echo*) is performed at baseline and immediately after termination of exercise. **B:** Flow diagram to demonstrate dobutamine echocardiography protocol. Wall motion is digitized at baseline (*1*), low-dose dobutamine (*2*), pre-peak dose (*3*), and peak dobutamine infusion with or without atropine.

echocardiography occasionally is used in conjunction with dobutamine stress.

INTERPRETATION

The interpretation of stress echocardiography is based primarily on the response of LV wall motion to stress (Table 8-3). Normally, with exercise or dobutamine infusion, LV wall motion becomes hyperdynamic (Fig. 8-5A). Worsening of wall motion abnormalities or the development of new ones is the hallmark of stress-induced myocardial ischemia (Fig. 8-5B and C). The lack of hyperdynamic motion may indicate ischemia, but it is less specific. If the lack of hyperdynamic motion is confined to a specific segment after adequate stress, it more strongly indicates ischemia. When the stress level is inadequate or the patient is taking a β-blocker, however, the entire LV segment still may contract normally without hyperdynamic motion. Other adjunctive diagnostic criteria for positive stress echocardiography include LV cavity dilatation, a decrease in global systolic function, diastolic dysfunction, and new or worsening mitral regurgitation; however, these adjunctive diagnostic criteria are more specific for detecting severe coronary artery disease and are not sensitive for detecting the presence of coronary artery disease. Also, it should be emphasized that the response to stress by dobutamine infusion is different from that due to exercise (8). Even in patients with severe coronary artery disease, including left main coronary artery disease, the LV cavity may not dilate and global systolic function may improve with dobutamine infusion despite new wall motion abnormalities due to severe coronary artery disease (Table 8-4). Comparison of exercise echocardiography with dobutamine stress echocardiography in patients with left main coronary artery disease showed cavity dilatation, decrease in systolic global function, and ECG evidence of ischemia (ST-segment depression) to be more common (87%) after exercise stress than after dobutamine infusion (17%). Comparison of stress wall motion with baseline resting wall motion is enhanced by reviewing digitized side-by-side cine-loop echocardiographic images; however, the digitized images alone may not be sufficient for complete regional wall motion analysis, and complete or selected videotape real-time images need to be reviewed to improve the diagnostic accuracy of stress echocardiography (9).

DIAGNOSTIC ACCURACY

The sensitivity and specificity of stress echocardiography, using the above criteria, are comparable to those of stress thallium or sestamibi single-photon emission computed tomography (10,11). In the largest comparison study (112 patients), Quinones et al. (10) reported that the overall sensitivity and specificity of exercise echocardiography were 85% and 88%, respectively, compared with 85% and 81% for exercise thallium. The sensitivity of exercise echocardiography and exercise thallium for coronary artery disease in patients with single-, double-, or triple-vessel involvement was also similar (58%, 86%, and 94% versus 61%, 86%, and 94%, respectively). The sensitivity of exercise echocardiography for predicting multivessel disease, however, is about 70% according to our experience (12). The diagnostic accuracy is affected by sex and verification bias because the stress test result is used to select patients for coronary angiography (13). When a diagnostic test is used routinely, the diagnostic accuracy depends on the patient population, the expertise of the interpreter, and the quality of the image.

MAYO CLINIC EXPERIENCE

Exercise Echocardiography

Of the first 2,000 consecutive exercise echocardiographic studies performed at the Mayo Clinic, the echocardiographic images were not adequate for analysis in 5% (3). The Bruce protocol was used in 82% of the studies and the Naughton protocol in 18%. The mean duration of the exercise test was 7 minutes, and the mean acquisition time for postexercise imaging was 1.4 ± 0.5 minutes. There was one death, which occurred immediately after exercise echocardiography; this patient subsequently was found to have had a massive pulmonary embolism. Of the first 127 patients who underwent coronary angiography after exercise echocardiography, the sensitivity and specificity of the tests for detecting a coronary stenosis >50% were 88% and 72%, respectively.

Dobutamine Stress Echocardiography

Of the first 1,000 consecutive patients to undergo dobutamine stress echocardiography, 94% had a physical lim-

---

TABLE 8-3. *Interpretation by regional wall motion (WM) analysis*

Rest		Stress	Interpretation
Normal WM and contractility	→	Hyperdynamic	Normal
Normal WM	→	New WM abnormality or lack of hyperdynamic WM[a]	Ischemia
WM abnormality	→	Worsening (hypokinesis → akinesis) (akinesis → dyskinesis)[b]	Ischemia
WM abnormality	→	Unchanged	Infarct
Akinetic WM	→	Improved to hypokinetic or to normal WM, biphasic response	Viable myocardium

[a] May not indicate ischemia in the setting of low workload or β-blockade.
[b] May not indicate ischemia.

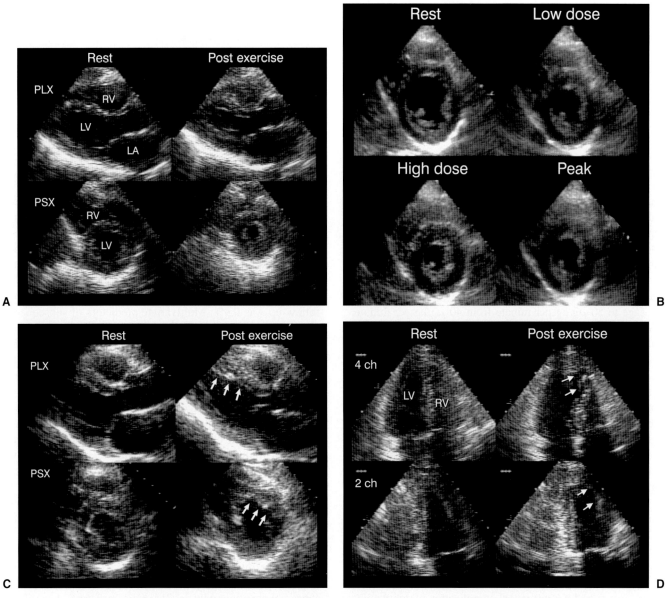

FIG. 8-5. A: Still frame of end-systolic parasternal views of normal exercise echocardiogram as shown in a quad-screen format. Left ventricular (*LV*) cavity is smaller and walls are hyperdynamic in postexercise period. *PLX,* parasternal long-axis; *PSX,* parasternal short-axis. **B:** Still frame of end-systolic PSX view of normal dobutamine stress echocardiogram. LV cavity becomes gradually smaller and walls are hyperdynamic with higher dose of dobutamine. **C:** Still frame of end-systolic parasternal views of positive exercise echocardiogram. Anteroseptum and anterior wall became severely hypokinetic (*arrows*) with exercise. **D:** Still frame of end-systolic apical views of positive exercise echocardiogram. Apical septum and anteroapex became akinetic to dyskinetic. *2 ch,* two-chamber view; *4 ch,* four-chamber view.

TABLE 8-4. *Ischemic manifestations of severe coronary artery disease*

	Exercise	Dobutamine
WM abnormality	Multiple	Multiple
LV cavity	Dilate	Usually not dilate
LV EF	Decrease	May not decrease
ST-segment depression	Common	Uncommon
Hypotension	Specific	Nonspecific

EF, ejection fraction; WM, wall motion.

itation that precluded conventional exercise testing (7). Of these patients, 295 (30%) had a contraindication to dipyridamole or adenosine infusion. The peak dose of dobutamine ranged from 10 to 50 μg/kg per minute, with a mean dose of 34 ± 9 μg/kg per minute, and the mean increase in heart rate was 51 beats/minute. Target heart rate was achieved in 56% of patients and increased to 61% after the addition of atropine and/or an increase of the dobutamine dosage to 50 μg/kg per minute from 40 μg/kg per minute. Atropine was administered in 20% of the total patient population (mean dose, 0.6 ± 0.3 mg) (14). Of the patients who were taking β-blockers, 49% were given atropine. Esmolol was required to treat symptoms and persistent tachycardia in 17% of the patients. Dynamic intracavitary obstruction as a result of hyperdynamic LV function (especially in the presence of LV hypertrophy) was present in approximately 20% of patients during dobutamine stress echocardiography (15). A subset of these patients developed hypotension. Therefore, hypotension during dobutamine infusion does not always indicate ischemia.

Dobutamine stress echocardiography is relatively safe and well tolerated, although mild side effects (chest pain, palpitations, tremor, headache, nausea, light-headedness, and shortness of breath) are frequently noted. Side effects were not more frequent after atropine administration, although it prolongs the duration of sinus tachycardia (14). The most feared but infrequent complication of dobutamine is malignant ventricular tachycardia. This complication may occur even after dobutamine infusion has been terminated; therefore, echocardiographic monitoring of wall motion should continue until stress-induced ischemia resolves and wall motion abnormality returns to baseline before the patient leaves the examination room. A paradoxical bradycardiac response occurs in 8% of patients (16). It usually is observed in patients with coronary artery disease, but it can be related to a vasodepressor effect mediated by the Bezold-Jarisch reflex. It is effectively reversed with atropine.

Atrial Pacing Stress Echocardiography

Atrial pacing provides another form of stress. It can be accomplished by swallowing a small electrode to be positioned behind the LA. With increasing heart rate, wall motion is monitored by echocardiography. In our preliminary study of 100 patients, a high concordance was found between dobutamine-induced and atrial pacing-induced regional wall motion abnormalities. A major advantage of this stress modality is the short duration of the test and that there is no need to administer a pharmacologic agent intravenously. Atrial capture by transesophageal pacing may not be possible in some patients, however.

Stress Echocardiography as a Prognostic Indicator

It is expected, and it has been established, that the prognosis for a patient is better if the stress echocardiographic findings are normal. The likelihood of a cardiac event (cardiac death, nonfatal infarct, or coronary revascularization) occurring after normal results are obtained on stress echocardiography is extremely low. Among 1,325 patients with normal findings on exercise echocardiography at the Mayo Clinic, the event rate over 3 years of follow-up was <3% (Fig. 8-6) (17). The cardiac event rate per person-years of follow-up was 0.9%. Multivariate predictors of subsequent cardiac events were angina during TMET, low workload (<7 METs for men and <5 METs for women), LV hypertrophy, and advancing age. Therefore, the interpretation of a normal exercise echocardiogram should take into consideration the patient's symptoms and workload.

The most common indication for dobutamine stress echocardiography is preoperative cardiac evaluation. In our experience, the risk of a cardiac event in patients who have abnormal findings on dobutamine stress echocardiography was increased 16-fold compared with the risk in patients with normal results (18). Perioperative risk is extremely low after negative findings on dobutamine stress echocardiography, but the risk is 25% to 30% if the results are positive.

The prognostic implications of stress echocardiography after acute myocardial infarction are emerging (19–21). Carlos and associates (22) performed graded dobutamine stress echocardiography in 214 patients 2 to 7 days after

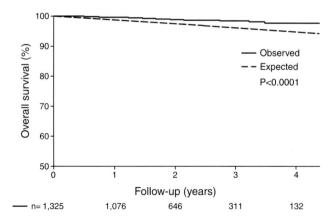

FIG. 8-6. Overall survival for 1,325 patients with normal exercise echocardiograms. Survival was better than expected. (From ref. 17, with permission.)

acute myocardial infarction, and the patients had follow-up of 494 ± 182 days. Multivariate analysis revealed that the only independent predictors of adverse outcome were ischemia at a distance and infarction-zone nonviability. Multivessel disease identified through dobutamine stress echocardiography was more predictive of adverse outcome than angiographically determined multivessel disease. Noninvasive stress testing in patients with uncomplicated myocardial infarction can select patients for coronary angiography without increasing the risk of these patients (23).

CAVEATS FOR TECHNICAL AND INTERPRETATION SKILLS

Stress echocardiography usually is performed by a well-trained sonographer, but final interpretation of the study is the responsibility of the echocardiologist. The following technical and interpretative caveats ensure the most satisfactory stress echocardiographic examination.

For the sonographer:

1. Be thoroughly familiar with the equipment. (There is no time to adjust variables during an examination, especially after exercise.)

2. Be aware of the most optimal transducer position. Obtain postexercise images from the easier window first. When both parasternal and apical windows are satisfactory, obtain the apical view first.

3. Be as prompt as possible in obtaining postexercise images, and record the time interval between the termination of exercise and the completion of imaging. (Optimal time interval, <1.0 minute.)

4. Record all images on videotape as well as digitize online.

5. Do not change field-depth during the entire examination.

6. Obtain images on videotape if chest pain develops or significant ECG changes occur during the recovery period.

For the cardiologist:

1. Ensure that the digitized images are adequate for wall motion analysis (satisfactory endocardial definition).

2. Ensure that the images are grabbed during systole and promptly after exercise.

3. Review the videotape images; this is usually necessary, especially in cases in which the digitized images are not satisfactory or there are other factors such as arrhythmia.

4. Report ancillary signs of ischemia, such as ventricular volume change and global contractility. The normal response is decreased end-systolic volume and increased contractility (or ejection fraction).

5. Be aware that normal systolic thickening of the LV wall is different from passive movement (''translational'' without thickening) of ischemic myocardium, which is pulled by adjacent healthy myocardium.

6. Be aware of possible

False-positive findings:

- Left bundle branch block exaggerates septal motion abnormalities
- Permanent pacemaker produces apical abnormality
- Hypertensive response may produce LV dilatation and systolic dysfunction
- Arrhythmias

False-negative findings:

- Long delay in capturing postexercise images
- Low workload or heart-rate response

7. Incorporate other clinical features (pretest probability) into the final interpretation.

DOPPLER STRESS HEMODYNAMICS IN VALVULAR HEART DISEASE

When there is a discrepancy between the severity of valvular heart disease and the clinical symptoms, an evaluation of valvular hemodynamics with exercise is helpful. A typical example is a symptomatic patient with a less-than-severe degree of mitral valve stenosis. Measurement of the mitral pressure gradient and pulmonary pressure (by tricuspid regurgitation velocity) with exercise often can be diagnostic. With increased heart rate, the mitral pressure gradient and pulmonary pressure increase, which can explain the symptoms. The results of one study revealed that symptoms correlated best with the degree of pulmonary hypertension (24). In this setting, patients may be treated with a β-blocker to decrease heart-rate response to exercise or with mitral valvotomy. An exercise Doppler study also may be useful in symptomatic patients who have hypertrophic cardiomyopathy and in asymptomatic patients who have severe aortic stenosis, although Otto and colleagues (25) demonstrated that exercise testing was not helpful in clinical decision making in asymptomatic patients with aortic stenosis. In this case, exercise testing should be monitored carefully. We do not recommend an exercise test for patients who have severe aortic stenosis and poor LV systolic function. If a patient has severe aortic stenosis and a low aortic gradient as a result of decreased cardiac output, dobutamine echocardiography with repeated hemodynamic measurements may be able to differentiate anatomically fixed severe aortic stenosis from functionally severe aortic stenosis. This subject is discussed in more detail in Chapter 9.

ASSESSMENT OF MYOCARDIAL VIABILITY

Akinetic wall segments seen on echocardiography do not always indicate scarred or irreversibly dysfunctional myocardium (Fig. 8-7). Because myocardial contractility ceases when 20% or more of the transmural thickness is involved

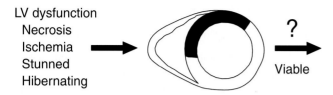

LV dysfunction
Necrosis
Ischemia
Stunned
Hibernating

Viable

FIG. 8-7. Diagram of parasternal short-axis view showing an akinetic segment at the septum and anterior wall (*black area*). Akinesis may result from a stunning or hibernating process as well as from permanent myocardial necrosis. Clinically, it is critical to identify the reason for the akinesis, because myocardial contractility may return to normal if the myocardium is still viable and decreased blood flow is restored to the myocardium.

by ischemia or infarction (26), a significant amount of myocardium still may be alive or viable even when no mechanical contractility is visualized. Therefore, it is important to determine whether akinetic myocardium is irreversible or is a manifestation of stunned or hibernating myocardium, with potential functional recovery.

1. *Stunned myocardium:* Reversible regional wall motion abnormalities after reperfusion of transient coronary artery occlusion (27,28). Reperfusion can occur spontaneously or after thrombolytic therapy or coronary angioplasty. Recovery of wall motion abnormalities may take days to weeks.

2. *Hibernating myocardium:* Chronically depressed myocardial function resulting from chronic myocardial ischemia; recovery of myocardial function after coronary revascularization is an example (29,30).

Thus, both stunned and hibernating myocardium are *viable*, with reversible LV dysfunction. Identification of myocardial viability is important clinically because coronary revascularization may lead to improved LV function and, hence, survival. Several diagnostic modalities can detect myocardial viability (Fig. 8-8). PET was the first imaging technique, and it remains the gold standard for detecting myocardial viability (31). It uses the perfusion indicator nitrogen-13-labeled ammonia ($^{13}NH_3$) and the metabolic tracer fluorine-18-deoxyglucose (^{18}FDG) to identify potentially viable myocardial tissue (Fig. 8-9). Resting two-dimensional echocardiography may help to identify viable myocardium by assessing myocardial wall thickness and evidence of fibrosis. Generally, a myocardial segment of normal or near-normal thickness is considered viable, whereas a thinned and echo-dense (fibrotic) segment is considered scarred. More frequently than not, however, it is difficult to distinguish viable from nonviable myocardium by simply assessing LV wall thickness.

It has been shown in animals that β-adrenergic stimula-

Myocardial Viability
Diagnostic Measures

Intact metabolism
(PET)

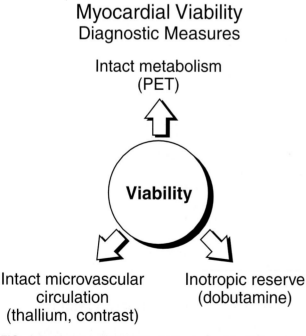

Viability

Intact microvascular circulation
(thallium, contrast)

Inotropic reserve
(dobutamine)

FIG. 8-8. Various diagnostic methods for identifying myocardial viability. Each method detects myocardial viability by assessing different properties of viable myocardium. *PET,* positron emission tomography.

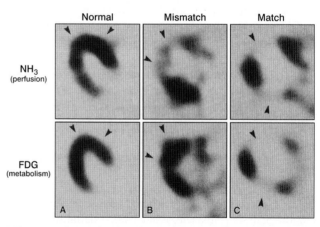

Normal   Mismatch   Match

NH₃
(perfusion)

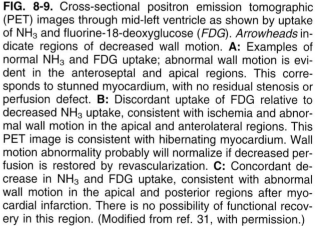

FDG
(metabolism)

A   B   C

FIG. 8-9. Cross-sectional positron emission tomographic (PET) images through mid-left ventricle as shown by uptake of NH₃ and fluorine-18-deoxyglucose (*FDG*). *Arrowheads* indicate regions of decreased wall motion. **A:** Examples of normal NH₃ and FDG uptake; abnormal wall motion is evident in the anteroseptal and apical regions. This corresponds to stunned myocardium, with no residual stenosis or perfusion defect. **B:** Discordant uptake of FDG relative to decreased NH₃ uptake, consistent with ischemia and abnormal wall motion in the apical and anterolateral regions. This PET image is consistent with hibernating myocardium. Wall motion abnormality probably will normalize if decreased perfusion is restored by revascularization. **C:** Concordant decrease in NH₃ and FDG uptake, consistent with abnormal wall motion in the apical and posterior regions after myocardial infarction. There is no possibility of functional recovery in this region. (Modified from ref. 31, with permission.)

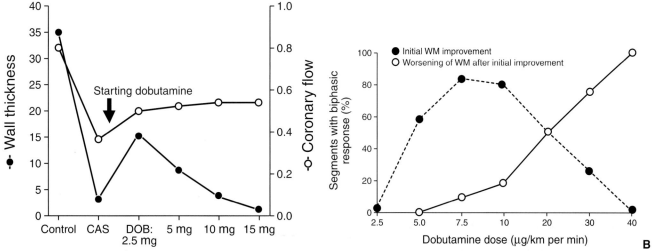

FIG. 8-10. A: Regional coronary blood flow and regional wall thickness with dobutamine (*DOB*) infusion in an animal model with significant coronary artery stenosis (*CAS*). With a low dose of dobutamine, regional coronary blood flow increases; however, it reaches a plateau and coronary blood flow does not increase further with a higher dose. Accordingly, regional wall thickness increases with a low dose of dobutamine but decreases with higher doses because of no change in coronary blood flow, although heart rate and inotropic properties increase. **B:** Graph demonstrating the percentage of myocardial segments with biphasic response, showing initial improvement and subsequent worsening of wall motion (*WM*) at various dobutamine doses. More than 80% of the segments exhibited an initial wall motion improvement at 7.5 mg/kg per minute dobutamine. Subsequent worsening began at a dose of 7.5 mg/kg per min in a small percentage of segments and was evident in 80% of segments at a dose of 30 mg/kg per min. (**A** modified from ref. 36, **B** from ref. 34, with permission.)

tion improves contractility of a chronically ischemic or postischemic myocardium with regional wall motion abnormalities, but it does not improve contractility in infarcted myocardium. Several human studies have demonstrated that a low dose of dobutamine (5 to 20 μg/kg per minute) induces contractility in viable myocardium, whether stunned or hibernating (32,33). Dobutamine-responsive wall motion improvement predicts subsequent improvement in regional LV wall thickening after coronary revascularization.

It has been shown that, at least in hibernating myocardium, a biphasic response best predicts recovery of myocardial function after revascularization (34,35). During infusion of a low dose of dobutamine, coronary blood flow increases and recruitment of contractile reserve improves wall motion of the dysfunctional myocardium (Fig. 8-10) (36). As the dobutamine dose is increased, coronary blood flow does not increase further and myocardial ischemia occurs because of stenosis of the coronary artery supplying

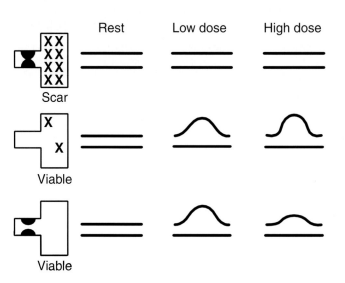

FIG. 8-11. Myocardial response to a low dose and a high dose of dobutamine in three different clinical scenarios, with resting akinetic segment. **Top:** When myocardium is scarred, with no myocardial viability, there is no myocardial thickening at rest with either a low dose or a high dose of dobutamine. **Middle:** If myocardium is viable with no stenosis of the coronary artery subtending the akinetic myocardium, myocardial contractility increases continuously with a low dose and a high dose of dobutamine. **Bottom:** If the myocardium is viable but the coronary artery that supplies the myocardium is severely stenotic, myocardial contractility improves initially with a low dose of dobutamine but worsens with a high dose. This is a typical biphasic response.

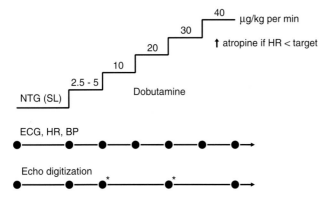

FIG. 8-12. Flowchart for a myocardial viability study. Sublingual (*SL*) nitroglycerin (*NTG*) may be used to detect increased myocardial thickening before giving a low dose (2.5 to 5 μg/kg per minute) of dobutamine. *Low-dose dobutamine image is obtained at a dobutamine dose between 5 and 20 μg/kg per minute. *BP*, blood pressure; *ECG*, electrocardiography; *HR*, heart rate.

the region, resulting in worsening of wall motion as compared with the previous lower dobutamine dose. Most of the initial improvement in wall motion takes place with a low dose of dobutamine, between 10 and 20 μg/kg per minute, and worsening occurs at a higher dose, 30 to 40 μg/kg per minute, or with atropine (Fig. 8-11).

Dobutamine is not as sensitive as thallium uptake or PET in detecting myocardial viability. Thallium uptake evaluates myocardial perfusion, and PET evaluates metabolic activity (37–39). Recovery of contractility of akinetic myocardium after revascularization is better predicted by increased contractility seen on dobutamine stress echocardiography than by thallium or PET, which are more sensitive in detecting a small area of metabolically viable myocardium that may not be large enough to produce contractility. Showing perfusion in the myocardium by using contrast echocardiography is another way to demonstrate potential myocardial viability. Microbubbles from the contrast agent opacify the myocardium, indicating integrity of the microvascular circulation. The presence of microvascular integrity may not necessarily indicate the presence of sufficient myocardium to restore myocardial contractility. Therefore, it appears that myocardial contrast echocardiography, like thallium perfusion, is less specific than dobutamine echocardiography in predicting functional recovery after revascularization (40–42). Therefore, dobutamine echocardiography may not demonstrate augmented contractility in a subset of myocardial segments in which myocardial contrast shows evidence of perfusion. Several studies, including a multicenter dobutamine viability registry, demonstrated that the outcome of patients with severe LV dysfunction and myocardial viability shown by dobutamine is better when they undergo revascularization (43). A dobutamine stress echocardiography protocol for detecting myocardial viability is shown in Fig. 8-12.

REFERENCES

1. Mayo Clinic Cardiovascular Working Group on Stress Testing. Cardiovascular stress testing: a description of the various types of stress tests and indications for their use. *Mayo Clin Proc* 1996;71:43–52.
2. Feigenbaum H. Digital recording, display, and storage of echocardiograms. *J Am Soc Echocardiogr* 1988;1:378–383.
3. Roger VL, Pellikka PA, Oh JK, Miller FA, Seward JB, Tajik AJ. Stress echocardiography. Part I. Exercise echocardiography: techniques, implementation, clinical applications, and correlations. *Mayo Clin Proc* 1995;70:5–15.
4. Hecht HS, DeBord L, Shaw R, et al. Digital supine bicycle stress echocardiography: a new technique for evaluating coronary artery disease. *J Am Coll Cardiol* 1993;21:950–956.
5. Sawada SG, Segar DS, Ryan T, et al. Echocardiographic detection of coronary artery disease during dobutamine infusion. *Circulation* 1991;83:1605–1614.
6. Picano E, Lattanzi F, L'Abbate A. Present application, practical aspects, and future issues on dipyridamole echocardiography. *Circulation* 1991;83(Suppl 3):III-111–III-115.
7. Pellikka PA, Roger VL, Oh JK, Miller FA, Seward JB, Tajik AJ. Stress echocardiography. Part II. Dobutamine stress echocardiography: techniques, implementation, clinical applications, and correlations. *Mayo Clin Proc* 1995;70:16–27.
8. Attenhofer CH, Pellikka PA, Oh JK, Roger VL, Sohn DW, Seward JB. Comparison of ischemic response during exercise and dobutamine echocardiography in patients with left main coronary artery disease. *J Am Coll Cardiol* 1996;27:1171–1177.
9. Attenhofer CH, Pellikka PA, Oh JK, et al. Is review of videotape necessary after review of digitized cine-loop images in stress echocardiography? A prospective study in 306 patients. *J Am Soc Echocardiogr* 1997;10:179–184.
10. Quinones MA, Verani MS, Haichin RM, Mahmarian JJ, Suarez J, Zoghbi WA. Exercise echocardiography versus ²⁰¹Tl single-photon emission computed tomography in evaluation of coronary artery disease. Analysis of 292 patients. *Circulation* 1992;85:1026–1031.
11. Pozzoli MM, Fioretti PM, Salustri A, Reijs AE, Roelandt JR. Exercise echocardiography and technetium-99m MIBI single-photon emission computed tomography in the detection of coronary artery disease. *Am J Cardiol* 1991;67:350–355.
12. Roger VL, Pellikka PA, Oh JK, Bailey KR, Tajik AJ. Identification of multivessel coronary artery disease by exercise echocardiography. *J Am Coll Cardiol* 1994;24:109–114.
13. Roger VL, Pellikka PA, Bell MR, Chow CW, Bailey KR, Seward JB. Sex and test verification bias: impact on the diagnostic value of exercise echocardiography. *Circulation* 1997;95:405–410.
14. Ling LH, Pellikka PA, Mahoney DW, et al. Atropine augmentation in dobutamine stress echocardiography: role and incremental value in a clinical practice setting. *J Am Coll Cardiol* 1996;28:551–557.
15. Pellikka PA, Oh JK, Bailey KR, Nichols BA, Monahan KH, Tajik AJ. Dynamic intraventricular obstruction during dobutamine stress echocardiography: a new observation. *Circulation* 1992;86:1429–1432.
16. Attenhofer CH, Pellikka PA, McCully RB, Roger VL, Seward JB. Paradoxical sinus deceleration during dobutamine stress echocardiography: description and angiographic correlation. *J Am Coll Cardiol* 1997;29:994–999.
17. McCully RB, Roger VL, Mahoney DW, et al. Outcome after normal exercise echocardiogram and predictors of subsequent cardiac events: follow-up of 1,325 patients. *J Am Coll Cardiol* 1998;31:144–149.
18. Pellikka PA, Roger VL, Oh JK, Seward JB, Tajik AJ. Safety of performing dobutamine stress echocardiography in patients with abdominal aortic aneurysm ≥ 4 cm in diameter. *Am J Cardiol* 1996;77:413–416.
19. Quintana M, Lindvall K, Ryden L, Brolund F. Prognostic value of predischarge exercise stress echocardiography after acute myocardial infarction. *Am J Cardiol* 1995;76:1115–1121.
20. Sicari R, Picano E, Landi P, et al. Prognostic value of dobutamine-atropine stress echocardiography early after acute myocardial infarction. Echo Dobutamine International Cooperative (EDIC) Study. *J Am Coll Cardiol* 1997;29:254–260.
21. Greco CA, Salustri A, Seccareccia F, et al. Prognostic value of do-

butamine echocardiography early after uncomplicated acute myocardial infarction: a comparison with exercise electrocardiography. *J Am Coll Cardiol* 1997;29:261–267.

22. Carlos ME, Smart SC, Wynsen JC, Sagar KB. Dobutamine stress echocardiography for risk stratification after myocardial infarction. *Circulation* 1997;95:1402–1410.
23. Smart SC, Knickelbine T, Stoiber TR, Carlos M, Wynsen JC, Sagar KB. Safety and accuracy of dobutamine-atropine stress echocardiography for the detection of residual stenosis of the infarct-related artery and multivessel disease during the first week after acute myocardial infarction. *Circulation* 1997;95:1394–1401.
24. Song JK, Kang DH, Lee CW, et al. Factors determining the exercise capacity in mitral stenosis. *Am J Cardiol* 1996;78:1060–1062.
25. Otto CM, Burwash IG, Legget ME, et al. Prospective study of asymptomatic valvular aortic stenosis: clinical, echocardiographic, and exercise predictors of outcome. *Circulation* 1997;95:2262–2270.
26. Lieberman AN, Weiss JL, Jugdutt BI, et al. Two-dimensional echocardiography and infarct size: relationship of regional wall motion and thickening to the extent of myocardial infarction in the dog. *Circulation* 1981;63:739–746.
27. Heyndrickx GR, Millard RW, McRitchie RJ, Maroko PR, Vatner SF. Regional myocardial functional and electrophysiological alterations after brief coronary artery occlusion in conscious dogs. *J Clin Invest* 1975;56:978–985.
28. Braunwald E, Kloner RA. The stunned myocardium: prolonged, post-ischemic ventricular dysfunction. *Circulation* 1982;66:1146–1149.
29. Matsuzaki M, Gallagher KP, Kemper WS, White F, Ross J Jr. Sustained regional dysfunction produced by prolonged coronary stenosis: Gradual recovery after reperfusion. *Circulation* 1983;68:170–182.
30. Rahimtoola SH. The hibernating myocardium. *Am Heart J* 1989;117:211–221.
31. Tillisch J, Brunken R, Marshall R, et al. Reversibility of cardiac wall-motion abnormalities predicted by positron tomography. *N Engl J Med* 1986;314:884–888.
32. Pierard LA, De Landsheere CM, Berthe C, Rigo P, Kulbertus HE. Identification of viable myocardium by echocardiography during dobutamine infusion in patients with myocardial infarction after thrombolytic therapy: Comparison with positron emission tomography. *J Am Coll Cardiol* 1990;15:1021–1031.
33. La Canna G, Alfieri O, Giubbini R, Gargano M, Ferrari R, Visioli O.
Echocardiography during infusion of dobutamine for identification of reversible dysfunction in patients with chronic coronary artery disease. *J Am Coll Cardiol* 1994;23:617–626.
34. Afridi I, Kleiman NS, Raizner AE, Zoghbi WA. Dobutamine echocardiography in myocardial hibernation. Optimal dose and accuracy in predicting recovery of ventricular function after coronary angioplasty. *Circulation* 1995;91:663–670.
35. Senior R, Lahiri A. Enhanced detection of myocardial ischemia by stress dobutamine echocardiography utilizing the ''biphasic'' response of wall thickening during low and high dose dobutamine infusion. *J Am Coll Cardiol* 1995;26:26–32.
36. Chen C, Li L, Chen LL, et al. Incremental doses of dobutamine induce a biphasic response in dysfunctional left ventricular regions subtending coronary stenoses. *Circulation* 1995;92:756–766.
37. Perrone-Filardi P, Pace L, Prastaro M, et al. Assessment of myocardial viability in patients with chronic coronary artery disease: rest-4-hour-24-hour ^{201}Tl tomography versus dobutamine echocardiography. *Circulation* 1996;94:2712–2719.
38. Di Carli MF, Asgarzadie F, Schelbert HR, et al. Quantitative relation between myocardial viability and improvement in heart failure symptoms after revascularization in patients with ischemic cardiomyopathy. *Circulation* 1995;92:3436–3444.
39. Bonow RO. Identification of viable myocardium. *Circulation* 1996;94:2674–2680.
40. Bolognese L, Antoniucci D, Rovai D, et al. Myocardial contrast echocardiography versus dobutamine echocardiography for predicting functional recovery after acute myocardial infarction treated with primary coronary angioplasty. *J Am Coll Cardiol* 1996;28:1677–1683.
41. Nagueh SF, Vaduganathan P, Ali N, et al. Identification of hibernating myocardium: comparative accuracy of myocardial contrast echocardiography, rest-redistribution thallium-201 tomography and dobutamine echocardiography. *J Am Coll Cardiol* 1997;29:985–993.
42. Meza MF, Kates MA, Barbee RW, et al. Combination of dobutamine and myocardial contrast echocardiography to differentiate postischemic from infarcted myocardium. *J Am Coll Cardiol* 1997;29:974–984.
43. Afridi I, Panza J, Zoghbi WA, Oh JK, Marwick TH. Dobutamine echocardiography predicts outcome in patients with coronary artery disease and severe ventricular dysfunction. *J Am Coll Cardiol (in press)*.

CHAPTER 9

Valvular Heart Disease

A major contribution of any new technology is to provide a safer, more reliable, and more cost-effective means of accomplishing the tasks performed by existing techniques. A good example is the use of two-dimensional (2D) Doppler echocardiography to evaluate valvular heart disease. Before the clinical application of Doppler and color-flow imaging, echocardiography was limited to providing qualitative morphological descriptions of valvular abnormalities. Most patients with severe valvular heart disease underwent cardiac catheterization before receiving surgical treatment. Today, however, hemodynamic variables such as pressure gradients across a stenotic valve, stenotic and regurgitant valve orifice area, cardiac output, regurgitant volume, and pulmonary artery pressures can be reliably measured with 2D Doppler echocardiography. This technique uses the same hydraulic formula used at cardiac catheterization to calculate valve area (*Gorlin equation*) (1), although flow velocities are used by Doppler instead of pressure gradients.

Doppler evaluation can be as, or even more, accurate than cardiac catheterization in assessing the hemodynamic state (2). For example, a pressure gradient across the mitral valve can be overestimated by cardiac catheterization when pulmonary capillary wedge pressure [instead of left atrial (LA) pressure] is used to measure the pressure gradient (2). Today, the evaluation of valvular regurgitation has become quantitative with the use of Doppler as well as color-flow imaging (3,4). Transesophageal echocardiography (TEE) allows clearer delineation of valvular morphology and provides easier access to a pulmonary vein physiology, which assists in determining the severity of mitral regurgitation, and to estimate diastolic filling pressures. Hence, in most patients with valvular heart disease, echocardiographic evaluation should provide comprehensive data regarding global left ventricular (LV) systolic function, valvular morphology, valvular hemodynamics, and pulmonary pressures. On the basis of this information, the patient's medical history, and the physical examination findings, physicians can better decide optimal treatment strategy, including the timing of surgical intervention.

The comprehensive echocardiographic and Doppler hemodynamic evaluation of valvular heart disease is discussed in this chapter.

EVALUATION OF VALVULAR STENOSIS

A stenotic valve generally is thickened and calcified, and its opening is restricted. All these features can be visualized on 2D echocardiography. Thus, a 2D echocardiographic examination is helpful in identifying the underlying cause of valvular stenosis, such as bicuspid aortic valve, rheumatic mitral valve, or carcinoid heart disease. It is also useful in measuring stenotic valve area directly by planimetry; however, 2D echocardiography allows limited hemodynamic assessment. To obtain comprehensive hemodynamic data, a complete Doppler examination should be performed on all patients with valvular stenosis.

All available transducer windows should be used to obtain the Doppler signal most parallel with the direction of the stenotic jet flow. This will provide the highest velocity with the most complete envelope. In comparison with a duplex transducer, a nonimaging continuous-wave Doppler transducer is smaller and thus easier to manipulate between the ribs and suprasternal notch. Color-flow imaging may be helpful in aligning the continuous-wave Doppler beam most parallel with the direction of the blood-flow jet.

The blood-flow velocity and pressure gradient increase as the valve becomes smaller. Blood-flow velocity (v) measured by Doppler echocardiography reliably reflects the pressure gradient according to the Bernoulli equation. In most clinical situations, transvalvular pressure gradients can be derived by a modified Bernoulli equation (see Chapter 6):

$$\text{Pressure gradient} = 4 \times v^2 \text{ or } (2 \times v)^2$$

The accuracy of a Doppler-derived instantaneous pressure gradient has been validated by simultaneous cardiac catheterization data (5–7). It should be emphasized that for a given valve area, the flow velocity and the pressure gradient vary with the change in cardiac output. Therefore, cardiac output or stroke volume should be taken into account in determining the severity of valvular stenosis. The continuity equation, which is derived from the same basic hydraulic formula as the Gorlin formula, can reliably estimate valve area by calculating stroke volume from another cardiac orifice (8). Excellent correlations have been obtained between echocardiographic-derived values and catheter-derived valve areas (8–10). Pressure half-time (PHT), which is the time interval required for the peak pressure gradient to reach one-half its initial value, is another useful Doppler variable to assess the severity of mitral stenosis (11).

The Doppler evaluation of pulmonary and tricuspid stenosis uses methods similar to those described for aortic and mitral stenosis, respectively. A comprehensive echocardiographic evaluation of an individual valvular stenosis is illustrated in the following section.

Aortic Stenosis

Two-Dimensional and M-Mode Echocardiography

A normal aortic valve has three thin cusps and an unrestrictive systolic opening. The normal aortic valve area is 3 to 4 cm², and the normal opening generally produces 2 cm of leaflet separation (Fig. 9-1A). The same degree of separation is maintained during most of systole unless the patient has low cardiac output (Fig. 9-1B) or LV outflow tract (LVOT) obstruction (Fig. 9-1C). The most common form of aortic stenosis is caused by degenerative valvular calcification. The leaflets are thickened and calcified, decreasing the systolic opening (Fig. 9-2). However, the M-mode echocardiogram may appear normal in patients with a noncalcific stenotic valve with systolic doming, as in congenital aortic stenosis, because the restriction of valve opening occurs at the distal portion with doming. Two-dimensional echocardiography visualizes the entire aortic valve structure and is helpful in identifying noncalcific, as well as calcific, aortic stenosis. Although occasionally it is difficult, the number of aortic cusps can be determined by 2D echocardiography, especially from the parasternal short-axis view at the level of the aortic valve (Fig. 9-3), or by TEE (Fig. 9-4). In addition, the degree of valvular calcification, the size of the aortic annulus and the supravalvular ascending aorta, and the presence of secondary subvalvular obstruction are easily evaluated. Furthermore, 2D echocar-

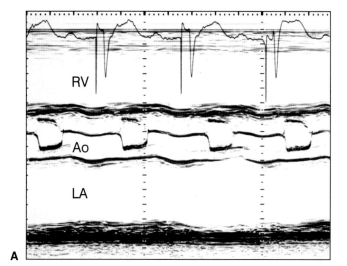

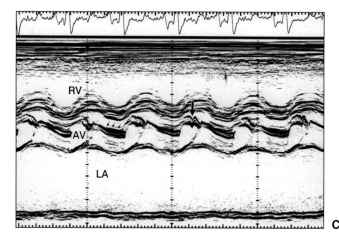

FIG. 9-1. M-mode echocardiograms of normal aortic valve. **A:** The normal aortic cusps are thin and their opening is not limited, having a maximal separation of 2 cm. Normally, the maximal opening is maintained throughout systole. **B:** The maximal opening tapers off during midsystole (*double arrowheads*) when cardiac output is severely reduced. **C:** In a 40-year-old patient with hypertrophic obstructive cardiomyopathy and endocarditis, the aortic valve (*AV*) opening is interrupted because of dynamic left ventricular (*LV*) outflow tract obstruction during midsystole [midsystolic closure (*large arrow*)] but reopens again at late systole. There is increased echo-density at the aortic cusps (*small arrows*) during diastole because of vegetation. *Ao*, aorta.

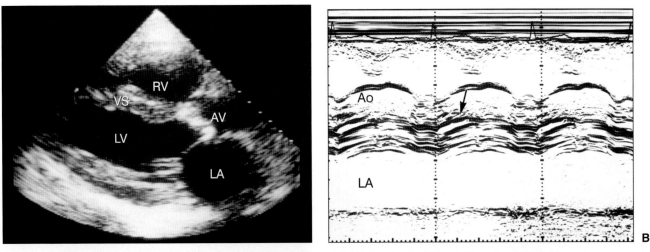

FIG. 9-2. Two-dimensional **(A)** and M-mode echocardiograms of a calcific aortic valve **(B)**. **A:** Parasternal long-axis view of systolic frame shows a calcified aortic valve (*AV*) with reduced opening. *VS*, ventricular septum. **B:** Aortic valve opening is only 4 mm, with thickened cusps. Also, multiple dense echoes (*arrow*) are noted in the aortic root during systole and diastole. These findings suggest significant aortic stenosis, but a Doppler study is required to determine how significant the stenosis is. *Ao*, aorta.

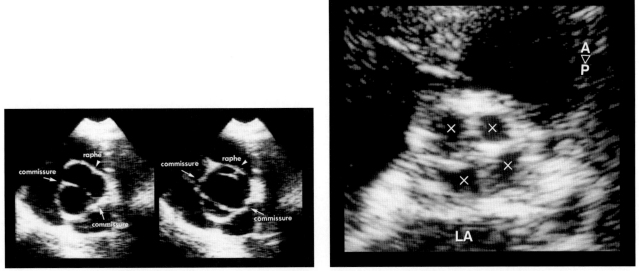

FIG. 9-3. Still-frame of two-dimensional echocardiogram of bicuspid **(A)** and quadricuspid **(B)** aortic valve. **A:** On the left is a diastolic frame showing commissures at 4 and 10 o'clock positions. On the right is a "fish-mouth" opening during systole. The raphe is at the 1 o'clock position. (From Brandenburg R Jr, Tajik AJ, Edwards WD, Reeder GS, Shub C, Seward JB. Accuracy of 2-dimensional echocardiographic diagnosis of congenitally bicuspid aortic valve: echocardiographic-anatomic correlation in 115 patients. *Am J Cardiol* 1983;51:1469–1473, with permission.) **B:** Diastolic frame showing four aortic cusps (*x*). *A*, anterior; *P*, posterior. (From Feldman BJ, Khandheria BK, Warnes CA, Seward JB, Taylor CL, Tajik AJ. Incidence, description and functional assessment of isolated quadricuspid aortic valves. *Am J Cardiol* 1990;65:937–938, with permission.)

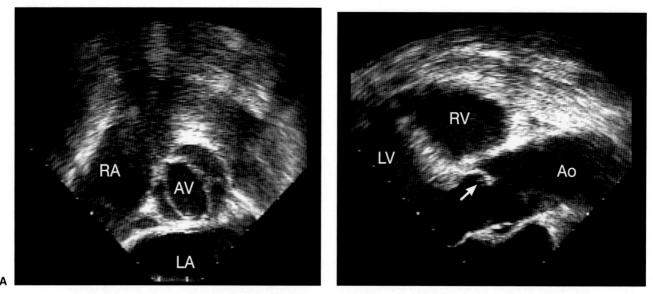

FIG. 9-4. Transesophageal echocardiographic image of bicuspid aortic valve from **(A)** short-axis view and **(B)** long-axis view. The short-axis view shows typical bicuspid aortic valve with the raphe at the 3 o'clock position and commissures at the 5 and 10 o'clock positions. From a long-axis view, the anterior cusp has a typical doming motion during systole (*arrow*). *Ao*, aorta; *AV*, aortic valve.

diography is useful in determining the degree of LV hypertrophy (wall thickness and mass), LA enlargement, ventricular function, and the integrity of the other valves.

Doppler Echocardiography

The hemodynamic severity of aortic stenosis determined by 2D and Doppler echocardiography is based on peak aortic flow velocity, mean pressure gradient, aortic valve area, and the LVOT-to-aortic valve (AoV) time velocity integral (TVI) ratio. A meticulous search for the maximal aortic velocity is essential because all the above variables are derived from the peak aortic flow velocity. The following steps are required to obtain these data:

Step 1. Determine stroke volume (SV) from LVOT diameter (D), and TVI (Fig. 9-5)

$$SV = \left(\frac{D}{2}\right)^2 \times \pi \times TVI$$

$$= (D)^2 \times 0.785 \times TVI$$

Step 2. Obtain the maximal aortic velocity by systematic search from multiple windows using continuous-wave Doppler (Fig. 9-6)

Step 3. Calculate the mean aortic pressure gradient and TVI by tracing the maximal velocity jet (Fig. 9-7 and 9-8); be familiar with three different pressure gradients: maximal instantaneous gradient, mean gradient, and peak-to-peak gradient (see Chapter 6)

Step 4. Calculate the aortic valve area (AVA) using the continuity equation (Fig. 9-9)

$$AVA = D^2 \times 0.785 \times \frac{TVI_{LVOT}}{TVI_{AoV}}$$

$$= \frac{SV}{TVI_{AoV}}$$

(For a detailed discussion of Doppler hemodynamics, see Chapter 6.)

Definition of Severe Aortic Stenosis

In patients with normal LV systolic function and cardiac output, aortic stenosis is usually severe when (10)

1. Peak aortic valve velocity is ≥4.5 m/sec (Fig. 9-10)
2. Mean pressure gradient is ≥50 mm Hg (Fig. 9-10)
3. Aortic valve area is ≤0.75 cm^2
4. LVOT/AoV TVI ratio is ≤0.25 (Fig. 9-11)

When LV systolic function and cardiac output are abnormally low or high, the following points should be considered: Peak velocity and mean aortic gradient vary with changes in stroke volume. If LV function or stroke volume is decreased, the peak aortic velocity and mean aortic pressure gradient may be less than 4.5 m/sec and 50 mm Hg, respectively, in patients with severe aortic stenosis. However, the velocity or TVI ratio (hence, aortic valve area) should be independent of any change in stroke volume because the LVOT and aortic valve velocities change proportionally (Fig. 9-12A). In patients with increased cardiac output across the aortic valve (as in aortic regurgitation or anemia), aortic stenosis may not be severe even when the peak velocity is 4.5 m/sec or greater, and the mean gradient

(text continues on page 111)

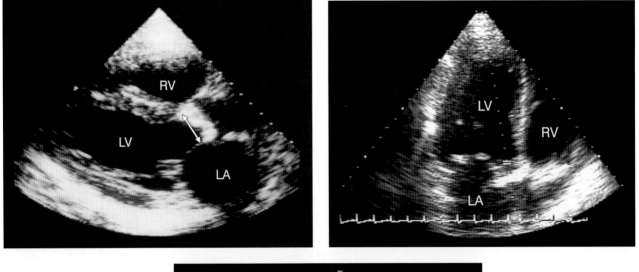

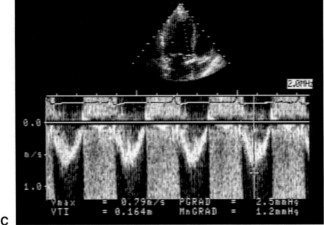

FIG. 9-5. Stroke volume across the aortic valve needs to be calculated to determine aortic valve area. This is done by measuring the left ventricular outflow tract (LVOT) diameter and flow velocity. **A:** Measurement of LVOT diameter (*double-headed arrow*): from the systolic freeze-frame of the parasternal long-axis view, the distance from where the anterior aortic cusp meets the ventricular septum to the point where the posterior cusp meets the anterior mitral leaflet. The line between the two cusps is almost perpendicular to the anterior wall of the aortic root. **B:** Measurement of LVOT velocity from the apical long-axis view. The pulsed-wave sample volume is located 3 to 5 mm below the aortic valve or at the aortic annulus. If the sample volume is too close to the aortic valve, prestenotic acceleration jet velocity may be recorded. **C:** Determination of LVOT time velocity integral [time velocity integral (*TVI*) or velocity time integral (*VTI*)]. TVI is determined by tracing the velocity envelope and is equal to the sum of individual velocities of the Doppler spectral envelope (TVI = 16 cm). After LVOT diameter (*D*) and TVI are determined, SV across the LVOT is calculated as follows:

$$LVOT\ SV = LVOT\ area \times LVOT\ TVI$$

$$= (D/2)^2 \times \pi \times LVOT\ TVI$$

$$= D^2 \times 0.785 \times LVOT\ TVI$$

The following table shows corresponding LVOT areas calculated from various LVOT diameters:

LVOT diameter (D), cm	Area (D² × 0.785), cm²	LVOT diameter (D), cm	Area (D² × 0.785), cm²
1.5	1.77	2.1	3.46
1.6	2.01	2.2	3.80
1.7	2.27	2.3	4.15
1.8	2.54	2.4	4.52
1.9	2.84	2.5	4.90
2.0	3.14		

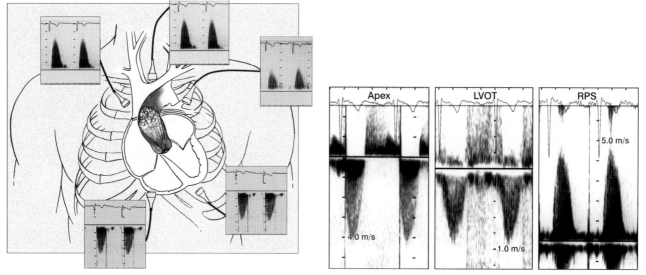

A

B

FIG. 9-6. **A:** Diagram of multiple transducer positions used to obtain aortic stenosis jet velocity. The maximal velocity is obtained most commonly (85% of the time) from the apical transducer position. The second most commonly successful position is the right parasternum. However, all the transducer positions should be used to ensure securing the maximal velocity. (Modified from Nishimura RA, Miller FA Jr, Callahan MJ, Benassi RC, Seward JB, Tajik AJ. Doppler echocardiography: theory, instrumentation, technique, and application. *Mayo Clin Proc* 1985;60:321–343, with permission. **B:** Continuous-wave Doppler recordings of the aortic velocity from the apex and right parasternal window (*RPS*) together with pulsed-wave Doppler recording of the left ventricular outflow tract (*LVOT*) in an elderly patient with severe aortic stenosis. Peak aortic flow velocity is higher (4.5 m/sec) from the RPS position than from the apex (4.0 m/sec). If continuous-wave Doppler was not performed from the RPS position, the severity of aortic stenosis would have been underestimated.

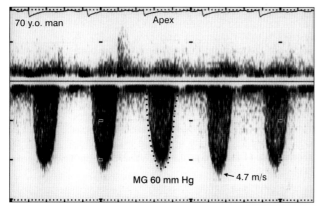

FIG. 9-7. Continuous-wave Doppler spectra from a 70-year-old man with severe aortic stenosis. The velocity was obtained from the apical window. The mean gradient (*MG*) was obtained by tracing a velocity signal.

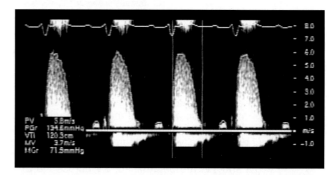

FIG. 9-8. Continuous-wave Doppler velocity signal of aortic stenosis from the right parasternal transducer position. The velocity signals were traced automatically, and the third velocity signal within two vertical lines was automatically interrogated for peak velocity (*PV*) (5.8 m/sec), peak gradient (*PGr*) (134 mm Hg), velocity time integral (*VTI*) (120 cm), mean velocity (*MV*) (3.7 m/sec), and mean gradient (*MGr*) (71.6 mm Hg).

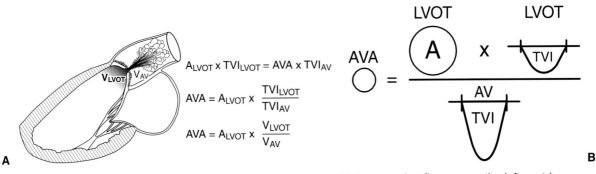

FIG. 9-9. **A:** Diagram illustrating the continuity equation, which states that flow across the left ventricular outflow tract (*LVOT*) is the same as flow across the aortic valve ("what goes in must come out"). Therefore,

$$Flow\ across\ LVOT = Flow\ across\ aortic\ valve$$

$$LVOT\ Area \times TVI_{LVOT} = AVA \times TVI_{AV}$$

$$LVOT\ (D)^2 \times 0.785 \times TVI_{LVOT} = AVA \times TVI_{AV}$$

$$AVA = LVOT\ D^2 \times 0.785 \times TVI_{LVOT}/TVI_{AV}$$

where *D* is the diameter, *AVA* is the aortic valve area, *AV* is the aortic valve, and *TVI* is the time velocity integral. Because flow duration across the LVOT and aortic valve is the same, the TVI ratio is similar to their peak velocity (*V*) ratio. Therefore, the continuity equation can be simplified as

$$AVA = D^2 \times 0.785 \times V_{LVOT}/V_{AV}$$

It is always preferable to use the TVI ratio. It should be noted that TVI or peak velocity ratio is inversely proportional to the area ratio of the LVOT and the aortic valve. For example, a TVI ratio of 0.3 indicates that the aortic valve area is about 30% of the LVOT area. This ratio is also useful in determining the severity of aortic stenosis (see Fig. 9-11). **B:** Continuity equation to calculate aortic valve area (*AVA*). *AV*, aortic valve; *LVOT*, LV outflow tract; *TVI*, time velocity integral.

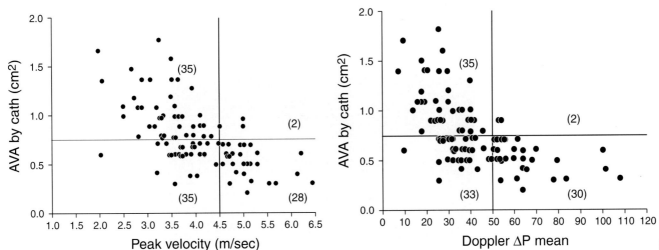

FIG. 9-10. Plot of catheter-derived aortic valve area (*AVA*) versus Doppler peak velocity **(A)** and Doppler-derived mean pressure (*ΔP*) gradients **(B)**. The aortic valve area is 0.75 cm² or smaller when the peak velocity and mean pressure gradient are at least 4.5 m/sec and 50 mm Hg, respectively, in essentially all patients. However, one-half of the patients with lower Doppler peak velocities and mean gradients also had an aortic valve area of 0.75 cm² or less, especially in the setting of low cardiac output. (From ref. 10, with permission.)

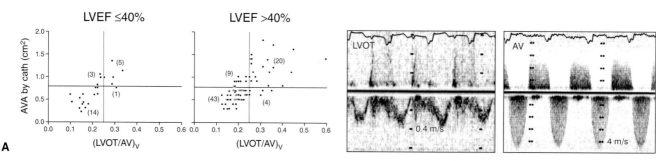

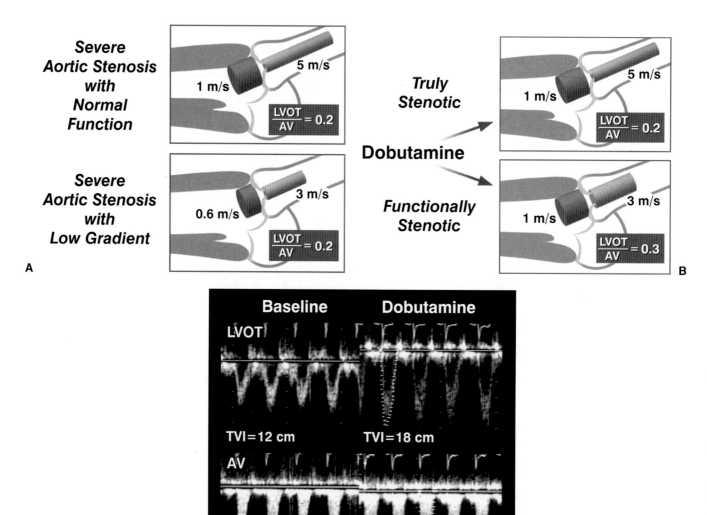

FIG. 9-11. A: Correlation of left ventricular outflow tract (*LVOT*)/aortic valve (*AV*) velocity ratio with catheter-derived aortic valve area (*AVA*). LVOT/AV velocity [(LVOT/AV)$_v$] or time velocity interval (TVI) ratio is inversely proportional to their area ratio. When the ratio is >0.25 (i.e., aortic valve area >25% of LVOT area), AVA is >0.75 cm^2. Most patients with a ratio <0.25 (i.e., AVA <25% of LVOT area) have severe aortic stenosis (i.e., AVA <0.75 cm^2), whether LV ejection fraction (*LVEF*) is >40% or ≤40%. **B:** Example of critical aortic stenosis in the setting of low cardiac output. The aortic valve (*AV*) velocity is 4.2 m/sec and *LVOT* flow velocity is 0.4 m/sec, indicating a marked decrease in cardiac output. The LVOT/AV velocity ratio is <0.1.

is 50 mm Hg or higher. Again, the LVOT/AoV TVI (or velocity) ratio and aortic valve area should be more helpful in determining the severity of aortic stenosis.

To calculate aortic valve area in the presence of significant aortic regurgitation, the following should be considered: flow across the aortic valve increases with aortic regurgitation, as does the aortic pressure gradient. The increased flow is reflected in the LVOT and aortic valve velocities proportionally; thus, the TVI ratio remains the same for a given aortic valve area. Cardiac catheterization is unreliable in this situation and tends to result in a lower calculated aortic valve area, mainly because of an underestimation of cardiac output.

Dobutamine Echocardiography in Severe Aortic Stenosis With Low Aortic Pressure Gradient

When LV systolic function is abnormal and cardiac output is reduced, aortic stenosis is probably severe if (a) the aortic valve area is $\leq$0.75 cm^2, and (b) the LVOT/AoV TVI (or velocity) ratio is $\leq$0.25.

In the setting of a low aortic gradient, the calculated aortic valve area may overestimate the true severity of aortic stenosis. Gradual infusion of a low dose of dobutamine (up to 20 μg/kg per minute) to increase stroke volume may be helpful in differentiating morphologically severe aortic stenosis from decreased effective orifice area caused by low cardiac output (pseudosevere aortic stenosis) (12). In patients with true severe aortic stenosis, dobutamine infusion increases the peak velocity and TVI of both the LVOT and the aortic valve proportionally (hence, the LVOT/AoV TVI ratio remains the same), whereas an increase in velocity and TVI of the LVOT is far greater than that of the aortic valve (whose area becomes larger with higher output); hence, the LVOT/AoV TVI ratio increases in patients with pseudo (or functionally) severe aortic stenosis (Fig. 9-12B and C). Dobutamine can be infused gradually from 5 μg/kg per minute in 5-μg increments every 3 minutes until the LVOT veloc-

ity or TVI reaches a normal value, 0.8 to 1.2 m/sec or 20 to 25 cm, respectively. Maximal velocity or stroke volume is usually obtained with 15 to 20 μg/kg per minute of dobutamine (13).

Caveats

1. The aortic stenosis jet must be differentiated from other systolic Doppler findings (Fig. 9-13), including mitral regurgitation, LVOT obstruction, tricuspid regurgitation, and pulmonary stenosis.

2. It may be difficult to measure LVOT diameter because of heavy calcification of the aortic valve and annulus. In this situation, another nonregurgitant orifice [right ventricular (RV) outflow tract or mitral valve] should be used to calculate stroke volume. In this case, the TVI ratio, not the peak velocity ratio, must be used because the flow ejection periods are different.

3. It may be difficult to obtain a satisfactory LVOT velocity because of coexisting LVOT obstruction from basal septal hypertrophy. Flow velocity proximal to the aortic valve may reach 2 m/sec, which can overestimate the aortic pressure gradient calculated from the modified Bernoulli equation.

4. If the patient's rhythm is other than sinus, the aortic and LVOT velocities will vary with each cardiac cycle, depending on the preceding RR interval. In this case, one should use the average velocities from five to ten cardiac cycles or match the RR intervals for LVOT and aortic valve velocity to obtain the TVI or velocity ratio.

5. Studies suggest that calculations of aortic valve area are affected by change in stroke volume (14,15). Hence, a slightly larger area determined with dobutamine echocardiography may be related to the continuity equation itself rather than be a true change in valve area. TEE planimetry of the aortic valve area may be helpful in this situation.

6. Aortic valve resistance is another hemodynamic index to represent the severity of aortic stenosis. It has a good

FIG. 9-12. A: Diagram demonstrating that aortic flow velocity (AV) can be deceptively low (<4.5 m/sec) in patients with severe aortic stenosis and low cardiac output. Cylinders represent stroke volume. Left ventricular outflow tract (LVOT) velocity is usually about 1 m/sec in patients with normal function **(top)** and decreases to 0.6 m/sec when stroke volume is decreased **(bottom)**. However, LVOT/AV velocity ratio is low (0.2) in both cases. **B:** When dobutamine is given to a patient with severe aortic stenosis and low stroke volume and gradient (or low velocity), AV may or may not increase as LVOT velocity increases. In truly anatomically severe aortic stenosis **(top)**, the AV velocity will increase in proportion to the increase in LVOT velocity. Hence, LVOT/AV remains low. In functionally (pseudo) severe aortic stenosis **(bottom)**, AV velocity does not increase in proportion to LVOT velocity, because aortic valve area increases with higher stroke volume. Hence, LVOT/AV increases. **C:** An example of dobutamine Doppler hemodynamic measurement in a patient with severe aortic stenosis and a low gradient. At baseline, LVOT TVI was low (12 cm), indicating a low stroke volume, and AV peak velocity was 3 m/sec, with TVI of 55 cm. TVI ratio between LVOT and AV was 0.22. With infusion of dobutamine up to 20 mg/kg per min, LVOT TVI increased to 18 cm, which is translated to a 50% increase in stroke volume, and AV TVI increased to a similar degree to 80 cm. TVI ratio was 0.23, similar to the baseline ratio. This result indicates that the aortic valve is truly stenotic, with a low gradient. The patient successfully underwent aortic valve replacement. *TVI,* time velocity integral.

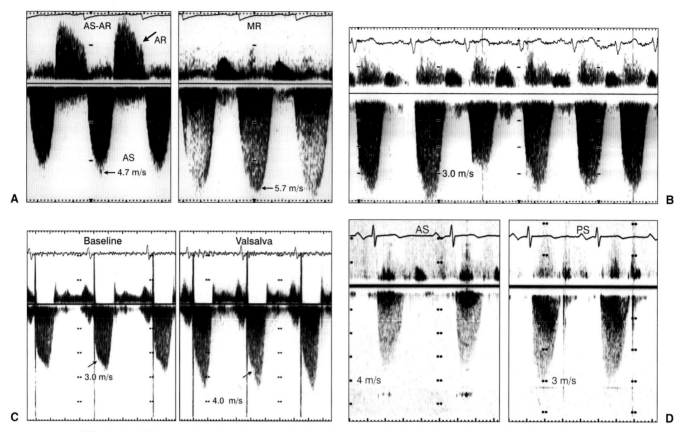

FIG. 9-13. Differentiation of aortic stenosis Doppler spectral velocity from other systolic Doppler spectra. Systolic flow velocities by continuous-wave Doppler echocardiography need to be analyzed on the following bases: (1) peak velocity, (2) flow duration or ejection time, (3) location of Doppler window, (4) accompanying diastolic flow signals, and (5) Doppler flow configuration. **A:** The duration of mitral regurgitation (*MR*) is longer than that of aortic stenosis (*AS*) because there is no ejection through the aortic valve during isovolumic relaxation and contraction, whereas regurgitation flow occurs during those periods. The mitral regurgitation jet is normally >4 to 5 m/sec unless LA pressure is markedly increased. The peak velocity of mitral regurgitation is always higher than that of aortic stenosis when they occur together in the same patient. The aortic regurgitation (*AR*) jet also is frequently recorded together with the AS velocity and not with mitral regurgitation. **B:** Tricuspid regurgitation velocity typically has respiratory variation, with a lower peak velocity during inspiration. **C:** The flow velocity of dynamic left ventricular outflow tract obstruction produces a late-peaking dagger-shaped (*arrow*) velocity envelope. Dynamic LV outflow velocity increases with Valsalva maneuver. **D:** The Doppler spectrum of pulmonary stenosis (*PS*) is almost identical to that of *AS*. The pulmonary stenosis signal is best obtained from the subcostal or left upper parasternal window, whereas an AS jet is usually obtained from the apex or right parasternal window.

correlation with aortic valve area (AVA) for a given aortic flow velocity.

Mean aortic valve resistance is calculated by using the mean aortic pressure gradient and a constant of 28 obtained by nonlinear regression analysis by Bermejo and his colleagues (16).

$$\text{Mean resistance} = \frac{28\sqrt{\text{Mean gradient}}}{\text{AVA}}$$

Aortic resistance appears to be affected less by change in flow. The index does not appear to provide more clinically valuable information than the other measurements noted above.

Natural Progression and Role of Exercise in Asymptomatic Patients With Aortic Stenosis

Patients with moderate to severe aortic stenosis may be asymptomatic. Understanding the natural progression of the severity of aortic stenosis is helpful in timing follow-up and surgical intervention. Otto and colleagues (17) repeated echocardiographic studies and correlated the results with the clinical outcome of asymptomatic patients with valvular aortic stenosis. Aortic jet velocity increased by 0.32 ± 0.34 m/sec per year and mean gradient by 7 ± 7 mm Hg per year, and valve area decreased by 0.12 ± 0.19 cm² per year. When peak aortic velocity was >4.0 m/sec, the likelihood of the patient remaining alive without valve replacement at 2 years was only 21% ± 18%. Exercise Doppler hemodynamics were not helpful in the management of individual patients.

TEE

When transthoracic Doppler echocardiography (TTE) is difficult to perform or there is dynamic LVOT obstruction, TEE can be used to measure aortic valve area by planimetry (18). A multiplane imaging probe is most satisfactory, with the transducer array rotated to 45 to 60 degrees to obtain the short-axis view of the aortic valve (Fig. 9-14). The number of aortic cusps can be determined confidently with TEE.

Many patients with severe aortic stenosis who undergo aortic valve replacement have mitral valve regurgitation, which is usually related to increased LV systolic pressure, without morphologic abnormality of the mitral valve. TEE frequently is used intraoperatively to evaluate the severity of mitral regurgitation before and after aortic valve replacement and to assess the need for mitral valve replacement or repair.

Clinical Implications

Echocardiography provides a comprehensive morphologic and hemodynamic evaluation of stenotic aortic valves, and on the basis of the information obtained with this technique, proper management decisions can be made. In patients with severe aortic stenosis (mean gradient > 50 mm Hg or aortic valve area ≤0.75 cm^2), we now perform and recommend aortic valve replacement after coronary angiography, but without LV angiography or invasive hemodynamic confirmation. In our current practice, more than 75% of patients undergo aortic valve replacement without invasive hemodynamic assessment (19). The change in our practice with regard to patients with severe aortic stenosis who have undergone aortic valve replacement is shown in Fig. 9-15.

Mitral Stenosis

Two-Dimensional and M-Mode Echocardiography

In almost all patients, valvular mitral stenosis is caused by rheumatic involvement of the mitral valve. Other uncommon causes include degenerative calcification, cafergot toxicity, hypereosinophilia, and vegetation. The typical M-mode and 2D echocardiographic features of rheumatic mitral stenosis include the following (Fig. 9-16):

1. Thickened and calcified mitral leaflets and subvalvular apparatus
2. Decreased E-F slope (M-mode)
3. "Hockey-stick" appearance of the anterior mitral leaflet in diastole (long-axis view)
4. Immobility of the posterior mitral leaflet (similar appearance can be seen in hypereosinophilia or ergot use)
5. "Fish-mouth" orifice in short-axis view
6. Increased LA size, with the potential for thrombus formation

Mitral valve area can be measured with planimetry from the parasternal short-axis view (Fig. 9-16D), which may be difficult in patients with a previous commissurotomy or heavy calcification. In patients undergoing mitral balloon valvuloplasty, an echocardiographic score based on valve thickness, calcification, mobility, and subvalvular thickening (Table 9-1) can be used to predict the outcome of the procedure (20). Patients with an echocardiographic score of 8 or less have a more favorable result from mitral balloon valvuloplasty than those with a higher score, but a score

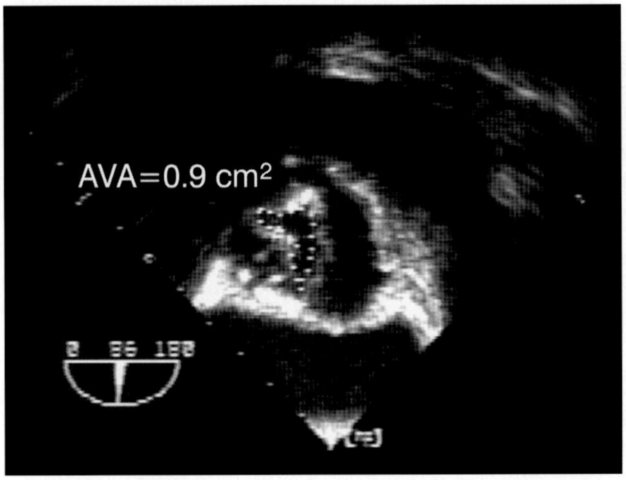

FIG. 9-14. Multiplane transesophageal echocardiographic short-axis view of the aortic valve. The opening of the aortic valve is well visualized, and planimetry of the aortic valve area (*AVA*) yields a measurement of 0.9 cm^2.

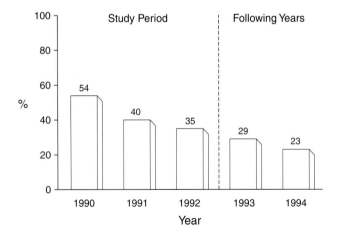

FIG. 9-15. Since the application of noninvasive Doppler hemodynamics, preoperative invasive measurement of aortic stenosis hemodynamics has continually declined. Currently, fewer than 25% of patients with aortic stenosis require an invasive hemodynamic assessment preoperatively. (From ref. 19, with permission.)

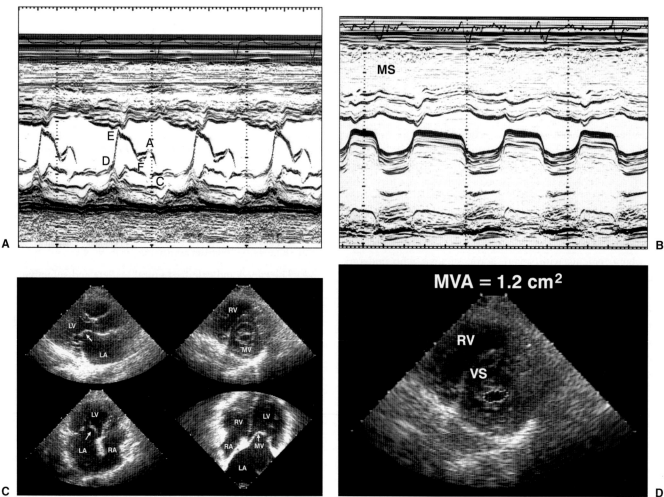

FIG. 9-16. A: M-mode echocardiogram of normal mitral valve. **B:** M-mode echocardiogram of typical mitral stenosis (*MS*). The mitral leaflet is thickened and the E–F slope is prolonged. **C:** Composite of two-dimensional echocardiogram of parasternal long-axis view, short-axis view, apical four-chamber view, and transesophageal transverse view during diastole in a patient with mitral stenosis. The mitral valve (*MV*) leaflets are thickened and have the typical "hockey-stick" appearance (*arrow*). Left atrium (*LA*) is enlarged. **D:** Two-dimensional echocardiogram of parasternal short-axis view showing the "fish-mouth" orifice (*dots*) of stenotic mitral valve. The orifice area (*MVA*) is measured by manual tracing. *VS*, ventricular septum.

TABLE 9-1. *Echocardiographic score used to predict outcome of mitral balloon valvuloplasty[a]*

Grade	Mobility	Subvalvular thickening	Thickening	Calcification
1	Highly mobile valve with only leaflet tips restricted	Minimal thickening just below the mitral leaflets	Leaflets near normal in thickness (4–5 mm)	A single area of increased echo brightness
2	Leaflet mid and base portions have normal mobility	Thickening of chordal structures extending up to one-third of the chordal length	Midleaflets normal, considerable thickening of margins (5–8 mm)	Scattered areas of brightness confined to leaflet margins
3	Valve continues to move forward in diastole, mainly from the base	Thickening extending to the distal third of the chords	Thickening extending through the entire leaflet (5–8 mm)	Brightness extending into the midportion of the leaflets
4	No or minimal forward movement of the leaflets in diastole	Extensive thickening and shortening of all chordal structures extending down to the papillary muscles	Considerable thickening of all leaflet tissue (>8–10 mm)	Extensive brightness throughout much of the leaflet tissue

[a] The total echocardiographic score was derived from an analysis of mitral leaflet mobility, valvular and subvalvular thickening, and calcification, which were graded from 0 (normal) to 4 according to the above criteria. This gave a total score of 0 to 16.

114

higher than 8 does not preclude the option of valvuloplasty. Commissural calcification or fusion is another important determinant of poor outcome after percutaneous valvuloplasty or valvotomy (21).

Doppler and Color-Flow Imaging

Doppler and color-flow imaging provides reliable quantitative and hemodynamic data about the severity of mitral stenosis. Because velocity and pressure gradient depend on the volume of flow across the mitral valve, they may not always be reliable predictors of severity. Calculation of mitral valve area is the most reliable means of determining the severity of mitral stenosis. There are several different methods for calculating mitral valve area in addition to visualization of the mitral valve with 2D echocardiography (22–24): continuity equation, PHT, and proximal isovelocity surface area (PISA) methods.

The following steps are required for comprehensive Doppler evaluation of mitral stenosis:

Step 1. Obtain the maximal velocity using continuous-wave Doppler from the apical and paraapical positions (Fig. 9-17)
Step 2. Determine the mean pressure gradient and TVI by tracing mitral flow velocity (Fig. 9-18A)
Step 3. Determine the mitral valve area (MVA) by the PHT method. Calculate MVA with the following equation after PHT is measured (Fig. 9-18B and C):

$$MVA = \frac{220}{PHT}$$

(This equation should not be used immediately after balloon valvuloplasty or in patients with severe aortic regurgitation.)

Step 4. Determine the MVA by the continuity equation. Determine the stroke volume from the LVOT diameter (D) and TVI. Calculate the MVA by dividing the LVOT stroke volume by mitral valve TVI (Fig. 9-19).

$$MVA = LVOT\ D^2 \times 0.785 \times \frac{TVI_{LVOT}}{TVI_{MV}}$$

(This equation cannot be used if there is significant aortic or mitral valve regurgitation.)

Step 5. Determine the MVA by the PISA method (Fig. 9-20A)
  a. Zoom the area of the mitral valve from the apical four-chamber view
  b. Color-flow imaging of mitral stenosis jet and upward shift of the zero baseline for color map (30- to 45-cm/sec aliasing velocity)
  c. Freeze color-flow images in a cine-loop and identify an optimal frame to measure radius (r) of PISA in the LA
  d. Determine the angle (α) between two mitral leaflets at the atrial surface and use the following formula:

$$MVA = \frac{6.28 \times r^2 \times Alias\ velocity}{Peak\ mitral\ stenosis\ velocity} \times \frac{\alpha°}{180°}$$

(Angle correction factor may not be necessary if the bottom surface of hemispheric PISA is relatively flat, which occurs if the aliasing velocity is set high; $\alpha = 180$ [Fig. 9-20B]).

Step 6. Determine the pulmonary artery pressure from the tricuspid regurgitant velocity (see Chapter 15). This may be repeated after exercise (Fig. 9-21).

Definition of Mitral Stenosis Severity

The following categorize the severity of mitral stenosis according to mitral valve area:

Normal, 4 to 6 cm^2
Mild, 1.6 to 2.0 cm^2
Moderate, 1.1 to 1.5 cm^2
Severe, 1.0 cm^2 or smaller

Mitral stenosis is considered severe when

1. Resting mean pressure gradient is $\geq$10 mm Hg
2. Mitral valve area $\leq$1.0 cm^2
3. PHT $\geq$220 msec

In summary, the mitral valve area can be determined (a) directly with planimetric measurements of 2D echocardiograms and the continuity equation and the PISA method or (b) indirectly with the PHT method. All four methods should be used in every patient.

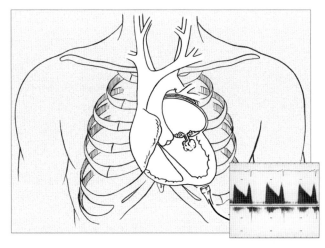

FIG. 9-17. Diagram of stenotic mitral valve and continuous-wave Doppler velocity measurement from the apex. Color-flow imaging occasionally is used to guide the continuous-wave Doppler beam to minimize the θ angle. (Modified from Nishimura RA, Miller FA Jr, Callahan MJ, Benassi RC, Seward JB, Tajik AJ. Doppler echocardiography: theory, instrumentation, technique, and application. *Mayo Clin Proc* 1985;60:321–343, with permission.)

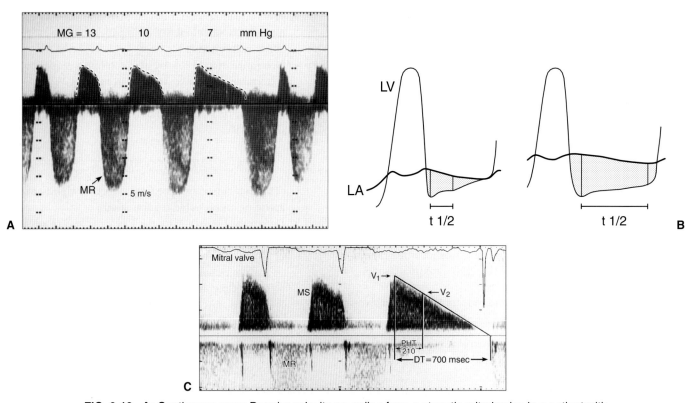

FIG. 9-18. A: Continuous-wave Doppler velocity recording from a stenotic mitral valve in a patient with rheumatic valvular disease and atrial fibrillation. Velocities above the baseline indicate mitral stenosis and ones below the baseline mitral regurgitation (*MR*). Mean gradient (*MG*) varies, depending on RR interval and diastolic filling periods. **B:** Schematic pressure drawings of left ventricle (*LV*) and left atrium (*LA*) in a normal subject **(left)** and in a patient with mitral stenosis **(right)**. With a smaller mitral valve orifice (*right*), the peak transmitral gradient is higher, and the time to reach half of the initial peak pressure gradient is prolonged [pressure half-time ($t_{1/2}$) is prolonged]. **C:** Pressure half-time (*PHT*) calculation from continuous-wave Doppler spectrum of mitral stenosis (*MS*). V_2 is where pressure gradient is one-half the peak pressure gradient at V_1 and is calculated as $V_1/1.4$. PHT is the interval from V_1 to V_2. PHT is always 29% (which can be rounded to 30%) of deceleration time (*DT*), which is the time for peak velocity (V_1) to reach baseline. In this example, DT is 700 msec, PHT is 210 msec (i.e., 700 × 0.3), mitral valve area is 220/210, which equals 1.05 cm² (≈1.1 cm²).

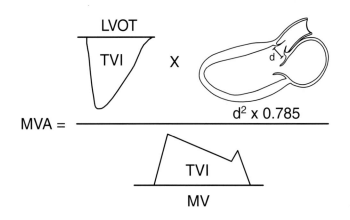

FIG. 9-19. Continuity equation to calculate mitral valve area (*MVA*). Note that time velocity integral (*TVI*) must be used (velocity cannot be substituted). *d*, LVOT diameter; *LVOT*, left ventricular outflow tract; *MV*, mitral valve.

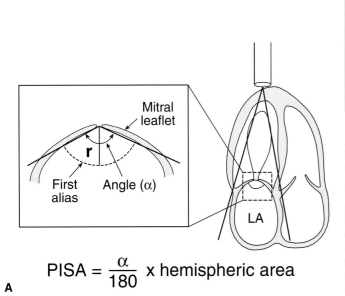

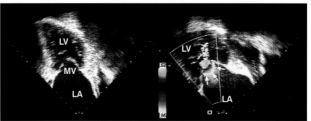

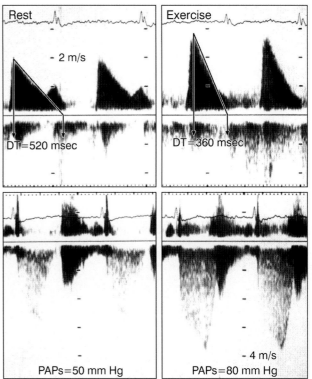

FIG. 9-20. A: Diagram of stenotic mitral valve and angle (α) between two leaflets. Because the proximal isovelocity surface area (*PISA*) is contained within two mitral leaflets, it is obtained by multiplying the hemispheric area by α/180. *r*, PISA radius. (Redrawn from Rodriguez L, Thomas JD, Monterroso V, et al. Validation of the proximal flow convergence method: calculation of orifice area in patients with mitral stenosis. *Circulation* 1993;88:1157–1165, with permission.) **B:** Longitudinal transesophageal view of a stenotic mitral valve (*MV*) demonstrating the PISA method with a relatively high aliasing velocity (52 cm/sec). PISA of the mitral stenosis has a complete hemisphere (*arrows*) with a flat bottom, hence α degrees = 180 degrees.

$$PISA = \frac{\alpha}{180} \times \text{hemispheric area}$$

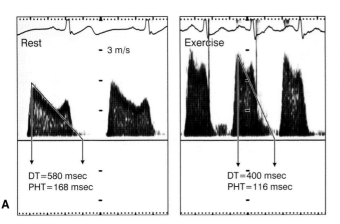

FIG. 9-21. A: Continuous-wave Doppler echocardiogram of patient at rest and after exercise. Heart rate increased from 65 to 110 beats/min. The peak and mean gradients increased, but the pressure half-time (*PHT*) became shorter (from 168 to 116 msec) with exercise. *DT*, deceleration time. **B:** Continuous-wave Doppler recordings of mitral and tricuspid valves in a patient with mitral stenosis and exertional dyspnea, at rest and with exercise (10 situps). By the PHT method, mitral stenosis is moderate in severity: PHT = 520 × 0.29 = 150 m/sec; mitral valve area = 220/150 = 1.47 cm². Systolic pulmonary artery pressure (*PAPs*) at rest is 50 mm Hg, because tricuspid regurgitation peak velocity = 3 m/sec. With mild exercise, mitral peak velocity increases to 3 m/sec (= 36 mm Hg) and tricuspid regurgitant velocity to 4 m/sec, producing a PAPs of about 80 mm Hg.

Caveats

1. Not all prolonged PHTs indicate mitral stenosis. Patients with abnormal myocardial relaxation have a prolonged PHT, but the peak E velocity is not increased and is usually lower than 1 m/sec.

2. Atrial fibrillation is common in patients with mitral stenosis. Hemodynamic variables should be averaged from five to ten cardiac cycles. PHT is best measured from a recording with adequate diastolic filling period.

3. Occasionally, there are two different deceleration slopes of mitral velocity. PHT should be measured from the slope with the longer duration.

4. The PHT is affected by concomitant aortic regurgitation or decreased LV compliance. A rapid increase in LV diastolic pressure in either of these conditions may shorten the PHT and underestimate the severity of mitral stenosis. In this case, the mitral valve area should be measured with 2D echocardiography planimetry, continuity equation, and the PISA method.

5. Concomitant mitral regurgitation can cause the severity of mitral stenosis to be overestimated when the continuity equation is used to calculate mitral valve area. Aortic regurgitation can cause an underestimation.

6. Patients with low cardiac output or bradycardia may have a low mean gradient even in the presence of severe mitral stenosis (and vice versa).

7. The mitral stenosis jet may be eccentric. It may be helpful to guide the continuous-wave Doppler beam by using color flow-imaging.

8. If the aliasing velocity is high (≥40 cm/sec), PISA becomes small enough not to be confined by mitral leaflets. In this case, angle correction may not be needed for calculating mitral valve area by the PISA method (Fig. 9-20B).

Exercise Hemodynamics

For patients who have mainly exertional symptoms and in whom resting hemodynamics do not clearly indicate severe mitral stenosis, it is helpful to perform the Doppler hemodynamic assessment during bicycle exercise or immediately after treadmill exercise. Although the mitral valve area does not change with exercise, the increase in cardiac output and heart rate will result in a significant increase in the transmitral gradient, LA pressure, and pulmonary artery pressure (Fig. 9-21). Song and colleagues (25) demonstrated that the duration of exercise in patients with mitral stenosis has an inverse correlation with tricuspid regurgitation velocity (i.e., systolic pulmonary artery pressure) but not with mitral valve area or transmitral gradient. Therefore, significant worsening of hemodynamics with exercise can be helpful in explaining the patient's symptoms in the setting of a mild to moderate resting hemodynamic abnormality.

TEE

The most frequent use of TEE in patients with mitral stenosis is to exclude LA or LA appendage thrombus if a patient sustains an embolic event or is considered for mitral balloon valvuloplasty. TEE occasionally is performed during mitral balloon valvuloplasty to guide transseptal puncture or position of a balloon (Fig. 9-22).

Clinical Implications

Echocardiography is the gold standard for evaluation of mitral stenosis, obviating cardiac catheterization. Because of the easy access of the mitral valve to apical transducer position, a Doppler signal can be obtained in nearly all patients. This noninvasive technique is well suited for serial

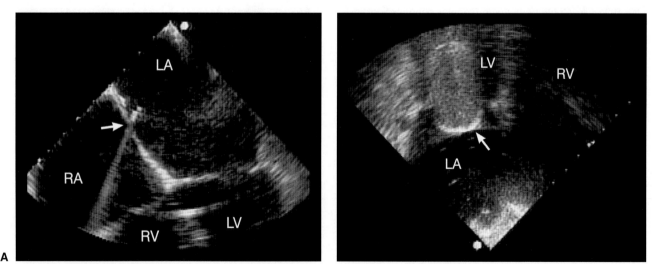

FIG. 9-22. Transesophageal echocardiography during transseptal catheterization **(A)** (*arrow* indicates satisfactory puncture of the atrial septum) and monitoring balloon inflation (*arrow*) during mitral valvotomy **(B)**.

examination to assess disease progression. The pressure gradient across the native or prosthetic mitral valve can be overestimated with cardiac catheterization when pulmonary capillary wedge pressure is used (instead of LA pressure by transseptal catheterization) to measure the transmitral pressure gradient (2).

Tricuspid and Pulmonary Stenosis

Tricuspid stenosis usually is caused by rheumatic fever. Other uncommon causes include carcinoid heart disease (which more commonly causes tricuspid regurgitation), tumor, vegetation, valvular damage from catheter or pacemaker leads, aneurysm of the sinus of Valsalva, and prosthesis obstruction. Two-dimensional echocardiography is valuable in determining the cause of tricuspid stenosis. The normal tricuspid inflow velocity is lower than 0.5 to 1 m/sec, with a mean gradient <2 mm Hg. There is a respiratory variation in tricuspid valve inflow velocity, and it is best to determine Doppler velocity while the patient holds his or her breath in expiration. The evaluation of tricuspid valve stenosis with Doppler echocardiography is similar to the method described for mitral stenosis, although the constant of 190 was proposed for the PHT method (26). Tricuspid stenosis is considered severe when the mean gradient is ≥7 mm Hg and PHT ≥190 ms.

Pulmonary Stenosis

Pulmonary stenosis occurs as an isolated lesion or as part of a complex congenital heart disease or syndrome. Pulmonary stenosis can also be an acquired disease caused by carcinoid heart disease, vegetation, or other (intracardiac or extracardiac) mass that obstructs or compresses the pulmonary outflow tract. Subvalvular pulmonary stenosis can occur as part of a congenital heart complex such as tetralogy of Fallot or as a result of hypertrophic obstructive cardiomyopathy involving the right side of the heart. The morphologic features of each of these lesions are easily identified on 2D echocardiography. Peak flow velocity and pressure gradient are obtained with continuous-wave Doppler echocardiography, usually best from the left upper sternal border or the subcostal position (see Fig. 9-13D). Pulmonary flow velocity must be determined in patients with increased tricuspid regurgitation velocity or unexplained systolic murmur.

Evaluation of Valvular Regurgitation

The evaluation of valvular regurgitation begins with 2D echocardiography and color-flow imaging. Cardiac structural changes demonstrated on 2D echocardiography alert physicians to the possibility of valvular regurgitation, such as mitral valve prolapse, flail segment of a valve, vegetation, or bicuspid aortic valve. Color-Flow imaging is the next step in estimating the amount of the regurgitant jet. The most widely used color-flow imaging criterion for se-

verity of valvular regurgitation is the comparison of the jet height or area with the dimension of the LVOT or the size of the LA for aortic valve or mitral valve regurgitation, respectively (27,28). This qualitative method has many pitfalls, however. It tends to underestimate the severity of regurgitation when the jet is eccentric and to overestimate it when the jet is central (usually functional regurgitation) (4,29). TEE is more helpful in delineating valvular structural abnormalities, but it is not necessarily more quantitative in judging the severity of valvular regurgitation. Thus, assessment of the severity of valvular regurgitation should be based not only on color-flow imaging but on hemodynamic data collected by continuous-wave and pulsed-wave Doppler echocardiography. Quantitative methods provide regurgitant volume, regurgitant fraction, and regurgitant orifice area. This integrated approach to the assessment of valvular regurgitation is discussed in detail in the following section.

Aortic Regurgitation

Two-Dimensional and M-Mode Echocardiography

The cause of aortic regurgitation varies widely and includes a congenitally abnormal valve, a dilated aortic root, Marfan syndrome, endocarditis, aortic dissection, prosthetic valve dysfunction, "Fen-Phen" valvulopathy, and, most commonly, a degenerative calcific aortic valve. These structural abnormalities are easily detected on 2D echocardiography. M-mode echocardiography is helpful in demonstrating premature mitral valve closure or diastolic opening of the aortic valve as a sign of severe, usually acute, aortic regurgitation and marked increase in LV diastolic pressure. It also demonstrates the fluttering motion of the anterior mitral leaflets caused by significant aortic regurgitation (Fig. 9-23) (see also Fig. 6-1).

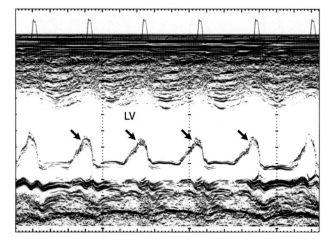

FIG. 9-23. M-mode echocardiogram of left ventricle (*LV*) and mitral valve showing a dilated LV with decreased function and the fluttering motion (*arrows*) of the anterior mitral leaflet caused by significant aortic valve regurgitation.

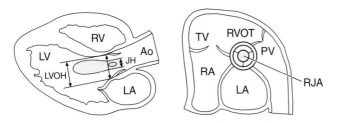

FIG. 9-24. Diagram of color-flow imaging to estimate severity of aortic regurgitation, from the parasternal long-axis **(left)** and short-axis **(right)** views. Left ventricular outflow height (*LVOH*) and jet height (*JH*) are determined from the parasternal long-axis view. Regurgitant jet area (*RJA*) is measured from the parasternal short-axis view at the aortic valve level. *Ao*, aorta; *PV*, pulmonary valve; *RVOT*, right ventricular outflow tract; *TV*, tricuspid valve. (Redrawn from ref. 27, with permission.)

Doppler and Color-Flow Imaging

Echocardiographic evaluation of aortic regurgitation requires color-flow imaging, continuous-wave Doppler of the regurgitant jet, and pulsed-wave Doppler of the descending thoracic aorta and mitral inflow. Color-flow imaging of aortic regurgitation is performed best from the parasternal long-axis and short-axis views (by the TTE window) or from the LVOT view (by the TEE window; 135-degree multiplane transducer position).

Comparison of color-flow imaging with aortic angiography showed the maximal extent or length of the regurgitant jet to be poorly correlated with the angiographic severity of aortic regurgitation. The regurgitant jet area obtained from the parasternal short-axis view relative to the short-axis area of the LVOT at the level of the aortic an-

nulus correlated best with the angiographic severity of aortic regurgitation (27). The width of the regurgitant jet at its origin relative to the dimension of the LVOT was also a good predictor of the angiographic severity of aortic regurgitation (Fig. 9-24). Other Doppler features that should be used in determining the severity of regurgitation (4,30–32) include PHT of the continuous-wave Doppler signal of the regurgitant jet, diastolic reversal flow in the descending aorta, and the deceleration time (DT) of the mitral flow E velocity. In severe aortic regurgitation, systemic diastolic pressure decreases quickly so that the aortic regurgitation signal (corresponding to the pressure difference between the aorta and the LV) has a shortened DT and, thus, PHT (Fig. 9-25). Diastolic retrograde flow can be demonstrated in the descending thoracic aorta (Fig. 9-26) and even in the abdominal aorta. In case of acute severe aortic regurgitation, LV diastolic pressure increases rapidly, resulting in a restrictive diastolic filling pattern in mitral inflow (Fig. 9-27). Regurgitant volume and fraction can be quantitated, as described in Chapter 6. If there is no significant mitral regurgitation, mitral valve (MV) inflow can be used to represent systemic stroke volume

$$MV\ flow\ =\ MV\ annulus\ area\ \times\ MV\ TVI$$

where *MV annulus area* is determined by annulus diameter squared (D^2) $\times$ 0.785 and *MV TVI* is determined by placing a sample volume at the MV annulus.

Regurgitant volume (*RegV*) is the difference between the stroke volume across the LVOT and MV

$$Aortic\ RegV\ =\ LVOT\ flow\ -\ MV\ flow$$
$$=\ (D^2\ \times\ 0.785\ \times\ TVI)\ LVOT$$
$$-\ (Annulus\ D^2\ \times\ 0.785\ \times\ TVI)\ MV$$

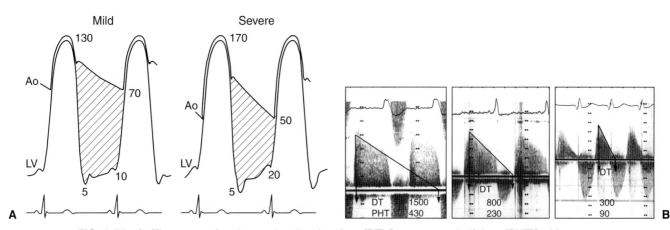

FIG. 9-25. A: The reason for shorter deceleration time (DT) [or pressure half-time (PHT)] with severe aortic regurgitation is shown in this diagram of LV and aortic (*Ao*) pressure traces. With more significant regurgitation, the aortic pressure decay is more rapid and associated with a rapid rise in diastolic left ventricular (*LV*) pressure. **B:** Continuous-wave Doppler spectra of aortic regurgitation from three patients illustrating decreased *PHT* with more severe aortic regurgitation. **Left panel** indicates mild regurgitation, with a PHT of 430 msec; **right panel** indicates severe regurgitation, with a PHT of 90 msec, and the **middle panel** indicates moderately severe regurgitation.

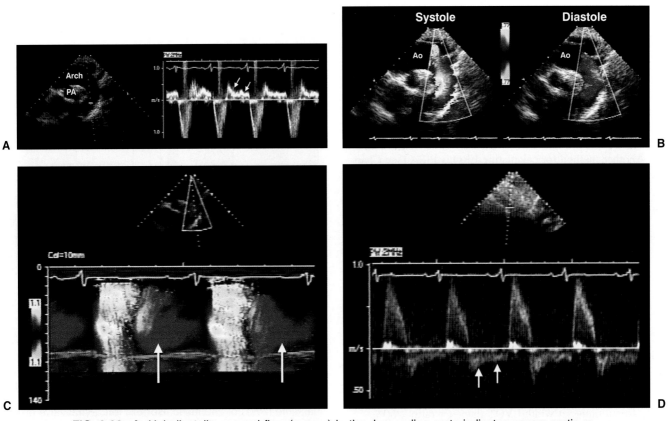

FIG. 9-26. A: Holodiastolic reversal flow (*arrows*) in the descending aorta indicates severe aortic regurgitation. Similar diastolic reversal can be seen in a descending thoracic aneurysm or shunt into the aorta during diastole (as in Blalock-Taussig shunt). The sample volume usually is located just distal to the takeoff of the left subclavian artery. *PA*, pulmonary artery. **B:** Two-dimensional color-flow imaging of the descending thoracic aorta during diastole. The orange-red flow in the descending aorta during diastole indicates flow toward the transducer, that is, reversal flow due to severe aortic regurgitation. *Ao*, aorta. **C:** Color M-mode from the descending thoracic aorta shows holodiastolic reversal flow (*arrows*). **D:** Pulsed-wave Doppler recording of abdominal aorta showing diastolic flow reversal (*arrows*) in severe aortic regurgitation.

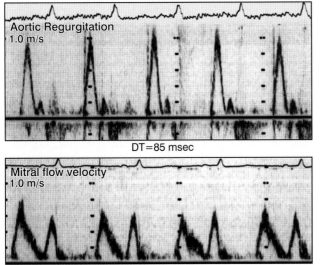

FIG. 9-27. Mitral inflow pulsed-wave Doppler in severe acute aortic regurgitation before **(top)** and after **(bottom)** aortic valve replacement. Note that left ventricular diastolic pressure increases quickly and produces a restrictive mitral inflow pattern with high E velocity, low A velocity, increased E/A ratio, and deceleration time (*DT*) of 85 msec with severe aortic regurgitation. This restrictive pattern normalizes after aortic valve replacement **(bottom)**.

Regurgitant fraction (*RF*) is obtained by the equation

$$RF = \frac{Aortic\ RegV}{LVOT\ stroke\ volume} \times 100\%$$

The aortic regurgitant orifice area can be calculated by two methods. Because flow volume is the product of area and TVI, the effective regurgitant orifice (ERO) area is calculated by dividing regurgitant volume by aortic regurgitant TVI.

Another method for calculating ERO is PISA (see Chapter 6). The regurgitant flow rate across the aortic valve is obtained from the flow rate of a proximal surface area with a known flow velocity.

$$Flow\ Rate = 2\pi\ (r)^2 \times Aliasing\ Velocity$$

$$ERO = \frac{Flow\ rate}{Peak\ AR\ velocity}$$

$$= \frac{6.28 \times r^2 \times Aliasing\ velocity}{Peak\ AR\ velocity}$$

On the basis of the data from 2D Doppler and color-flow imaging, the severity of aortic regurgitation is determined as follows:

Severe aortic regurgitation (Fig. 9-28)

1. Regurgitant jet width/LVOT diameter ratio ≥60%
2. Regurgitant jet area/LVOT area ratio ≥60%
3. Aortic regurgitation PHT ≤250 msec
4. Restrictive mitral flow pattern (usually in acute setting)
5. Holodiastolic flow reversal in the descending aorta
6. Dense continuous-wave Doppler signal
7. Regurgitant fraction ≥55%
8. Regurgitant volume ≥60 mL
9. LV diastolic dimension ≥7.5 cm (chronic aortic regurgitation)
10. Effective regurgitant orifice ≥0.30 cm²

Mild aortic regurgitation

1. Regurgitant jet width/LVOT diameter ratio ≤30%
2. Regurgitant jet area/LVOT diameter ≤30%
3. Aortic regurgitation PHT ≥400 msec
4. Mild early diastolic flow reversal in the descending aorta
5. Faint continuous-wave Doppler signal
6. Regurgitant fraction <30%
7. LV diastolic dimension (chronic) <6.0 cm
8. Effective regurgitant orifice <0.10 cm²

Mitral Regurgitation

Two-Dimensional and M-Mode Echocardiography

As in aortic regurgitation, 2D echocardiography and M-mode echocardiography are useful in detecting the underlying cause of mitral regurgitation, such as mitral valve

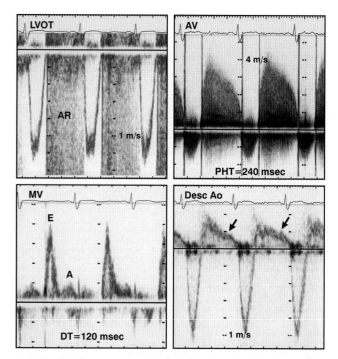

FIG. 9-28. Composite of typical Doppler velocity signals found in severe aortic regurgitation. **Top left:** left ventricular outflow tract (*LVOT*) velocity is high (1.3 m/sec). **Top right:** Aortic valve (*AV*) regurgitation velocity has a short pressure half-time (*PHT*) of 240 msec. **Bottom left:** Mitral valve (*MV*) inflow is restrictive (E/A = 4.0, DT = 120 msec). **Bottom right:** There is holodiastolic reversal flow (*arrows*) in the descending thoracic aorta (*Desc Ao*). AR, aortic regurgitation. DT, deceleration time of E velocity.

prolapse, flail mitral leaflet, ruptured chordae, mitral annulus calcification, papillary muscle dysfunction or rupture, rheumatic valve, ''fen-phen'' valvulopathy, cleft mitral valve, endocarditis, or perforation.

Mitral Valve Prolapse

Mitral valve prolapse is a common indication for echocardiography. It usually is suspected because of a midsystolic click and mid-to-late systolic murmurs. Initially, the diagnosis of mitral valve prolapse was based on M-mode criteria (Fig. 9-29A): late or holosystolic bowing of a mitral valve leaflet 3 mm or more below the C–D line. With the application of 2D echocardiography, which visualizes mitral valve motion in real time, however, this method has a higher sensitivity in the diagnosis of mitral valve prolapse. Now that it is known that the mitral annulus is saddle shaped, the echocardiographic diagnosis of mitral valve prolapse is based on the parasternal long-axis view (33). *Mitral valve prolapse* is defined as systolic displacement of one or both mitral leaflets into the LA, below the plane of

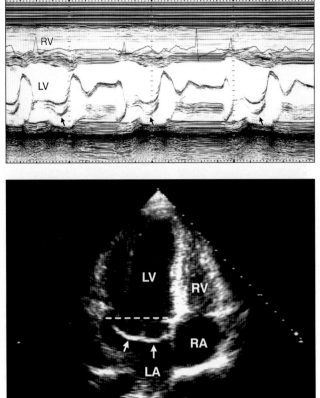

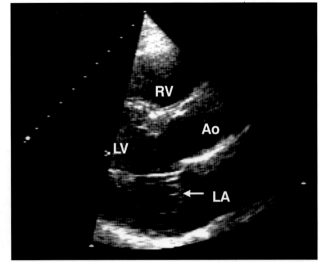

FIG. 9-29. A: M-mode and two-dimensional echocardiographic features of mitral valve prolapse. Mitral leaflets are thickened, and there is late systolic bowing of the posterior mitral leaflet below the C–D line (*arrows*). **B:** From the parasternal long-axis view, there is systolic displacement of the anterior mitral leaflet (*arrow*) into the left atrium (*LA*) beyond the plane of the mitral annulus. *Ao*, aorta. **C:** Apical four-chamber view showing prolapse of both mitral leaflets (*arrows*). *Dotted lines* indicate the plane of the mitral annulus. In general, the apical view should not be used to make the diagnosis of mitral valve prolapse.

the mitral annulus (Fig. 9-29B). The diagnosis is more certain when the mitral leaflets are thickened (*myxomatous*). This classic pattern of mitral valve prolapse is associated with an increased risk of serious complications such as endocarditis, severe mitral valve regurgitation, and mitral valve repair or replacement (34–36). Auscultatory findings are not good enough to identify a high-risk group of patients with mitral valve prolapse. The myxomatous nature of mitral valve prolapse most likely represents a biochemical defect involving connective tissue. In long-term follow-up (mean, 6.2 years) of 237 patients with mitral valve prolapse documented by M-mode echocardiography, the presence of redundant mitral valve leaflet was the only variable associated with sudden death and infectious endocarditis (34). The risk of an embolic event or stroke has not been found to be related to leaflet thickness or redundancy.

Doppler and Color-Flow Imaging

In color-flow imaging of mitral regurgitation, the area of the regurgitant jet relative to the size of the LA is most predictive of regurgitant severity determined with angiography (Fig. 9-30) (37). Color-flow imaging of valvular regurgitation depends on the gain setting, pulsed repetition frequency, field depth, direction of jet, and loading conditions. Adjacent cardiac walls influence the size of the regurgitant color flow if the regurgitant jet is eccentric. A flow jet directed against the atrial wall appears smaller than a free jet of the same regurgitant volume (*Coanda effect*). Therefore, jet size on color-flow imaging should be interpreted in the context of jet geometry and the surrounding solid boundaries (38).

In mitral regurgitation, antegrade flow (*mitral inflow*) velocity may increase with severe regurgitation (especially with a prosthesis with a fixed orifice area) and the continuous-wave Doppler spectrum may have a characteristic configuration (due to the V wave) with increased intensity. On Doppler echocardiography, the velocity of mitral regurgitation tends to be lower (<5 m/sec) with increasing severity because the increase in LA pressure reduces the transmitral systolic gradient (Fig. 9-31), unless the LV pressure is markedly increased (as in aortic stenosis or hypertrophic obstructive cardiomyopathy). In severe mitral regurgitation, there may be a systolic flow reversal in the

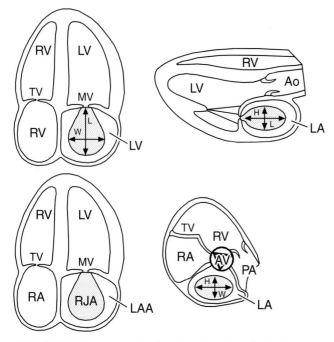

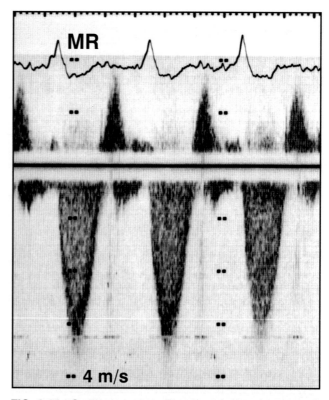

FIG. 9-30. Diagrams of color-flow imaging of mitral regurgitation from apical four-chamber and parasternal long- and short-axis views. Left atrial area (*LAA*) and regurgitant jet area (*RJA*) are measured by planimetry. *Ao,* aorta; *AV,* aortic valve; *H,* height; *L,* length; *MV,* mitral valve; *PA,* pulmonary artery; *TV,* tricuspid valve; *W,* width. (Redrawn from ref. 28, with permission.)

FIG. 9-31. Continuous-wave Doppler velocity of severe mitral regurgitation (*MR*). MR peak velocity is 3.5 m/sec (equivalent to a transmitral gradient of 49 mm Hg). This was obtained in a patient with cardiogenic shock due to severe MR and severe left ventricle (*LV*) systolic dysfunction. Pulmonary capillary wedge pressure was 54 mm Hg, and systolic blood pressure was 100 mm Hg.

pulmonary vein (Fig. 9-32) (39); however, the absence of systolic flow reversal in the pulmonary vein does not exclude severe mitral regurgitation.

Most recently, vena contracta width by color-flow mapping correlates well with other quantitative measures for mitral regurgitation severity (40). Vena contracta is the narrowest portion of the mitral regurgitation jet downstream from the orifice. A biplane vena contracta width ≥0.5 cm (the average of vena contracta widths from two apical views) was always associated with a regurgitant volume >60 mL and an effective regurgitant orifice >0.4 cm².

Regurgitant volume, fraction, and orifice area can be calculated by the volumetric or PISA method to assess the severity of mitral regurgitation (41).

Volumetric Method

In the absence of significant aortic regurgitation, the difference between flow across the MV and the LVOT is the mitral regurgitant volume (RegV) (Fig. 9-33). Flow across the mitral valve is calculated by the product of the area of the mitral annulus area and the TVI of flow obtained by placing the sample volume at the mitral annulus. Flow across the LVOT is calculated by the product of the area of the aortic annulus and the TVI of flow obtained by placing the sample volume at the aortic annulus. The regurgitant

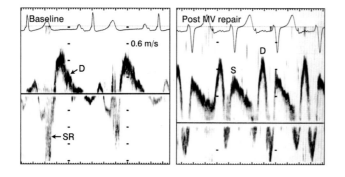

FIG. 9-32. Pulmonary vein pulsed-wave Doppler using transesophageal echocardiography in the operating room. The baseline study **(left)** is consistent with severe mitral regurgitation, with decreased and reversed systolic pulmonary vein flow (*SR*). This pattern is normalized **(right)** after mitral valve (*MV*) repair. The systolic (*S*) forward flow in the pulmonary vein remains slightly lower than diastolic (*D*) flow.

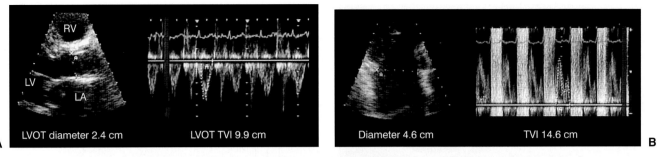

A LVOT diameter 2.4 cm   LVOT TVI 9.9 cm

Diameter 4.6 cm   TVI 14.6 cm **B**

FIG. 9-33. Volumetric method of calculating mitral regurgitant volume. Mitral regurgitant volume is obtained by subtracting left ventricle outflow tract (*LVOT*) stroke volume from the mitral inflow stroke volume. **A:** Still frame of the parasternal long-axis view demonstrating measurement of LVOT diameter **(left)** and pulsed-wave Doppler recording of LVOT velocity **(right)**. *LVOT stroke volume = LVOT diameter²* × 0.785 × *LVO TVI* = 2.4² × 0.785 × 9.9 = 4.5 cm² × 9.9 cm = 45 cc. *TVI,* time velocity integral. **B:** Demonstration of how to calculate mitral valve inflow stroke volume. Apical four-chamber view with a zoom to the mitral annulus area, with a diameter of 4.6 cm **(left)**, and pulsed-wave Doppler flow velocity at the mitral annulus with TVI of 14.6 cm **(right)**. Mitral inflow stroke volume is obtained by multiplying mitral annulus area by mitral inflow TVI. Therefore, mitral inflow stroke volume = mitral annulus diameter² × 0.785 × mitral inflow TVI = 4.6² × 0.785 × 14.6 = 243 cc. Thus, the mitral regurgitant volume is equal to 243 − 45 cc = 198 cc. Regurgitant fraction is obtained by dividing regurgitant volume by mitral inflow stroke volume. Mitral valve regurgitant fraction = 198 ÷ 243 × 100 = 81%.

fraction (RF) is calculated by dividing RegV by flow across MV and multiplying by 100.

$$MV\ RegV = MV\ flow - LVOT\ flow$$

$$= (Annulus\ D^2 \times 0.785 \times TVI)_{MV}$$

$$- (D^2 \times 0.785 \times TVI)_{LVOT}$$

$$MV\ RF = \frac{MV\ RegV}{MV\ flow} \times 100(\%)$$

The ERO area is estimated by dividing the RegV by the TVI of mitral regurgitation (MR) velocity recorded by continuous-wave Doppler echocardiography

$$ERO_{MV} = \frac{MR_{RegV}}{MR_{TVI}}$$

Proximal Isovelocity Surface Area Method

The PISA method is based on the principle of conservation of flow and the continuity equation (41–44). The amount of blood flow across a regurgitant orifice can be estimated with the PISA method. As blood in the LV converges toward the mitral regurgitant orifice, blood-flow velocity increases and forms a series of hemispheric waves, whose surface has the same velocity (*isovelocity*) (Fig. 9-34). Color-flow imaging can identify a PISA in the LV because the red-blue aliasing interface corresponds to the surface of the hemisphere and the flow velocity at the surface is the same as the aliasing velocity. Therefore, the flow rate at the surface of a hemispheric PISA is calculated as area of hemisphere times aliasing velocity. Aliasing velocity needs to be lowered to create a larger PISA (for flow away from the apical transducer), because the further the flow is from

the regurgitant orifice, the slower the velocity. Aliasing velocity can be altered by downward shift of the zero baseline (in case of transthoracic imaging of MR) so that an optimal (hemispheric) PISA can be identified. The flow rate at the PISA is equal to the flow rate across the regurgitant orifice.

Flow rate at PISA = Flow rate across regurgitant orifice

$$2\pi\ (r^2) \times Alias\ velocity = ERO \times MR\ velocity$$

$$ERO = 6.28\ r^2 \times \frac{Alias\ Velocity}{MR\ Velocity}$$

After ERO has been calculated, mitral RegV is calculated as

$$MR\ RegV = ERO \times MR\ TVI$$

The stepwise method of obtaining mitral regurgitation flow rate, ERO area, and mitral regurgitant volume using the PISA method is as follows:

Step 1. Optimize color-flow imaging of mitral regurgitation from an apical window (Figs. 9-35 and 9-36A)

Step 2. Expand the image of the regurgitant mitral valve by using zoom or regional expansion selection (RES) mode (Figs. 9-35 and 9-36B).

Step 3. Shift the color-flow zero baseline downward to increase hemispheric PISA; the negative aliasing velocity is usually 20 to 40 cm/sec (Figs. 9-35B and 9-36B). Zero baseline shift of the color-flow map is toward the direction of desired color-flow jet. The baseline shift is upward (toward the transducer) if TEE is used

Step 4. Use cine-mode to scroll through several cardiac cycles to select the most satisfactory hemispheric PISA, which occurs at midsystole

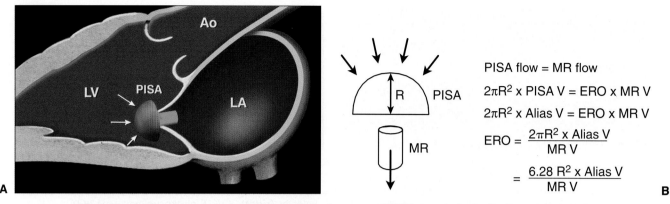

FIG. 9-34. A: Diagram of proximal isovelocity surface area (*PISA*) (*arrows*) of mitral regurgitation. As blood flow converges toward the mitral regurgitant orifice, blood-flow velocity increases gradually and forms multiple isovelocity hemispheric shells. The flow rate calculated at the surface of the hemisphere is equal to the flow rate going through the mitral regurgitant orifice. *Ao*, Aorta. **B:** Calculation and derivation of effective regurgitant orifice (*ERO*) area of mitral regurgitation (*MR*) using the PISA method. *R*, PISA radius; *V*, velocity.

Step 5. From a frame with an ideal PISA, measure the radius (r in cm) of the PISA at midsystole (Figs. 9-35B and 9-36C) along the direction of the ultrasound beam

Step 6. Measure mitral regurgitation velocity with continuous-wave Doppler to obtain peak mitral regurgitation velocity and TVI (Fig. 9-36C)

Step 7. Calculate mitral flow rate, ERO, and mitral regurgitation volume, as described.

Simplification of the PISA Method

The PISA method can be simplified, which is especially helpful when the peak velocity of the mitral regurgitation jet cannot be obtained. Also, simplification is helpful in determining the severity of mitral regurgitation intraoperatively when a surgical decision needs to be made without delay. There are several different ways to simplify the PISA method, and all the methods are based on the same formula.

1. If the aliasing velocity is about 30 cm/sec and the mitral regurgitation velocity is assumed to be about 500 cm/sec (Fig. 9-37).

$$\text{ERO} = \frac{6.28 \times r^2 \times 30 \text{ cm/sec}}{500 \text{ cm/sec}}$$

ERO becomes 0.38 cm^2 when r = 1 cm. Hence, a PISA radius $\geq$1 cm indicates severe mitral regurgitation when the aliasing velocity is $\geq$30 cm/sec. Because the peak mitral regurgitation velocity is assumed to be 500 cm/sec, this simplification will overestimate the ERO if systemic blood pressure is increased, which would result in a mitral regurgitation peak velocity much higher than 500 cm/sec.

2. If aliasing velocity is about 40 cm/sec, and the mitral regurgitation velocity is assumed to be 500 cm/sec

$$\text{ERO} = \frac{6.28 \times r^2 \times 40 \text{ cm/sec}}{500 \text{ cm/sec}} = \frac{251 \times r^2}{500} = \frac{r^2}{2}$$

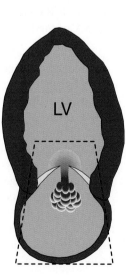

- Optimize 2-D color flow (apical view)
- Zoom or RES
- Freeze in cine-loop

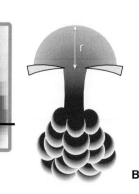

- Obtain mid-systolic frame
- Color flow baseline shift to blue aliasing velocity of 20-40 cm/s
- Measure PISA radius (r)

FIG. 9-35. A,B: Diagrams of how to obtain aliasing velocity and proximal isovelocity surface area (*PISA*) radius (*r*). *V*, velocity; *RES*, regional expansion selection.

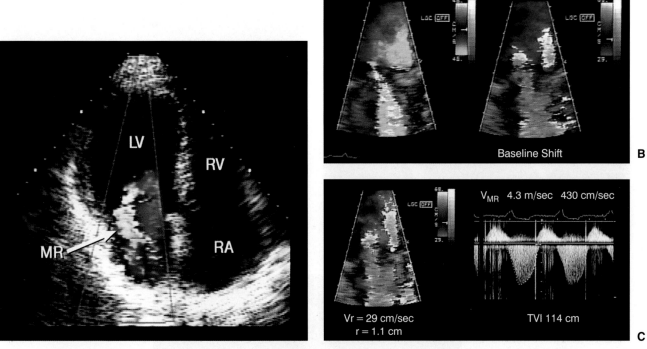

FIG. 9-36. A: Apical four-chamber view and color-flow imaging of mitral regurgitation (*MR*). **B:** Mitral regurgitant orifice and mitral regurgitation jet were zoomed. **Left:** In this figure, aliasing velocity is 46 cm/sec to either direction. Baseline for color-flow map has not been shifted. **Right:** Color-flow map baseline is shifted downward so that the negative aliasing velocity was reduced from 46 cm/sec to 29 cm/sec. The downward baseline shift makes the change of color flow farther from the mitral regurgitant orifice, because blood flow converging toward the mitral regurgitant orifice has a lower velocity further away from the regurgitant orifice. Therefore, a downward baseline shift makes the radius of the identified proximal isovelocity surface area (*PISA*) larger. **C:** The measured radius (*r*) was 1.1 cm, with an aliasing velocity (*Vr*) of 29 cm/sec. Mitral regurgitation velocity (V_{MR}) was obtained by continuous-wave Doppler from the apex, and the peak velocity was 4.3 m/sec (430 cm/sec) with a time velocity integral (*TVI*) of 114 cm. From the data of PISA radius, color-flow map aliasing velocity, mitral regurgitation peak velocity and mitral regurgitation TVI, mitral regurgitation effective regurgitant orifice (*ERO*) and regurgitant volume can be calculated.

$$ERO = \frac{6.28 \times (1.1)^2 \times 29}{430} = 0.51 \text{ cm}^2$$

Regurgitant volume = ERO × MR TVI = 0.51 × 114 = 58 cc

ERO becomes half of the r^2 value.

3. The relationship between TVI and peak velocity of mitral regurgitation has been shown to be relatively constant (45). Usually

$$\frac{MR_{TVI}}{MR_{Velocity}} = \frac{1}{3.25}$$

Therefore,

Mitral RegV = ERO × Mitral regurgitation TVI

$$= \frac{6.28 \times r^2 \times \text{Alias Velocity} \times MR_{TVI}}{MR_{Velocity}}$$

$$= 6.28 \times r^2 \times \text{Alias Velocity} \times \frac{MR_{TVI}}{MR_{Velocity}}$$

Therefore,

$$MR \text{ RegV} = \frac{6.28 \times r^2 \times \text{Alias Velocity}}{3.25}$$

$$= 2 r^2 \times \text{Alias Velocity}$$

The following criteria indicate or suggest severe mitral regurgitation:

1. Definite
   a. 2D echocardiographic evidence of disruption of the mitral valve apparatus (papillary muscle rupture, flail mitral leaflet)
   b. ERO ≥ 0.40 cm²
   c. Mitral regurgitation volume ≥ 60 cc
   d. Regurgitation fraction ≥ 55%

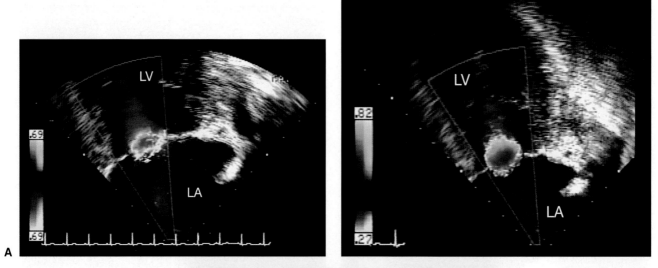

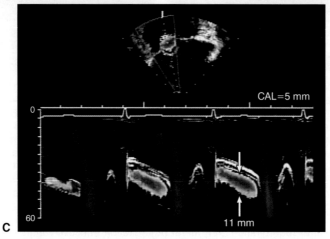

FIG. 9-37. Transesophageal long-axis view showing the mitral valve and mitral valve regurgitation at baseline **(A)** and with a baseline shift toward the transducer **(B)**. The patient has a visible proximal isovelocity surface area (PISA) even at the baseline, but the radius (r) increases to 1.1 cm when the aliasing velocity is decreased to 27 cm/sec. **C:** Color M-mode echocardiogram of PISA is helpful in measuring PISA radius and midsystole (*arrows*). If mitral regurgitation peak velocity cannot be measured, a simplified method can be used to calculate effective regurgitant orifice (ERO) and mitral regurgitation volume as follows: This simplified method ($0.38 \times r^2 = ERO$) works if the aliasing velocity is 30 ± 5 cm/sec (this example, 27 cm/sec), and the mitral regurgitation velocity is assumed to be approximately 500 cm/sec.

$$ERO = 0.38 \times 1.1^2 = 0.46 \text{ cm}^2$$

Mitral regurgitant volume can be calculated in a simplified manner ($2 \times r^2 \times v$).

$$\textit{Mitral regurgitant volume} = 2 \times 1.1^2 \times 27 = 66 \text{ cc}$$

Both ERO and mitral regurgitant volume calculated by these simplified methods are consistent with severe mitral valve regurgitation. CAL, calibration.

e. Pulmonary vein systolic flow reversals
f. Mitral regurgitation color flow jet reaching the posterior wall of the LA (with a high aliasing velocity of color map)
2. Suggestive
   a. Color-flow area ≥40% of LA size
   b. Eccentric mitral regurgitation jet reaching the posterior wall of the LA
   c. Dense continuous-wave Doppler signal
   d. Increased E velocity (≥1.5 m/sec for native valve and 2 m/sec for prosthesis)
   e. LV dimension ≥7 cm (along with color flow evidence of mitral regurgitation)
   f. LA size ≥5.5 cm

TEE

Mitral regurgitation is the valvular heart disease that most often requires TEE evaluation. It is difficult to assess the cause and occasionally the magnitude of mitral regurgitation with TTE because the mitral valve is some distance from the chest wall and the mitral regurgitation jet is directed away from the transducer. TEE visualizes the mitral valve apparatus clearly in all patients and can determine the cause and severity of mitral regurgitation with color-flow imaging and pulsed-wave Doppler. When the onset of severe mitral regurgitation is acute (as in the setting of acute myocardial infarction), the patient becomes hemodynamically unstable and precordial echocardiography may be even more difficult. TEE often provides invaluable clinical information in this particular setting. When the mitral regurgitation color jet (mosaic turbulent jet) reaches the posterior wall of the LA, the regurgitation is usually severe. The jet area may not be large if it is eccentric and hugs the atrial septum or the lateral wall of the LA. The PISA method is the same as described for TTE except that the zero baseline for a color-flow map is shifted upward to reduce the aliasing velocity of flow toward the transducer (see Fig. 9-37). M-mode of PISA is helpful in measuring its radius at midsystole (see Fig. 9-37). When the peak velocity of a mitral regurgitation jet cannot be obtained, a simplified method may be sufficient to establish the severity of the regurgitation, especially during an intraoperative examination. When the aliasing velocity is set at 30 ± 5 cm/sec, the PISA radius correlates well with the severity of the mitral regurgitation determined by double-sampling dye curves intraoperatively (46). When the PISA radius is ≥1 cm, the percent of dye concentration in the LA is usually greater than 20% of that in the aorta after dye is injected into the LV.

Tricuspid Regurgitation

Two-Dimensional and M-Mode Echocardiography

Two-dimensional and M-mode echocardiography detect the underlying cause of tricuspid regurgitation, such as rheumatic valve, prolapse, carcinoid involvement (Fig. 9-38), Ebstein anomaly, annular dilatation, RV infarct, and tricuspid valve rupture.

Doppler and Color-Flow Imaging

The Doppler features mentioned above for mitral regurgitation should be looked for systematically and applied to tricuspid regurgitation. Instead of flow reversal in the pulmonary vein, however, severe tricuspid regurgitation results in systolic flow reversal in the hepatic veins (Fig. 9-39). The tricuspid continuous-wave Doppler signal is characteristic when the regurgitation is severe: increased forward flow velocity, relatively decreased tricuspid regurgitation velocity, and concave late systolic configuration of tricuspid regurgitation due to a large right atrial V wave (Fig. 9-39).

The following criteria suggest severe tricuspid regurgitation:

1. Color-flow regurgitant jet area ≥30% of RA area
2. Dense continuous-wave Doppler signal
3. Annulus dilatation (≥4 cm) or inadequate cusp coaptation
4. Late systolic concave configuration of continuous-wave signal
5. Increased tricuspid inflow velocity (≥1.0 m/sec)
6. Systolic flow reversals in the hepatic vein

Drug-Induced Valvular Heart Disease

Ergot preparations and "fen-phen" appetite suppressant induce valvular abnormalities similar in echocardiographic

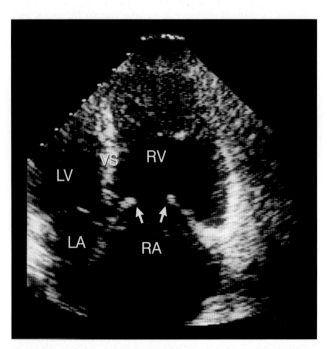

FIG. 9-38. Right ventricle (*RV*) inflow view showing a systolic frame of the tricuspid valve (*arrows*). The valve leaflets are held in a fixed open position because of the sclerosing effect of carcinoid syndrome. *VS*, ventricular septum.

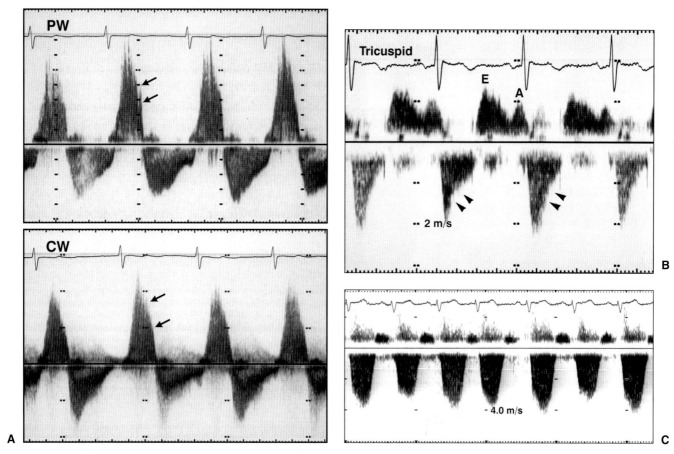

FIG. 9-39. A: Hepatic vein pulsed-wave (*PW*) and continuous-wave (*CW*) Doppler showing marked systolic reversal (*arrows*) caused by severe tricuspid regurgitation. **B:** Doppler spectrum of tricuspid valve in a patient with severe tricuspid regurgitation. Forward inflow velocity is increased (*E* = 1.4 m/sec) and tricuspid regurgitation peak velocity is relatively decreased because of a small pressure gradient between the right ventricle and right atrium. A large V wave makes the Doppler spectrum dented during mid to late systole (*arrowheads*). **C:** In comparison, continuous-wave Doppler velocity spectrum from a patient with pulmonary hypertension and moderate tricuspid regurgitation shows increased peak velocity but with a rounded configuration.

appearance to carcinoid heart disease or rheumatic valvular disease (47). (See Chapter 13 for more details.)

Valvular Regurgitation in Normal Subjects

It should be pointed out that trivial to mild degrees of valvular regurgitation are common in the normal population, and its prevalence increases with age. The Doppler color-flow imaging technique is so sensitive that it detects trivial to mild degrees of valvular regurgitation not frequently appreciated even with careful auscultation. Klein and colleagues (48) used comprehensive color-flow imaging to assess the age-related prevalence of valvular regurgitation in 118 normal volunteers. Regurgitation of mitral, aortic, tricuspid, and pulmonary valves was detected in 48%, 11%, 65%, and 31% of subjects, respectively. Aortic regurgitation was not present in persons younger than 50 years. There was no influence of sex on the frequency of valvular regurgitation. Although not important hemodyn-

amically, Doppler detection of valvular regurgitation is useful in estimating intracardiac pressures. Trivial regurgitation detected by color-flow imaging does not warrant prophylaxis for bacterial endocarditis.

CLINICAL IMPACT

When a patient undergoes an echocardiographic evaluation for valvular heart disease, the variables listed below should be assessed using the integrated approach of 2D, continuous-wave and pulsed-wave Doppler, and color flow imaging. In some patients, TEE may be necessary.

1. LV dimension and systolic function
2. LV wall thickness and mass
3. Valvular morphology
4. Regurgitant jet area and extent
5. Valvular hemodynamics
   a. Stroke volume and cardiac output

b. Pressure gradients

c. Stenotic valve area

d. Effective regurgitant orifice area

e. Regurgitant volume and regurgitant fraction

f. Systolic flow reversal in pulmonary or hepatic vein

6. Pulmonary artery pressure

It should be emphasized that the determination of the severity of valvular lesions is based on all the available echocardiographic data (*integrated approach*). Any discrepancies between different measures of severity should be explained; for example, in a patient with a mean aortic pressure gradient of 55 mm Hg, the aortic valve does not appear to be severely stenotic on 2D imaging. Further evaluation shows that cardiac output is increased because of significant anemia, as reflected in an increase in LVOT velocity and TVI. The integrated echocardiographic approach should provide a complete assessment of valvular heart disease in most patients. When surgical intervention is needed, patients with suspected coronary artery disease or those at high risk will need coronary angiography. Hemodynamic evaluation by cardiac catheterization is necessary only when 2D echocardiography, Doppler hemodynamics, and color-flow imaging are not adequate (in about 5% of patients) or when there is a discrepancy between the clinical and 2D and Doppler echocardiographic findings in decision making and the discrepancy is not resolved by a repeat study and examination by a more experienced echocardiographer and physician.

Timing of Surgery for Valvular Disease

Patients with symptoms related to severe valvular heart disease usually require surgical or catheter-based intervention. It is easier to determine the timing of intervention in patients with stenotic lesions because the symptoms are an important factor in making this clinical decision. It is uncommon for asymptomatic patients with severe valvular stenosis to experience sudden death; however, it may be difficult to ascertain the extent of a patient's symptoms on the basis of the clinical history alone. It now is common clinical practice that the timing of surgery is determined by echocardiographic hemodynamic findings. If aortic stenosis is severe, with aortic velocity >5 m/sec, mean gradient >60 mm Hg, or aortic valve area <0.7 cm², it is reasonable to offer aortic valve replacement even in an asymptomatic, otherwise healthy patient because aortic stenosis continues to progress, with an average of 0.3 m/sec increase in aortic flow velocity each year (49). The timing of surgery is more difficult to determine in asymptomatic patients with severe valvular regurgitation; traditionally, surgical timing was based on LV dimension (LV end-systolic dimension ≥55 mm) or the development of LV systolic dysfunction (or both). This LV dimension criterion was found to be inappropriate for the timing of surgery in women because they rarely met this criterion (50). The dimension criterion was

derived from men, and women usually develop symptoms before reaching that degree of LV dilatation. Therefore, it is recommended that surgical correction of aortic regurgitation be considered at an earlier stage in women.

In patients with organic mitral regurgitation (structural abnormality of the mitral valve as opposed to functional mitral valve regurgitation), LV ejection fraction measured by echocardiography was the most powerful predictor of late survival, suggesting early surgical treatment even in the absence of symptoms, before LV dysfunction occurs (51), especially in patients with a flail mitral leaflet diagnosed on echocardiography. Ling and colleagues (52) at our institution demonstrated that patients with a flail leaflet who were treated medically had a significantly higher than expected mortality rate. At 10 years, the mean rate of heart failure, atrial fibrillation, and death or surgery was 63%, 30%, and 90%, respectively. Surgical correction of mitral regurgitation was associated with a decreased mortality rate. Therefore, in addition to the clinical history of patients with severe valvular heart disease, echocardiographic findings (hemodynamic or structural) have a decisive role in determining the timing of surgical intervention.

REFERENCES

1. Gorlin R, Gorlin SG. Hydraulic formula for calculation of the area of the stenotic mitral valve, other cardiac valves, and central circulatory shunts. I. *Am Heart J* 1951;41:1–29.

2. Nishimura RA, Rihal CS, Tajik AJ, Holmes DR Jr. Accurate measurement of the transmitral gradient in patients with mitral stenosis: a simultaneous catheterization and Doppler echocardiographic study. *J Am Coll Cardiol* 1994;24:152–158.

3. Enriquez-Sarano M, Bailey KR, Seward JB, Tajik AJ, Krohn MJ, Mays JM. Quantitative Doppler assessment of valvular regurgitation. *Circulation* 1993;87:841–848.

4. Enriquez-Sarano M, Tajik AJ, Bailey KR, Seward JB. Color flow imaging compared with quantitative Doppler assessment of severity of mitral regurgitation: influence of eccentricity of jet and mechanism of regurgitation. *J Am Coll Cardiol* 1993;21:1211–1219.

5. Callahan MJ, Tajik AJ, Su-Fan Q, Bove AA. Validation of instantaneous pressure gradients measured by continuous-wave Doppler in experimentally induced aortic stenosis. *Am J Cardiol* 1985;56:989–993.

6. Currie PJ, Seward JB, Reeder GS, et al. Continuous-wave Doppler echocardiographic assessment of severity of calcific aortic stenosis: a simultaneous Doppler-catheter correlative study in 100 adult patients. *Circulation* 1985;71:1162–1169.

7. Hegrenaes L, Hatle L. Aortic stenosis in adults: non-invasive estimation of pressure differences by continuous wave Doppler echocardiography. *Br Heart J* 1985;54:396–404.

8. Skjaerpe T, Hegrenaes L, Hatle L. Noninvasive estimation of valve area in patients with aortic stenosis by Doppler ultrasound and two-dimensional echocardiography. *Circulation* 1985;72:810–818.

9. Zoghbi WA, Farmer KL, Soto JG, Nelson JG, Quinones MA. Accurate noninvasive quantification of stenotic aortic valve area by Doppler echocardiography. *Circulation* 1986;73:452–459.

10. Oh JK, Taliercio CP, Holmes DR Jr, et al. Prediction of the severity of aortic stenosis by Doppler aortic valve area determination: prospective Doppler-catheterization correlation in 100 patients. *J Am Coll Cardiol* 1988;11:1227–1234.

11. Hatle L, Brubakk A, Tromsdal A, Angelsen B. Noninvasive assessment of pressure drop in mitral stenosis by Doppler ultrasound. *Br Heart J* 1978;40:131–140.

12. deFilippi CR, Willett DL, Brickner ME, et al. Usefulness of dobutamine echocardiography in distinguishing severe from nonsevere val

vular aortic stenosis in patients with depressed left ventricular function and low transvalvular gradients. *Am J Cardiol* 1995;75:191–194.

13. Pellikka PA, Roger VL, McCully RB, et al. Normal stroke volume and cardiac output response during dobutamine stress echocardiography in subjects without left ventricular wall motion abnormalities. *Am J Cardiol* 1995;76:881–886.

14. Rask LP, Karp KH, Eriksson NP. Flow dependence of the aortic valve area in patients with aortic stenosis: assessment by application of the continuity equation. *J Am Soc Echocardiogr* 1996;9:295–299.

15. Burwash IG, Thomas DD, Sadahiro M, et al. Dependence of Gorlin formula and continuity equation valve areas on transvalvular volume flow rate in valvular aortic stenosis. *Circulation* 1994;89:827–835.

16. Bermejo J, Garcia-Fernandez MA, Torrecilla EG, et al. Effects of dobutamine on Doppler echocardiographic indexes of aortic stenosis. *J Am Coll Cardiol* 1996;28:1206–1213.

17. Otto CM, Burwash IG, Legget ME, et al. Prospective study of asymptomatic valvular aortic stenosis: clinical, echocardiographic, and exercise predictors of outcome. *Circulation* 1997;95:2262–2270.

18. Hoffmann R, Flachskampf FA, Hanrath P. Planimetry of orifice area in aortic stenosis using multiplane transesophageal echocardiography. *J Am Coll Cardiol* 1993;22:529–534.

19. Roger VL, Tajik AJ, Reeder GS, et al. Effect of Doppler echocardiography on utilization of hemodynamic cardiac catheterization in the preoperative evaluation of aortic stenosis. *Mayo Clin Proc* 1996;71:141–149.

20. Abascal VM, Wilkins GT, Choong CY, et al. Echocardiographic evaluation of mitral valve structure and function in patients followed for at least 6 months after percutaneous balloon mitral valvuloplasty. *J Am Coll Cardiol* 1988;12:606–615.

21. Cannan CR, Nishimura RA, Reeder GS, et al. Echocardiographic assessment of commissural calcium: a simple predictor of outcome after percutaneous mitral balloon valvotomy. *J Am Coll Cardiol* 1997;29:175–180.

22. Nakatani S, Masuyama T, Kodama K, Kitabatake A, Fujii K, Kamada T. Value and limitations of Doppler echocardiography in the quantification of stenotic mitral valve area: comparison of the pressure half-time and the continuity equation methods. *Circulation* 1988;77:78–85.

23. Rifkin RD, Harper K, Tighe D. Comparison of proximal isovelocity surface area method with pressure half-time and planimetry in evaluation of mitral stenosis. *J Am Coll Cardiol* 1995;26:458–465.

24. Faletra F, Pezzano A Jr, Fusco R, et al. Measurement of mitral valve area in mitral stenosis: four echocardiographic methods compared with direct measurement of anatomic orifices. *J Am Coll Cardiol* 1996;28:1190–1197.

25. Song JK, Kang DH, Lee CW, et al. Factors determining the exercise capacity in mitral stenosis. *Am J Cardiol* 1996;78:1060–1062.

26. Fawzy ME, Mercer EN, Dunn B, al-Amri M, Andaya W. Doppler echocardiography in the evaluation of tricuspid stenosis. *Eur Heart J* 1989;10:985–990.

27. Perry GJ, Helmcke F, Nanda NC, Byard C, Soto B. Evaluation of aortic insufficiency by Doppler color flow mapping. *J Am Coll Cardiol* 1987;9:952–959.

28. Helmcke F, Nanda NC, Hsiung MC, et al. Color Doppler assessment of mitral regurgitation with orthogonal planes. *Circulation* 1987;75:175–183.

29. McCully RB, Enriquez-Sarano M, Tajik AJ, Seward JB. Overestimation of severity of ischemic/functional mitral regurgitation by color Doppler jet area. *Am J Cardiol* 1994;74:790–793.

30. Teague SM, Heinsimer JA, Anderson JL, et al. Quantification of aortic regurgitation utilizing continuous wave Doppler ultrasound. *J Am Coll Cardiol* 1986;8:592–599.

31. Samstad SO, Hegrenaes L, Skjaerpe T, Hatle L. Half time of the diastolic aortoventricular pressure difference by continuous wave Doppler ultrasound: a measure of the severity of aortic regurgitation? *Br Heart J* 1989;61:336–343.

32. Oh JK, Hatle LK, Sinak LJ, Seward JB, Tajik AJ. Characteristic Doppler echocardiographic pattern of mitral inflow velocity in severe aortic regurgitation. *J Am Coll Cardiol* 1989;14:1712–1717.

33. Levine RA, Triulzi MO, Harrigan P, Weyman AE. The relationship of mitral annular shape to the diagnosis of mitral valve prolapse. *Circulation* 1987;75:756–767.

34. Nishimura RA, McGoon MD, Shub C, Miller FA Jr, Ilstrup DM, Tajik AJ. Echocardiographically documented mitral-valve prolapse. Long-term follow-up of 237 patients. *N Engl J Med* 1985;313:1305–1309.

35. Marks AR, Choong CY, Sanfilippo AJ, Ferre M, Weyman AE. Identification of high-risk and low-risk subgroups of patients with mitral-valve prolapse. *N Engl J Med* 1989;320:1031–1036.

36. Zuppiroli A, Rinaldi M, Kramer-Fox R, Favilli S, Roman MJ, Devereux RB. Natural history of mitral valve prolapse. *Am J Cardiol* 1995;75:1028–1032.

37. Spain MG, Smith MD, Grayburn PA, Harlamert EA, DeMaria AN. Quantitative assessment of mitral regurgitation by Doppler color flow imaging: angiographic and hemodynamic correlations. *J Am Coll Cardiol* 1989;13:585–590.

38. Cape EG, Yoganathan AP, Weyman AE, Levine RA. Adjacent solid boundaries alter the size of regurgitant jets on Doppler color flow maps. *J Am Coll Cardiol* 1991;17:1094–1102.

39. Castello R, Pearson AC, Lenzen P, Labovitz AJ. Effect of mitral regurgitation on pulmonary venous velocities derived from transesophageal echocardiography color-guided pulsed Doppler imaging. *J Am Coll Cardiol* 1991;17:1499–1506.

40. Hall SA, Brickner E, Willett DL, Irani WN, Afridi I, Grayburn PA. Assessment of mitral regurgitation severity by Doppler color flow mapping of the vena contracta. *Circulation* 1997;95:636–642.

41. Enriquez-Sarano M, Seward JB, Bailey KR, Tajik AJ. Effective regurgitant orifice area: a noninvasive Doppler development of an old hemodynamic concept. *J Am Coll Cardiol* 1994;23:443–451.

42. Gorlin R, Dexter L. Hydraulic formula for the calculation of the cross-sectional area of the mitral valve during regurgitation. *Am Heart J* 1952;43:188–205.

43. Recusani F, Bargiggia GS, Yoganathan AP, et al. A new method for quantification of regurgitant flow rate using color Doppler flow imaging of the flow convergence region proximal to a discrete orifice. An in vitro study. *Circulation* 1991;83:594–604.

44. Enriquez-Sarano M, Sinak LJ, Tajik AJ, Bailey KR, Seward JB. Changes in effective regurgitant orifice throughout systole in patients with mitral valve prolapse: a clinical study using the proximal isovelocity surface area method. *Circulation* 1995;92:2951–2958.

45. Rossi A, Dujardin KS, Bailey KR, Seward JB, Enriquez-Sarano M. Rapid estimation of regurgitant volume by the proximal isovelocity surface area method in mitral regurgitation: can continuous-wave Doppler echocardiography be omitted? *J Am Soc Echocardiogr* 1998;11:138–148.

46. Horn RA, Oh JK, Click RL, et al. Intraoperative transesophageal echo determination of the severity of mitral regurgitation using proximal isovelocity surface area: correlation with double sampling dye curve. *J Am Soc Echocardiogr* 1996;9:374(abst).

47. Connolly HM, Crary JL, McGoon MD, et al. Valvular heart disease associated with fenfluramine-phentermine. *N Engl J Med* 1997;337:581–588.

48. Klein AL, Burstow DJ, Tajik AJ, et al. Age-related prevalence of valvular regurgitation in normal subjects: a comprehensive color flow examination of 118 volunteers. *J Am Soc Echocardiogr* 1990;3:54–63.

49. Roger VL, Tajik AJ. Progression of aortic stenosis in adults: new insights provided by Doppler echocardiography. *J Heart Valve Dis* 1993;2:114–118.

50. Klodas E, Enriquez-Sarano M, Tajik AJ, Mullany CJ, Bailey KR, Seward JB. Surgery for aortic regurgitation in women. Contrasting indications and outcomes compared with men. *Circulation* 1996;94:2472–2478.

51. Enriquez-Sarano M, Tajik AJ, Schaff HV, Orszulak TA, Bailey KR, Frye RL. Echocardiographic prediction of survival after surgical correction of organic mitral regurgitation. *Circulation* 1994;90:830–837.

52. Ling LH, Enriquez-Sarano M, Seward JB, et al. Clinical outcome of mitral regurgitation due to flail leaflet. *N Engl J Med* 1996;335:1417–1423.

CHAPTER 10

Prosthetic Valve Evaluation

Valve replacement usually is required for severe valvular heart disease, although increasingly valve repair is performed for a regurgitant lesion. No prosthetic valve is perfect, and a significant portion of cardiology practice is dedicated to following patients who have a prosthetic valve and to evaluating prosthetic valvular dysfunction when the patients present with cardiovascular symptoms. Prosthetic valves can be classified as either *tissue* or *mechanical* valves (Fig. 10-1). A tissue prosthesis is an actual valve or one made of biologic tissue from an animal (*bioprosthesis* or *heterograft)* or human (*homograft* or *allograft)* source. A mechanical valve is made of a nonbiologic material [e.g., pyrolitic carbon, polymeric silicone substances (Silastic), or titanium], as in a ball-cage (Starr-Edwards) or tilting-disk (St. Jude Medical) valve. Blood flow characteristics, hemodynamics, durability, and thromboembolic tendency vary depending on the type and size of each prosthesis and, more importantly, on patient characteristics. The physical examination of patients with a prosthetic valve is different from that of those with native valves, because prosthetic valves are inherently stenotic and may produce additional prosthetic sounds (caused by ball movement or disk closure). Therefore, it can be a clinical challenge to distinguish between abnormal and normal prosthetic valve sounds. The evaluation of prosthetic valves requires a thorough knowledge of the unique makeup and hemodynamic profiles of the different prostheses. Dysfunction of a native valve is usually suspected on the basis of abnormal findings on two-dimensional (2D) echocardiography, but it is more difficult to identify an abnormality of a prosthetic valve with transthoracic 2D echocardiography alone. At the Mayo Clinic, we rely more on Doppler and color-flow imaging as well as on transesophageal echocardiography (TEE) to detect dysfunction of prosthetic valves.

TWO-DIMENSIONAL ECHOCARDIOGRAPHY

Two-dimensional echocardiography can identify gross structural abnormalities of a prosthesis, such as dehiscence, vegetation, thrombus, or degeneration of a tissue prosthesis,

but its sensitivity for cardiac prosthetic dysfunction is hampered by difficulty in visualizing structures around and behind the cardiac prosthesis. Echo reflectance of the prosthetic material, attenuation of the ultrasound beam, and multiple ultrasound reverberations from the prosthesis result in difficulties in interpretation. Normally, it is easier to image a tissue prosthesis than a mechanical prosthesis. To identify the structural abnormalities associated with a prosthesis, it is important to understand the characteristics of the prosthesis and the surgical technique (Fig. 10-2).

DOPPLER AND COLOR-FLOW IMAGING

Doppler echocardiography reliably detects flow velocity across a prosthetic valve, thus permitting the determination of pressure gradients by using the modified Bernoulli equation (*Pressure gradient = 4 × Velocity*^{2}). An excellent correlation has been shown between Doppler and invasive dual-catheter pressure measurements made simultaneously across various prosthetic valves (Fig. 10-3) (1); however, several *in vitro* models of a normal disk prosthesis have demonstrated an overestimation of aortic prosthetic gradients determined by Doppler velocities in comparison with

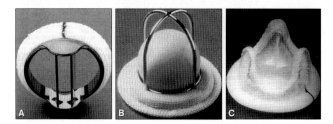

FIG. 10-1. Three popular types of valve prostheses. **A:** Bi-leaflet St. Jude prosthesis in fully opened position (there are two lateral major flow orifices and a minor central orifice). **B:** Starr-Edwards prosthesis (model 6120). **C:** Porcine heterograft (frame-mounted glutaraldehyde-preserved). (From Schaff HV. Prosthetic valves. In: Giuliani ER, Gersh BJ, McGoon MD, Hayes DL, Schaff HV, eds. *Mayo Clinic practice of cardiology,* 3rd ed. St. Louis: Mosby, 1996:1484–1496, with permission.)

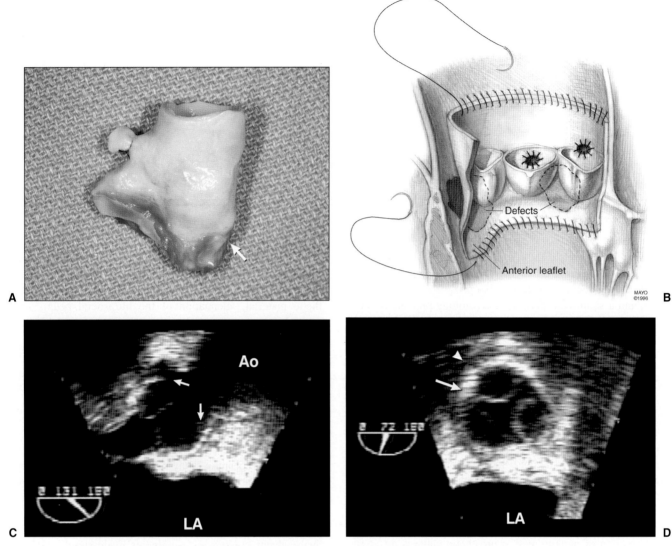

FIG. 10-2. A: Photograph of an aortic homograft specimen. *Arrow* indicates area of aortic annulus. A portion of coronary artery has a tie around it. **B:** Diagram of surgical technique for placement of an aortic homograft. Both the proximal and distal portions of the homograft are sutured to the native aorta, providing a potential space between the two structures. The allograft aortic valve is used as an intraaortic cylinder. In this diagram, the allograft anterior mitral leaflet is used to repair the defects created by endocarditis. **C:** Transesophageal echocardiographic appearance of normal aortic homograft. **Left:** Longitudinal view (131 degrees). **Right:** Short-axis view (72 degrees). This has a cylinder-in-cylinder appearance due to insertion of homograft (*arrows*) within the patient's aortic root (*arrowhead*). *Ao*, aorta. (**B** from Dearani JA, Orszulak TA, Schaff HV, Daly RC, Anderson BJ, Danielson GK. Results of allograft aortic valve replacement for complex endocarditis. *J Thorac Cardiovasc Surg* 1997;113:285–291, with permission.)

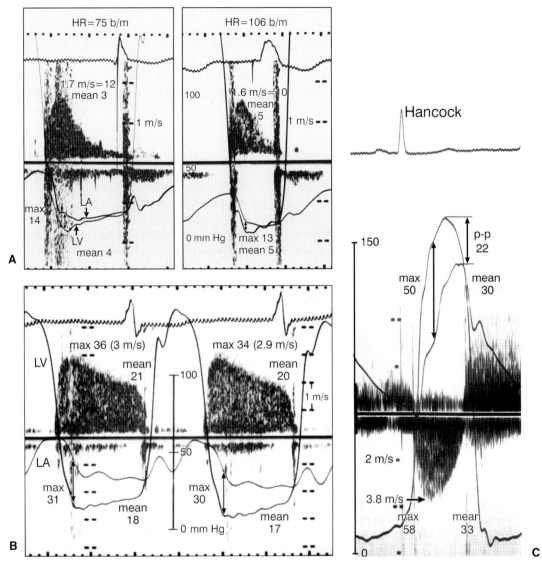

FIG. 10-3. A: Simultaneous Doppler and catheterization study of a normal mechanical mitral prosthesis. The correlation between the two techniques at different heart rates (*HR*) is good. *b/m*, beats per minute. **B:** Simultaneous continuous-wave Doppler and catheter pressure measurements [left ventricle (*LV*) and left atrium (*LA*)] in a patient with an obstructed Hancock mitral prosthesis. The maximal (36 versus 31 mm Hg) and mean (21 versus 18 mm Hg by Doppler and catheter, respectively) gradients derived from these two techniques correlate well. **C:** Simultaneous Doppler and catheterization study in a patient with a Hancock aortic prosthesis. The correlation between Doppler-derived and catheter-derived maximal (58 versus 50 mm Hg) and mean (33 versus 30 mm Hg) pressure gradients is good. A good correlation also was noted for the mechanical aortic prosthesis. Note that the peak-to-peak (*p-p*) gradient, which is a nonphysiologic assessment, underestimates the severity of obstruction (p-p gradient, 22 mm Hg; catheter-derived mean gradient, 30 mm Hg). (**B** and **C** from ref. 1, with permission.)

catheter-derived gradients (2,3). The highest catheter-derived gradient was found within the central orifice of the St. Jude prosthesis, and it decreased rapidly when the catheter was moved downstream (*pressure recovery phenomenon*). The discrepancy is smaller in a prosthesis with a larger ring and in a tissue prosthesis. The potential source of difference between Doppler-derived and catheter-derived prosthetic pressure gradients should be considered, but it has not been a major problem in the evaluation of a dysfunctional prosthesis. The continuity equation can be used to estimate the functional orifice area of prosthetic aortic and mitral valves (Chapter 9) (4–6). The *pressure half-time* (PHT) method used for stenosis of a native mitral valve *overestimates the area of mitral prosthesis* (4). The prosthetic valve is inherently stenotic in varying degrees in comparison with the respective native valve; therefore, flow velocity across a normal prosthetic valve is higher than that expected for a native valve. Normal prosthetic flow velocity (hence, maximal and mean pressure gradients) varies based on the type and size of the prosthesis, the location, and the cardiac output. Hence, it is important to know the normal ranges of flow velocities across a particular prosthesis for comparison with measured values. The Mayo echocardiography laboratory determined prospectively a range of normal Doppler values for each type of aortic, mitral, and tricuspid prosthesis in a large number of patients: 609, 456, and 82, respectively (Tables 10-1, 10-2, and 10-3) (7–9). Because the hemodynamics of a prosthesis depend on various factors, it is recommended that a baseline Doppler study be done in the early postoperative period ("fingerprint") so that it can be used as a reference for later comparison with later studies (10).

Regurgitation and obstruction both result in increased flow velocities across a prosthesis (Fig. 10-4). The increase in flow velocity indicates a smaller orifice when the prosthesis is obstructed or increased flow across the prosthesis when there is significant regurgitation. Other helpful Doppler features differentiate obstruction from regurgitation (Table 10-4). When a prosthesis is obstructed, flow velocities increase and the PHT is prolonged (for mitral and tricuspid valve prostheses). The increase in flow velocity across the obstructed aortic prosthesis is not accompanied by increased LV outflow tract (LVOT) velocity, but it is with a severe regurgitation. When the velocity across the mitral or tricuspid prosthesis is increased because of severe regurgitation, PHT is normal or shortened and LVOT velocity is decreased because forward flow is decreased (Fig. 10-5). High cardiac output state also increases velocity across a prosthesis, and it can be confirmed by recording increased flow velocities across all cardiac orifices (LVOT, atrioventricular valve, RV outflow tract).

OBSTRUCTION

When a prosthetic valve becomes obstructed, the motion of the disk, ball, or leaflets decreases; however, it is difficult to visualize and yet more difficult to quantitate the restriction of excursion by surface 2D echocardiographic examination. TEE may be able to visualize normal and abnormal (Fig. 10-6A) prosthetic valve motion. The most accurate method for detecting and quantitating the degree of prosthetic obstruction is Doppler echocardiography (Fig. 10-6B and 10-7). The Doppler study must be performed with various transducer positions to ensure that the maximal jet velocity across the stenosed prosthesis is recorded. From the Doppler velocity tracing, maximal and mean pressure gradients and the effective valve area can be calculated using the same formulae and equations described for the native valve (see Chapter 9). It is important to remember, however, that increased flow velocity *per se* does not always indicate prosthetic obstruction. The velocity can be increased without stenosis, in a high-output state, and in the presence of severe prosthetic regurgitation (Table 10-4). In patients with a mitral prosthesis, PHT is useful for determining whether increased velocity (i.e., gradient) is secondary to increased flow or to obstruction. PHT as well as peak flow velocity are expected to increase when a mitral or tricuspid prosthesis is obstructed (see Fig. 10-4).

If an aortic prosthesis is obstructed, flow velocity (hence, pressure gradient) increases unless cardiac output decreases. Increased flow velocity across an aortic prosthesis is also expected with severe prosthetic regurgitation (hence, increased flow through the aortic prosthesis). With aortic obstruction (as in aortic stenosis), however, LV flow velocity is normal to slightly decreased and increases with aortic regurgitation. The LVOT and aortic prosthesis velocity or

TABLE 10-1. *Doppler hemodynamic profiles of 609 normal aortic valve prostheses*

Type of prosthesis	No. of prostheses	Peak velocity (m/sec)	Mean gradient (mm Hg)	LVOT TVI/AV TVI
Heterograft	214	2.4 ± 0.5	13.3 ± 6.1	0.44 ± 0.21
Ball-cage	160	3.2 ± 0.6	23.0 ± 8.8	0.32 ± 0.09
Björk-Shiley	141	2.5 ± 0.6	13.9 ± 7.0	0.40 ± 0.10
St. Jude Medical	44	2.5 ± 0.6	14.4 ± 7.7	0.41 ± 0.12
Homograft	30	1.9 ± 0.4	7.7 ± 2.7	0.56 ± 0.10
Medtronic-Hall	20	2.4 ± 0.2	13.6 ± 3.3	0.39 ± 0.09
Total	609	2.6 ± 0.7	15.8 ± 8.3	0.40 ± 0.16

AV, aortic valve; LVOT, left ventricular outflow tract; TVI, time velocity integral.
From ref. 7, with permission.

TABLE 10-2. *Doppler hemodynamic profiles of 456 normal mitral valve prostheses*

Type of prosthesis	No. of prostheses	Peak velocity (m/sec)	Mean gradient (mm Hg)	Effective area (cm^2)
Heterograft	150	1.6 ± 0.3	4.1 ± 1.5	2.3 ± 0.7
Ball-cage	161	1.8 ± 0.3	4.9 ± 1.8	2.4 ± 0.7
Björk-Shiley	79	1.7 ± 0.3	4.1 ± 1.6	2.6 ± 0.6
St. Jude Medical	66	1.6 ± 0.4	4.0 ± 1.8	3.0 ± 0.8

From ref. 8, with permission.

TABLE 10-3. *Doppler hemodynamic profiles of 82 normal tricuspid valve prostheses*

Type of prosthesis	No. of prostheses	Peak velocity (m/sec)	Mean gradient (mm Hg)	Pressure half-time (m/sec)
Heterograft	41	1.3 ± 0.2	3.2 ± 1.1	146 ± 39
Ball-cage	33	1.3 ± 0.2	3.1 ± 0.8	144 ± 46
St. Jude Medical	7	1.2 ± 0.3	2.7 ± 1.1	108 ± 32
Björk-Shiley	1	1.3	2.2	144
Total	82	1.3 ± 0.2	3.1 ± 1.0	142 ± 42

From ref. 9, with permission.

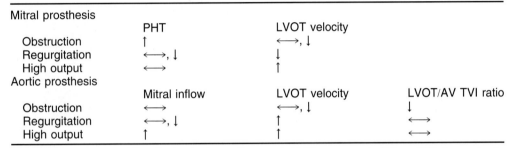

TABLE 10-4. *Interpretation of increased prosthesis flow velocity*

Mitral prosthesis

	PHT	LVOT velocity	
Obstruction	↑	⟷, ↓	
Regurgitation	⟷, ↓	↓	
High output	⟷	↑	

Aortic prosthesis

	Mitral inflow	LVOT velocity	LVOT/AV TVI ratio
Obstruction	⟷	⟷, ↓	↓
Regurgitation	⟷, ↓	↑	⟷
High output	↑	↑	⟷

AV, aortic valve; LVOT, left ventricular outflow tract; PHT, pressure half-time; TVI, time velocity integral. ↑, increased; ↓, decreased; ⟷, no change.

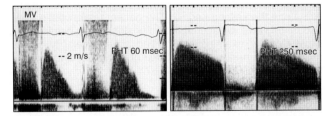

FIG. 10-4. Continuous-wave Doppler examination of regurgitant **(left)** and obstructed **(right)** mitral valve (*MV*) prostheses. In both regurgitant and obstructive prostheses, velocities increase and are higher than 2 m/sec, hence increased mean gradient. However, pressure half-time (*PHT*) from the regurgitant mitral prosthesis was not prolonged (PHT, 60 msec) but was prolonged to 250 msec in the obstructed prosthesis.

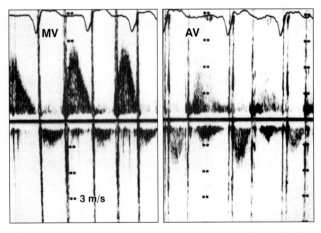

FIG. 10-5. Continuous-wave Doppler spectra in a patient with severe mitral valve prosthetic regurgitation who has mitral and aortic prostheses. **Left:** The mitral velocity is increased to 3 m/sec, but its pressure half-time is normal (60 msec), indicating increased flow across the mitral prosthesis without obstruction. **Right:** The velocity through the aortic prosthesis is relatively low (1.6 m/sec), indicating that the increased mitral flow velocity is due to mitral valve regurgitation rather than to a high systemic cardiac output. If mitral flow velocity is increased because of increased systemic cardiac output, peak velocity across the aortic prosthesis is expected to increase as well. *AV*, aortic valve; *MV*, mitral valve.

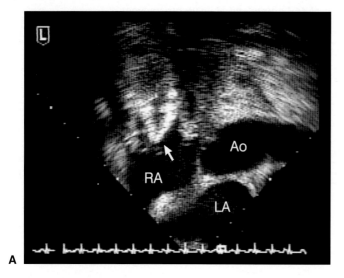

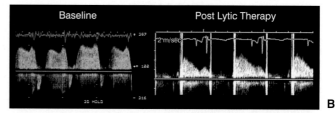

FIG. 10-6. A: Longitudinal transesophageal view of a St. Jude Medical tricuspid valve prosthesis (*arrow*). The disks of the prosthesis failed to move because of thrombotic obstruction. *Ao*, aorta. **B:** Continuous-wave Doppler echocardiographic examination from the apex showed peak velocity across the tricuspid valve prosthesis to be close to 2 m/sec, with a slight respiratory variation that is typical for a tricuspid valve prosthesis. The velocity and mean gradient returned to baseline after 2 days of treatment with continuous infusion of streptokinase. After thrombolytic therapy, peak velocity was 1 m/sec, with a mean gradient of 4 mm Hg.

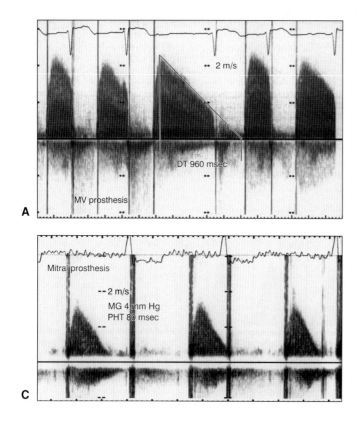

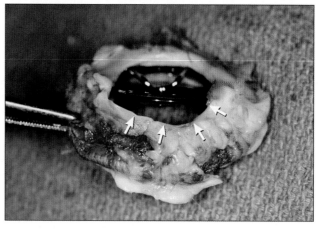

FIG. 10-7. A: Continuous-wave Doppler examination of an obstructed mechanical mitral valve (*MV*) prosthesis. Peak velocity was 2.2 m/sec, with a pressure half-time of 290 msec. *DT*, deceleration time. **B:** At the time of operation, thrombus as well as pannus formation (*arrows*) was identified along the sewing ring. **C:** The patient underwent a second mitral valve replacement, and postoperative continuous-wave Doppler examination showed a peak velocity of 1.6 m/sec, with a mean gradient (*MG*) of 4 mm Hg and a pressure half-time (*PHT*) of 80 ms.

time velocity integral (TVI) ratio are helpful in differentiating increased flow velocity across an aortic prosthesis due to a prosthetic obstruction (the ratio decreases, ≤0.2) from increased velocity due to regurgitation (the ratio remains normal, ≥0.3) (Table 10-4).

CALCULATION OF EFFECTIVE PROSTHETIC ORIFICE AREA

The PHT method overestimates the area of a mitral prosthesis. The constant 220 was derived for stenotic lesions of a native mitral valve and not for calculating the effective orifice area of a mitral prosthesis. When there is no significant aortic or mitral regurgitation, the continuity equation is a valid and better method for determining the area of mitral and aortic prostheses (4).

$$MP\ area = LVOT\ area \times (LVOT\ TVI/MP\ TVI)$$

$$= LVOT\ diameter^2$$

$$\times\ 0.785 \times LVOT\ TVI/MP\ TVI$$

where MP is mitral prosthesis, *LVOT TVI* is *LVOT* time velocity integral, and *MP TVI* is time velocity integral of mitral prosthesis inflow velocity obtained by continuous-wave Doppler echocardiography.

The area of an aortic prosthesis can be estimated by the product of the TVI ratio (between LVOT and aortic prosthesis) and the area of the LVOT, using the continuity equation.

$$AP\ area = LVOT\ area \times (LVOT\ TVI/AP\ TVI)$$
$$= SROD^2 \times 0.785 \times LVOT\ TVI/AP\ TVI$$

where AP is aortic prosthesis, and SROD is sewing-ring outer diameter.

LVOT area is calculated from the outer diameter of the sewing ring. Aortic prosthesis TVI is obtained from continuous-wave Doppler velocity of the aortic prosthesis. Effective prosthesis area and (LVOT TVI/AP TVI) calculated from normal mitral and aortic prostheses, respectively, are shown in Tables 10-1–10-3.

THROMBOLYTIC THERAPY FOR OBSTRUCTION OF PROSTHETIC VALVES

Formation of thrombus is responsible for 90% of obstructive prosthetic valves with or without additional pannus formation. Thrombus may be visualized with TEE, and its size is important in deciding on an optimal treatment strategy. Unless there is a large thrombus (>5 mm), thrombolytic therapy appears to be a reasonable treatment for left-sided as well as right-sided heart prosthetic valve obstruction (11). The initial success rate is 80% to 85%, and the rate of recurrent obstruction is 18% according to metaanalysis (12). The efficacy of different thrombolytic agents for valve obstruction and their risks are listed in Tables 10-5 and 10-6. The decision of whether to treat with thrombolysis or surgery should be made on the basis of each patient's clinical condition, functional status, valve location, and comorbid status.

REGURGITATION

Color-flow imaging is the principal technique used to detect prosthetic valvular regurgitation. The same criteria used for native valvular regurgitation are used for semi-quantitation of prosthetic valvular regurgitation. However, color-flow imaging of a mitral or tricuspid prosthesis with the transthoracic approach frequently is unsatisfactory (especially for a mechanical prosthesis) because of the marked attenuation of the ultrasound beam by the prosthesis and reverberations in the atrium. TEE circumvents these limitations.

It should be noted that a small amount of "built-in" regurgitation is normal for all types of prostheses (closing volume). On transthoracic color-flow imaging, regurgitant flow is detected in about 30% of normally functioning prostheses. The detection rate increases to 44% and 95% for aortic and mitral prostheses, respectively, when transesophageal color-flow imaging is used. The normal prosthetic regurgitant flow has the following features (13):

1. Regurgitant jet area <2 cm^2 and jet length <2.5 cm in the mitral position.
2. Jet area <1 cm^2 and length <1.5 cm in the aortic position.
3. Characteristic flow pattern (one central jet for Medtronic-Hall, two curved side jets for Starr-Edwards, two unequal side jets for Björk-Shiley, and two side and one central jet for St. Jude Medical), as shown in Fig. 10-8.

Pathologic regurgitation should be distinguished from the "normal" regurgitation of a prosthetic valve using the above criteria, the morphology of the valve, and the number and location of regurgitant jets.

As in the assessment of regurgitation of native valves, an integrated approach is required for the evaluation of prosthetic valvular regurgitation, with color-flow imaging being one of several determinants. Because transthoracic color-flow imaging has more limitations with prosthetic valves, it is essential to obtain complete hemodynamic data using pulsed-wave and continuous-wave Doppler before considering TEE. For aortic prosthetic regurgitation, the following should be determined: PHT of the jet, mitral inflow pattern, diastolic reversal flow in the descending thoracic aorta, and regurgitant fraction. For mitral prosthetic regurgitation, the following should be determined: mitral

TABLE 10-5. *Efficacy of thrombolytic agents used for valve obstruction, stratified by valve position*

	Agent					
	Streptokinase		Urokinase		Tissue-type plasminogen activator	
Position	No.[a]	%	No.[a]	%	No.[a]	%
Mitral	75/88	85	10/23	43	7/11	64
Aortic	24/32	75	11/15	73	1/1	100
Tricuspid	18/20	90	3/5	60	2/3	67
Pulmonary	5/5	100	1/1	100	—	—
Total	122/145	84[b]	25/44	57	10/15	67

[a] Number of patients in whom therapy was successful of total number treated.
[b] P < 0.5 for streptokinase versus urokinase.
From ref. 12, with permission.

TABLE 10-6. *Mortality and morbidity with thrombolytic therapy for valve obstruction, stratified by valve position*

Position	No. of valves	Death		Embolism		Stroke		Nondisabling bleed	
		No.	%	No.	%	No.	%	No.	%
Mitral	122	9	7	12	10	5	4	9/85	11
Aortic	51	3	6	5	10	1	2	2/24	8
Tricuspid	28	0	0	1	4	0	0	9/28	32
Pulmonary	6	0	0	0	0	0	0	0/6	0
Total	207	12[a]	6	18	9	6	3	20/143	14[b]

[a] Seven deaths were attributed to failed thrombolytic therapy, and five were directly related to the induced lytic state.
[b] Includes those not categorized by valve position.
From ref. 12, with permission.

inflow peak velocity and PHT, intensity of the mitral regurgitant continuous-wave Doppler signal, and regurgitant fraction. The proximal isovelocity surface area (PISA) method described for a native mitral valve may be helpful in assessing the severity of prosthetic mitral regurgitation. Although a regurgitant jet in the LA may not be detected with surface echocardiography, proximal flow can be visualized clearly enough that the PISA method can be used. These variables can be assessed and interpreted as for native valves (Chapter 9). The following variables indicate severe aortic prosthetic regurgitation:

1. PHT of regurgitant jet ≤250 m/sec
2. Restrictive mitral inflow pattern (in acute aortic regurgitation)
3. Holodiastolic reversals in the descending thoracic aorta
4. Regurgitant fraction ≥55%

The following variables indicate severe mitral prosthetic regurgitation:

1. Increased mitral inflow peak velocity (≥2.5 m/sec) and normal mitral inflow PHT (≤150 m/sec)

2. Dense mitral regurgitant continuous-wave Doppler signals
3. Regurgitant fraction ≥55%
4. Effective regurgitant orifice ≥0.35 cm^2
5. Systolic flow reversals in the pulmonary vein

TRANSESOPHAGEAL ECHOCARDIOGRAPHY

Prosthetic valve stenosis (or obstruction) is usually diagnosed by detecting increased flow velocity with precordial continuous-wave Doppler; it is difficult to visualize the decreased motion of the prosthetic valve by precordial 2D echocardiography. The motion of the prosthetic valve, especially that of mitral and tricuspid prosthetic valves, is more clearly seen with TEE. A TEE view of decreased disk-opening motion in a patient with obstruction of a mitral disk prosthesis is shown in Fig. 10-9. Disk motion may become intermittently abnormal, and prolonged TEE observation may be necessary if such intermittent abnormality is suspected clinically (Fig. 10-10). All TEE probes are equipped with continuous-wave Doppler and are able to measure reliably transmitral flow velocities and pressure gradients.

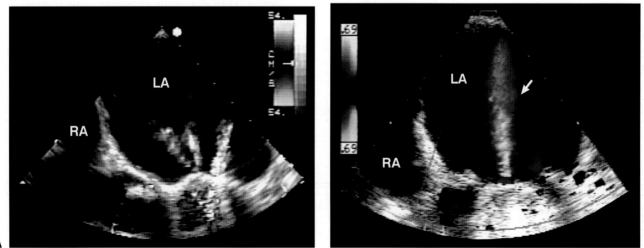

FIG. 10-8. Transesophageal echocardiographic examination of normal mitral prostheses with closing volume. Three jets **(left)** in St. Jude prosthesis and a large central jet *(arrow)* in Medtronic-Hall prosthesis **(right)**.

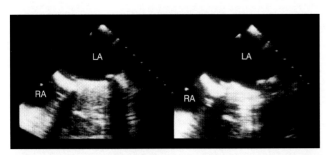

FIG. 10-9. Transesophageal echocardiographic (horizontal basal view or zero-degree) examination of an obstructed mitral disk prosthesis. The systolic **(left)** and diastolic **(right)** frames demonstrate a marked decrease in the opening angle of the mitral disk (approximately 30 degrees). Normally, an angle of 60 degrees is expected.

TEE is essential in the evaluation of mitral and tricuspid prosthetic regurgitation and, sometimes, aortic prosthetic regurgitation (14–16). The transesophageal view of the atria is not hindered by the prosthesis, and the origin and extent of mitral or tricuspid prosthetic regurgitation are clearly demonstrated by TEE. When aortic prosthetic regurgitation originates from the posterior aspect of the prosthesis, TEE is also quite helpful, but anteriorly located aortic prosthetic regurgitation may not be seen from the transesophageal window, especially in the presence of a mitral prosthesis.

TEE is also useful in the evaluation of dehiscence, endocarditis, ring abscess, and intracardiac (especially atrial) mass or thrombi in the presence of a prosthetic valve (17) (Fig. 10-11 to 10-13). These applications are discussed separately in other chapters (Chapters 9 and 14). Hemolysis is an uncommon but alarming complication of mitral valve replacement or repair. It is associated with distinct patterns of mitral regurgitation flow disturbance. Collision of a mitral regurgitation jet against a cardiac structure with rapid deceleration is the most common reason for hemolysis (Fig. 10-14). TEE has demonstrated that regurgitation through a small orifice is associated with greater hemolysis (18).

CLINICAL IMPACT

Hemodynamic cardiac catheterization is rarely necessary anymore to evaluate prosthetic valvular dysfunction. With 2D, Doppler, color flow, and transesophageal imaging, if necessary, a comprehensive evaluation of prosthetic valves is feasible. However, it should be emphasized that the integrated approach is key for the most comprehensive evaluation (by transthoracic and TEE examination) to provide the following information:

1. Ventricular size and function
2. Structural integrity of the prosthesis
3. Hemodynamic data
   a. Peak flow velocity
   b. Maximal and mean gradients
   c. PHT or deceleration time

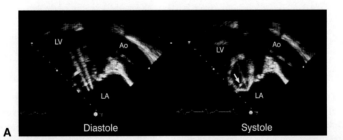

FIG. 10-10. Intermittent failure to close one of the mitral prosthesis disks, resulting in intermittent severe mitral regurgitation detected with transesophageal echocardiography. **A:** Normal motion of a St. Jude mitral prosthesis seen from the transesophageal longitudinal plane. During diastole, the two disks are almost parallel. Each disk moves about 85 degrees toward the left atrium (*LA*) during systole. A small echo-dense structure (*arrow*) is seen. **B:** Intermittently, one of the disks failed to close during systole (*arrow*). **C:** Color-flow imaging during normal closure **(left)** showed a mild degree of periprosthetic regurgitation (*arrow*), but during a failed closure **(right)**, there was severe prosthetic mitral regurgitation (*arrows*). At surgery, a small fibrin-thrombus material was found caught between the two disks. The prosthesis was replaced with a Starr-Edwards prosthesis. *Ao*, aorta.

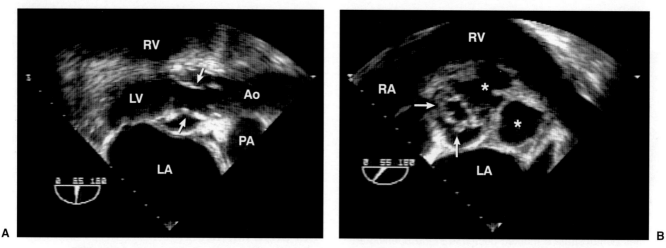

FIG. 10-11. A: Long-axis view of abnormal aortic homograft by multiplane transesophageal imaging during systole. The aortic homograft (inside cylinder) is compressed (*arrows*) by blood flow in the space between the native aorta and the homograft because of the dehiscence of the proximal anastomosis. *Ao*, aorta; *PA*, pulmonary artery. **B:** Short-axis multiplane transesophageal view of the same homograft during systole. The allograft aortic valve (*arrows*) is compressed and surrounded by aneurysmal cavities (*asterisk*). Continuous-wave Doppler examination demonstrated a high-velocity (4.5 m/sec) jet across the compressed homograft.

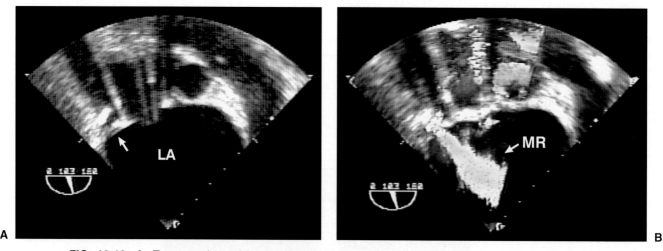

FIG. 10-12. A: Transesophageal long-axis view of the dehisced sewing ring (*arrow*) of a St. Jude mitral prosthesis from the lateral mitral annulus. **B:** Color-flow imaging shows severe mitral regurgitation (*MR*) from the dehiscence.

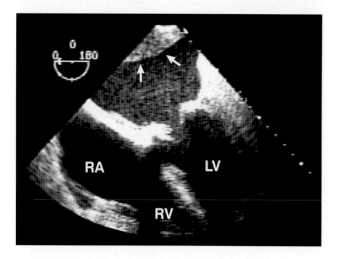

FIG. 10-13. Large thrombus (*arrows*) in the left atrium in a patient with a mitral bioprosthesis. The left atrium is dilated and filled with spontaneous echocontrast.

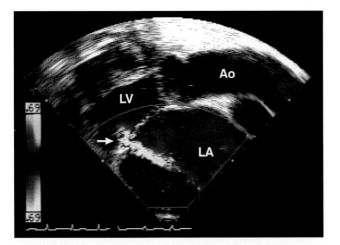

FIG. 10-14. Longitudinal transesophageal view of repaired mitral valve with mitral regurgitation in a patient in whom hemolytic anemia developed. Blood flow hits a portion of the annulus ring (*arrow*) and is reflected acutely into the left atrium (*LA*). At surgery, the annulus ring was found to be torn at that location. *Ao,* aorta.

d. Effective valve area
e. Pulmonary artery pressure
f. Diastolic filling profile
g. Color-flow jet area
h. Pulmonary vein (for mitral regurgitation) or descending aorta (for aortic regurgitation) or hepatic vein (for tricuspid regurgitation) flow reversals
i. Regurgitant fraction

With all the data obtained from a comprehensive echocardiographic examination, the most appropriate management strategy can be formulated for most patients with prosthetic valves.

CAVEATS

Occasionally, the discrepancy between Doppler-derived and catheter-derived pressure gradients across a prosthetic valve is significant (1). A catheter-derived gradient may overestimate the actual transmitral gradient. When pulmonary capillary wedge pressure is used as a surrogate of LA pressure instead of transseptal catheterization for direct measurements of LA pressure, the transmitral pressure gradient may be overestimated because of a phase shift and dampened contour. For an aortic disk prosthesis, the Doppler-derived maximal instantaneous gradient may be higher than the catheter-derived maximal gradient because the pressure within the prosthetic orifice is higher than that in the ascending aorta (pressure recovery). The duration of

peak Doppler velocity is quite short, however, and the mean pressure gradient determined by the two methods should be similar.

REFERENCES

1. Burstow DJ, Nishimura RA, Bailey KR, et al. Continuous wave Doppler echocardiographic measurement of prosthetic valve gradients: a simultaneous Doppler-catheter correlative study. *Circulation* 1989;80: 504–514.
2. Baumgartner H, Khan S, DeRobertis M, Czer L, Maurer G. Discrepancies between Doppler and catheter gradients in aortic prosthetic valves *in vitro*: a manifestation of localized gradients and pressure recovery. *Circulation* 1990;82:1467–1475.
3. Stewart SF, Nast EP, Arabia FA, Talbot TL, Proschan M, Clark RE. Errors in pressure gradient measurement by continuous wave Doppler ultrasound: type, size and age effects in bioprosthetic aortic valves. *J Am Coll Cardiol* 1991;18:769–779.
4. Dumesnil JG, Honos GN, Lemieux M, Beauchemin J. Validation and applications of mitral prosthetic valvular areas calculated by Doppler echocardiography. *Am J Cardiol* 1990;65:1443–1448.
5. Dumesnil JG, Honos GN, Lemieux M, Beauchemin J. Validation and applications of indexed aortic prosthetic valve areas calculated by Doppler echocardiography. *J Am Coll Cardiol* 1990;16:637–643.
6. Chafizadeh ER, Zoghbi WA. Doppler echocardiographic assessment of the St. Jude Medical prosthetic valve in the aortic position using the continuity equation. *Circulation* 1991;83:213–223.
7. Miller FA, Callahan JA, Taylor CL, Larson-Keller JJ, Seward JB. Normal aortic valve prosthesis hemodynamics: 609 prospective Doppler examinations. *Circulation* 1989;80(Suppl 2):II–169(abst).
8. Lengyel M, Miller FA Jr, Taylor CL, Larson-Keller JJ, Seward JB, Tajik AJ. Doppler hemodynamic profiles of 456 clinically and echonormal mitral valve prostheses. *Circulation* 1990;82 Suppl 3:III–43(abst).
9. Connolly HM, Miller FA Jr, Taylor CL, Naessens JM, Seward JB, Tajik AJ. Doppler hemodynamic profiles of 82 clinically and echocardiographically normal tricuspid valve prostheses. *Circulation* 1993;88:2722–2727.
10. Wiseth R, Hegrenaes L, Rossvoll O, Skjaerpe T, Hatle L. Validity of an early postoperative baseline Doppler recording after aortic valve replacement. *Am J Cardiol* 1991;67:869–872.
11. Silber H, Khan SS, Matloff JM, Chaux A, DeRobertis M, Gray R. The St. Jude valve: thrombolysis as the first line of therapy for cardiac valve thrombosis. *Circulation* 1993;87:30–37.
12. Hurrell DG, Schaff HV, Tajik AJ. Thrombolytic therapy for obstruction of mechanical prosthetic valves. *Mayo Clin Proc* 1996;71:605–613.
13. Mohr-Kahaly S, Kupferwasser I, Erbel R, Oelert H, Meyer J. Regurgitant flow in apparently normal valve prostheses: improved detection and semiquantitative analysis by transesophageal two-dimensional color-coded Doppler echocardiography. *J Am Soc Echocardiogr* 1990;3:187–195.
14. Nellessen U, Schnittger I, Appleton CP, et al. Transesophageal two-dimensional echocardiography and color Doppler flow velocity mapping in the evaluation of cardiac valve prostheses. *Circulation* 1988;78:848–855.
15. Taams MA, Gussenhoven EJ, Cahalan MK, et al. Transesophageal Doppler color flow imaging in the detection of native and Björk-Shiley mitral valve regurgitation. *J Am Coll Cardiol* 1989;13:95–99.
16. Khandheria BK, Seward JB, Oh JK, et al. Value and limitations of transesophageal echocardiography in assessment of mitral valve prostheses. *Circulation* 1991;83:1956–1968.
17. Garcia MJ, Vandervoort P, Stewart WJ, et al. Mechanisms of hemolysis with mitral prosthetic regurgitation: study using transesophageal echocardiography and fluid dynamic simulation. *J Am Coll Cardiol* 1996;27:399–406.
18. Khandheria BK. Transesophageal echocardiography in the evaluation of prosthetic valves. *Cardiol Clin* 1993;11:427–436.

CHAPTER 11

Infective Endocarditis

Infective endocarditis is an uncommon but potentially fatal illness with nonspecific symptoms and signs. The incidence of endocarditis in Olmsted County, Minnesota, was 4.9 per 100,000 person-years (1). The incidence is higher among patients who have valvular heart disease (rheumatic valve, bicuspid aortic valve, mitral valve prolapse), congenital heart disease, or a prosthetic valve and among intravenous drug users. The hydraulics of the blood stream is important in the pathogenesis of endocarditis. It is associated with a high-pressure source (i.e., aorta, left ventricle) that drives blood at a high velocity through a narrow orifice (coarctation, ductus arteriosus, ventricular septal defect, regurgitant aortic or mitral valve) into a low-pressure chamber (2). Most commonly, the mitral and aortic valves are involved with endocarditis, but right-side cardiac valve involvement is not uncommon in intravenous drug users. Because the consequence of untreated endocarditis is devastating and often fatal, it is of utmost importance that the underlying infection and its complications be recognized promptly and treated appropriately.

Since the first M-mode echocardiographic observation of valvular vegetation in 1973 (3), the role of echocardiography in diagnosing infective endocarditis has grown in conjunction with improvements in resolution and technologic advances, including Doppler, color-flow imaging, and transesophageal echocardiography (TEE). Currently, echocardiography is the diagnostic procedure of choice in detecting valvular vegetation. A patient with endocarditis may have negative findings on blood culture if the infection is partially treated or caused by an esoteric or fastidious organism. Therefore, the diagnosis of infective endocarditis may be suggested on the basis of echocardiography, even in the absence of positive blood culture (or before such positive culture is reported).

NEW DIAGNOSTIC CRITERIA

Since 1981, the diagnosis of endocarditis has been based on Von Reyn criterion (4) according to which, a definite diagnosis of infective endocarditis is possible only from direct histologic examination of the involved tissue or positive findings on bacteriologic studies. Therefore, even in patients who show the symptoms and signs typical of the acute stage of infection, the diagnosis of infective endocarditis cannot be made without positive findings on blood culture. At the time Von Reyn criterion was established, the diagnostic capability of echocardiography was not fully appreciated because modalities other than transthoracic M-mode and two-dimensional (2D) imaging were not available. With further advances in echocardiography, including TEE, that improved the detection of vegetation, abscesses, and other complications of endocarditis, echocardiography currently provides major diagnostic information. Certain characteristics of valvular masses seen with echocardiography are sometimes as diagnostic as the detection of typical organisms in blood culture, such as HACEK (*Haemophilus* spp., *Actinobacillus actinomycetemcomitans, Cardiobacterium hominis, Eikenella* spp., and *Kingella kingae*) (Table 11-1).

To improve the sensitivity and specificity of diagnostic criteria for infective endocarditis, new major and minor criteria (Duke criteria) have been proposed (5). The two major and six minor criteria are listed in Table 11-1. The diagnosis of infective endocarditis is definite if a patient meets two major criteria, or one major criterion plus three minor criteria, or five minor criteria (Table 11-2). Echocardiographic evidence typical for endocarditis is one of the major criteria, and it can be used to diagnose infective endocarditis definitely in combination with three minor criteria, even in the absence of typical positive blood culture results. These new Duke criteria were compared with the Von Reyn criterion by Bayer et al. (6), in 63 febrile patients with suspected infective endocarditis. More cases were classified as "definite" with the Duke criteria, and the detection of vegetation with echocardiography was important in the diagnosis of endocarditis in 57% of patients.

ECHOCARDIOGRAPHIC APPEARANCE

The echocardiographic features typical for infective endocarditis are (a) an oscillating intracardiac mass on a valve

TABLE 11-1. *Definition of terms used in the proposed diagnostic criteria*

Major criteria
 Positive blood culture for infective endocarditis
  Typical microorganisms for infective endocarditis from two separate blood cultures
   Viridans streptococci, *Streptococcus bovis,* HACEK group *or*
   Community-acquired *Staphylococcus aureus* or enterococci, in the absence of a primary focus, *or*
  Persistently positive blood culture, defined as microorganism consistent with infective endocarditis from
   Blood cultures drawn more than 12 hours apart *or*
   All of three, or majority of four or more, separate blood cultures, with first and last drawn at least 1 hour apart
 Evidence of endocardial involvement
  Positive echocardiogram for infective endocarditis:
   Oscillating intracardiac mass on valve or supporting structures or in the path of regurgitant jets or on iatrogenic devices, in the absence of an alternative anatomical explanation *or*
   Abscess *or*
   New partial dehiscence of prosthetic valve *or*
  New valvular regurgitation (worsening or changing of preexisting murmur not sufficient)
Minor criteria
 Predisposition: predisposing heart condition or intravenous drug use
 Fever: ≥38.0°C
 Vascular phenomena: arterial embolism, septic pulmonary infarcts, mycotic aneurysm, intracranial hemorrhage, Janeway lesions
 Immunologic phenomena: glomerulonephritis, Osler nodes, Roth spots
 Echocardiogram: consistent with infective endocarditis but not meeting major criterion as noted above
 Microbiologic evidence: positive blood culture but not meeting major criterion as noted above or serologic evidence of active infection with organism consistent with infective endocarditis

HACEK, *Haemophilus* spp., *Actinobacillus actinomycetemcomitans, Cardiobacterium hominis, Eikenella* spp., and *Kingella kingae.*

TABLE 11-2. *New criteria for diagnosis of infective endocarditis*

Definite infective endocarditis
 Pathologic criteria
  Microorganisms: demonstrated by culture or histology in a vegetation, or in a vegetation that has embolized, or in an intracardiac abscess
                 or
  Pathologic lesions: vegetation or intracardiac abscess present, confirmed by histology showing active endocarditis
 Clinical criteria (see definitions of terms in Table 11-1)
  2 major criteria *or*
  1 major and 3 minor criteria *or*
  5 minor criteria
Possible infective endocarditis
 Findings consistent with infective endocarditis that fall short of "definite" but not "rejected"
Rejected
 Firm alternate diagnosis explaining evidence of infective endocarditis
                 or
 Resolution of infective endocarditis syndrome, with antibiotic therapy for 4 d or less,
                 or
 No pathologic evidence of infective endocarditis at surgery or autopsy, with antibiotic therapy for 4 d or less

or supporting structure or in the path of a regurgitation jet or on an iatrogenic device, (b) abscesses, (c) new partial dehiscence of a prosthetic valve, or (d) new valvular regurgitation. The initial attachment site to the mitral and tricuspid valve is usually on the atrial side, but an aortic vegetation usually starts from the ventricular surface (Fig. 11-1). Vegetation appears as an echogenic (mobile) mass or masses attached to the valve, endocardial surface, or prosthetic materials in the heart (Fig. 11-2 to 11-4). Vegetations can be linear, round, irregular, or shaggy, and they frequently show high-frequency flutter or oscillations (7). The sensitivity of 2D echocardiography for the detection of vegetation depends on its size, location, and the echocardiographic window used. The sensitivity of detecting vegetation with transthoracic 2D echocardiography is 65% to 80% and 95% with TEE (8–11). The diagnostic yield of

transthoracic echocardiography (TTE) is especially poor in prosthetic valve endocarditis; however, the sensitivity for TEE in this clinical setting is 90%. Patients with suspected endocarditis should have a baseline echocardiographic examination and serial studies as dictated by their clinical and hemodynamic status. The vegetations in endocarditis on the right side are larger (Fig. 11-2) than those in endocarditis on the left side, with an average diameter of 70 mm (12).

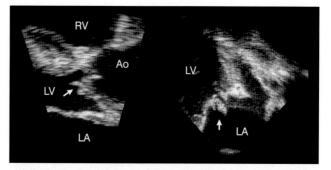

FIG. 11-1. Transesophageal echocardiograms of aortic **(left)** and mitral **(right)** valve demonstrating typical attachment sites for vegetation. The initial attachment site to the aortic valve is usually on the ventricular surface (*left arrow*), and for the mitral and tricuspid valves, it is on the atrial side (*right arrow*). It results from the high-velocity blood jet from the high-pressure chamber to the low-pressure chamber. When the regurgitation jet is eccentric, as in mitral valve prolapse, satellite vegetation lesions can develop along the direction of the mitral regurgitation jet, as shown in Fig. 11-3. *Ao,* aorta.

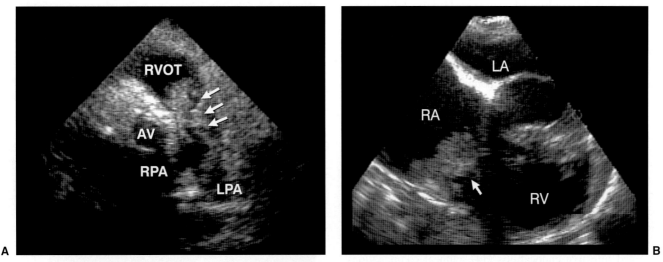

FIG. 11-2. A: Transthoracic echocardiogram of the pulmonary valve involved with a large *Candida* vegetation (*arrows*) in a young patient who had been chronically ill after aortic valve replacement. **B:** Transverse view of transesophageal echocardiographic imaging of the tricuspid valve with large vegetation (*arrow*). *AV*, aortic valve; *LPA*, left pulmonary artery; *RPA*, right pulmonary artery; *RVOT*, right ventricular outflow tract.

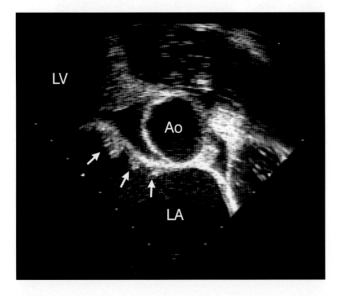

FIG. 11-3. Transesophageal echocardiogram of the left atrium (*LA*) and the anterior mitral leaflet with multiple polypoid satellite lesions (*arrows*) of endocarditis in a 64-year-old man with *Staphylococcus aureus* endocarditis and flail posterior mitral leaflet. He presented with stroke. The satellite lesions are related to the eccentric mitral regurgitant jet from the infected flail posterior leaflet. *Ao*, aorta.

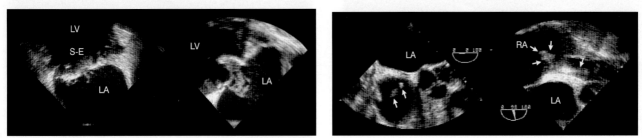

FIG. 11-4. Transesophageal echocardiography (TEE) improves the detection of valvular vegetation, especially when associated with a prosthetic valve **(A)** and intracardiac devices **(B)**. **A:** TEE of vegetation attached to the atrial side of a mitral prosthesis. The left image shows a linear mobile vegetation attached to the Starr-Edwards (*S-E*) mitral prosthesis and the right frame shows a large mobile vegetation attached to the mitral bioprosthesis. **B:** Transverse **(left)** and longitudinal **(right)** multiplane TEE of a patient with vegetations associated with the pacemaker wires (*arrows*).

In the study by San Roman et al. (12), TEE did not improve on the diagnostic accuracy of TTE in detecting vegetations associated with right-sided endocarditis. Vegetations frequently persist after successful medical treatment of endocarditis (13); however, persistent vegetations are not independently associated with late complications.

COMPLICATIONS

The complications of endocarditis arise primarily from vegetations, destruction of valvular or intracardiac structures (Figs. 11-5 to 11-12), and subsequent hemodynamic deterioration (Table 11-3). Therefore, the presence and characteristics of vegetations affect the prognosis and clinical course of patients with infective endocarditis. In a comprehensive prospective study of 204 patients with documented infective endocarditis (14), clinical complications were correlated with TTE findings and characteristics of vegetations. When no significant valvular abnormalities were detected on echocardiography, no patient developed congestive heart failure, required valve replacement, or failed to have improvement with antibiotic treatment; however, peripheral and cerebral emboli occurred in 15% of patients who had no detectable vegetations. In left-side valve endocarditis, the frequency of clinical complications increases with the greater mobility, extent, consistency (less calcific), and size of a vegetation. When vegetation size was larger than 11 mm, 50% of patients or more developed at least one complication of infective endocarditis. In patients with tricuspid valve endocarditis, pulmonary embolism was the most common complication (69%).

Mügge and colleagues (9), using TEE, also noted that the patients with a large (>10 mm) vegetation involving the mitral valve or attached to it were at increased risk for embolic events, but vegetation size was not correlated with the degree of heart failure and patient survival. Hence, echocardiography is useful not only in diagnosing endocarditis but, by characterizing valvular vegetation, in predicting potential complications. Valve replacement is re-

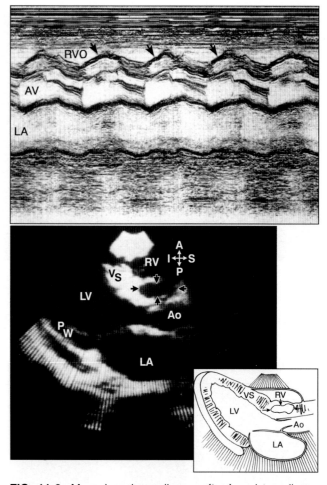

FIG. 11-6. M-mode echocardiogram **(top)** and two-dimensional (2D) parasternal long-axis view **(bottom)** showing an aortic root abscess. **Top:** An echo-free space (*arrows*) anterior to the aortic valve (*AV*) is recorded. **Bottom:** 2D echo image shows a cavity in the anterior aortic root extending into the upper ventricular septum (*VS*). A small pericardial effusion is present behind the posterior wall (*PW*); this occurs frequently with the cardiac abscess. *Ao,* aorta.

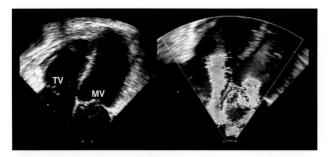

FIG. 11-5. Transesophageal view of abnormal mitral (*MV*) and tricuspid (*TV*) valves due to *Staphylococcus aureus* endocarditis. No active vegetations are present, but the anterior mitral leaflet has a perforation and aneurysmal cavity, and the septal tricuspid leaflet has a flail segment, with severe regurgitation from MV and TV.

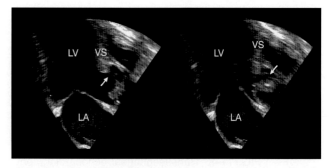

FIG. 11-7. Transesophageal echocardiogram of abscess cavity (*arrow*) extending from the infected aortic valve to the ventricular septum (*VS*). This 44-year-old patient developed high-grade atrioventricular block. The organism was *Staphylococcus aureus*.

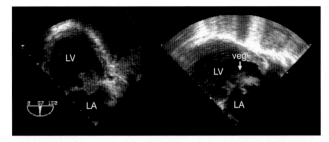

FIG. 11-8. Transesophageal echocardiography (TEE) in a 28-year-old woman with *Staphylococcus aureus* endocarditis. Note the vegetation (*veg*) attached to the mitral valve, specifically the anterior leaflet of the mitral valve. As a complication, the anterior leaflet of the mitral valve with the vegetation was dehisced (*arrow*) from the mitral annulus, causing severe mitral regurgitation. The patient suddenly developed pulmonary edema and a loud murmur during the treatment of endocarditis, and TEE demonstrated the dehiscence as a complication of the endocarditis.

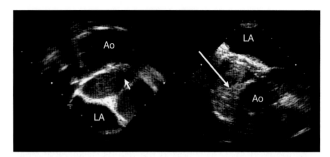

FIG. 11-11. Similar process as in Fig. 11-9 in a patient with an aortic prosthesis complicated by endocarditis and a large abscess cavity filled with infectious materials (*arrow*). *Ao*, aorta.

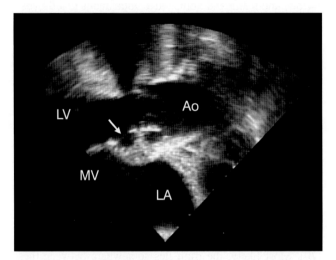

FIG. 11-9. Transesophageal long-axis view showing a small abscess cavity (*arrow*) at the aortic and mitral valve intervalvular fibrosa. The increased echodensity in the region posterior to the aortic valve is consistent with an infectious process. *Ao*, aorta; *MV*, mitral valve.

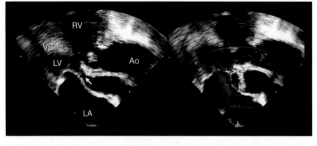

FIG. 11-12. Transesophageal echocardiogram of an aortic prosthesis and a large pseudoaneurysm in an asymptomatic patient who was treated for aortic prosthesis endocarditis. Routine follow-up examination showed a large pseudoaneurysmal cavity that communicates with the left ventricular (*LV*) outflow tract (*arrow*). *Ao*, aorta.

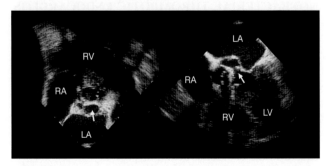

FIG. 11-10. Transesophageal echocardiogram of an aortic prosthesis with endocarditis complicated by an abscess cavity in the mitral-aortic intervalvular fibrosa. **Left:** Short-axis view of the aortic prosthesis shows an echo-free space (*arrow*) between the aortic prosthesis and LA, consistent with an abscess cavity. **Right:** Transverse view shows the communication (*arrow*) between the echo-free aneurysmal space and the left ventricular (*LV*) outflow tract.

TABLE 11-3. *Complications of endocarditis*

Structural
  Cusp or leaflet rupture/flail
Perforation
Abscess
Aneurysm
Fistula
Dehiscence of prosthetic valve
Pericardial effusion (more frequent with abscess)
Hemodynamic compromise
  Valvular regurgitation
  Acute mitral regurgitation
  Acute aortic regurgitation
  Premature mitral valve closure
  Restrictive mitral inflow pattern
  Valvular stenosis
  Shunt
  Congestive heart failure
Embolization
  Systemic
  Cerebral
  Pulmonary

quired in one-third of patients with endocarditis on the left side and in less than 10% of those with involvement of the right side. Therefore, detection of valvular vegetation does not necessarily indicate valvular replacement. Surgery is indicated when a patient's hemodynamic condition deteriorates, high-degree conduction abnormalities develop, mobile vegetation persists after an embolic event, the vegetation becomes larger while being treated with antibiotics, or an abscess cavity develops.

Mullany et al. (15) reported the results of surgical treatment of culture-positive active endocarditis in 151 patients between 1961 and 1991 at the Mayo Clinic. The operative mortality was 26%. The most important determinants of mortality were abscess and renal failure. On multivariate analysis, the most important adverse determinants of long-term survival were heart failure, renal failure, and prosthetic valve endocarditis. The risk of reoperation was 23% and 36% at 5 and 10 years, respectively.

TRANSESOPHAGEAL ECHOCARDIOGRAPHY

Because of improved resolution, the sensitivity of TEE for detecting vegetations or complications of endocarditis is much higher than that of TTE. It has been suggested that TEE should be performed in all patients in whom endocarditis is suspected or diagnosed, but the clinical impact of such an approach requires further evaluation. The sensitivity of TTE in detecting the complications of endocarditis is not optimal, and TEE improves the diagnostic sensitivity of detecting these complications (see Figs. 11-6 to 11-12) (16–18). TEE should be performed in all patients suspected to have such abnormalities (these patients usually have persistent fever, heart failure without a demonstrable cause, persistent positive findings on blood cultures) or in whom TTE findings are nondiagnostic.

Anatomic complications of endocarditis were found to be more common than previously thought when consecutive patients with aortic valve endocarditis were examined with TEE (17,18). Of patients with aortic valve endocarditis, 44% had involvement of subaortic structures: mitral-aortic intervalvular fibrosa aneurysm (see Figs. 11-9 and 11-10) or perforation with communication into the left atrium (LA), aortic annular abscess, or perforation of the mitral leaflet. This observation is important because these complications may be responsible for unexplained hemodynamic compromise. The subaortic complications were suggested by TTE examination in only one-half of these patients.

Occasionally, endocarditis involves the aortic wall, resulting in a mycotic aneurysm. An example visualized by TEE is shown in Fig. 11-13.

TRANSESOPHAGEAL ECHOCARDIOGRAPHY OR NO TRANSESOPHAGEAL ECHOCARDIOGRAPHY

The optimal use and timing of TEE in patients with suspected or documented infective endocarditis have been de-

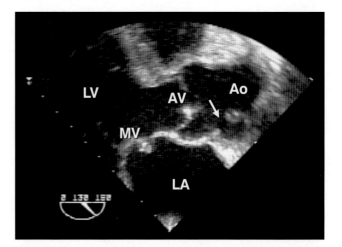

FIG. 11-13. Longitudinal view (130-degree transducer position) of multiplane transesophageal echocardiography demonstrating a mycotic aneurysm in the ascending aorta (*arrow*) and mitral and aortic valve vegetations in a 59-year-old man with *Enterococcus* endocarditis. *Ao*, aorta; *AV*, aortic valve; *MV*, mitral valve.

bated intensively. The conservative view is that TEE should not be used to make a diagnosis of endocarditis in patients with a low clinical probability of the disease; it is recommended only for patients with a prosthetic valve and in whom a TTE examination was either technically inadequate or indicated an intermediate probability of endocarditis (19). The other and more liberal view is that almost all patients who have suspected or known endocarditis and no contraindication to TEE should undergo the procedure because both positive and negative test results are important to the management and outcome of a patient's condition (20). Most likely, the truth lies somewhere between these views. Currently, TEE is the diagnostic procedure of choice for excluding vegetation and for detecting complications of infective endocarditis.

NONBACTERIAL THROMBOTIC ENDOCARDITIS

When the endocardial surface is traumatized, a series of events may lead to platelet deposition, thus creating a nonsterile platelet fibrin thrombus that causes nonbacterial thrombotic endocarditis. Libman and Sacks (21) described four cases of valvular and mural lesions of verrucous appearance designated as *atypical verrucous*. This condition usually involves the mitral valve and is found most commonly on the basal portion of the mitral valve, but it can extend to the chordal structure or papillary muscles. These lesions are difficult to see on TTE. The important condition associated with nonbacterial thrombotic endocarditis is antiphospholipid syndrome. The diagnostic criteria for this syndrome were proposed in 1987 and include one episode of thrombosis or two miscarriages plus anticardiolin levels greater than 200 units or a positive test for lupus anticoagulants on two occasions more than 8 weeks apart.

Many of these patients have a cerebral embolic event, and endocardial valvular lesions are noted on echocardiography (see Chapter 13). Other cardiac involvement includes pericardial effusion and myocardial dysfunction. The mitral valve is usually involved, causing regurgitation; the aortic valve is involved less frequently. The usual nonbacterial thrombotic vegetations accumulate at the distal tip of the mitral leaflet, most likely with endothelial trauma. The mitral vegetation in a patient with antiphospholipid syndrome reportedly disappeared after 9 months of treatment with warfarin (22). A metastatic tumor also can involve cardiac valves and produce lesions similar to those in Libman-Sacks endocarditis. This is called *marantic endocarditis* and occurs most commonly with Hodgkin disease and adenocarcinoma of the lung, pancreas, stomach, and colon.

CLINICAL CAVEATS

The echocardiographic detection of valvular vegetation has several limitations and pitfalls. Other valvular lesions, such as marked myxomatous degeneration of the mitral valve, nonbacterial thrombotic endocarditis, or tumor thrombus attached to the valve (i.e., papilloma), may simulate or mask vegetations. When a valve is sclerotic, calcified, or prosthetic, it is more difficult to visualize a vegetation. TEE may be useful under these circumstances. Because vegetations are usually mobile and may not be seen in certain imaging planes, multiple tomographic planes should be used. Clinical presentation, laboratory data (blood culture results and sedimentation rate), and systemic symptoms need to be incorporated into the interpretation of the echocardiographic findings. A healed vegetation is more fibrotic and refractile than a new active one.

REFERENCES

1. Steckelberg JM, Melton LJ III, Ilstrup DM, Rouse MS, Wilson WR. Influence of referral bias on the apparent clinical spectrum of infective endocarditis. *Am J Med* 1990;88:582–588.
2. Rodbard S. Blood velocity and endocarditis. *Circulation* 1963;27:18–28.
3. Dillon JC, Feigenbaum H, Konecke LL, Davis RH, Chang S. Echocardiographic manifestations of valvular vegetations. *Am Heart J* 1973;86:698–704.
4. Von Reyn CF, Levy BS, Arbeit RD, Friedland G, Crumpacker CS. Infective endocarditis: an analysis based on strict case definitions. *Ann Intern Med* 1981;94:505–518.
5. Durack DT, Lukes AS, Bright DK, Duke Endocarditis Service. New criteria for diagnosis of infective endocarditis: utilization of specific echocardiographic findings. *Am J Med* 1994;96:200–209.
6. Bayer AS, Ward JI, Ginzton LE, Shapiro SM. Evaluation of new clinical criteria for the diagnosis of infective endocarditis. *Am J Med* 1994;96:211–219.
7. Roy P, Tajik AJ, Giuliani ER, Schattenberg TT, Gau GT, Frye RL. Spectrum of echocardiographic findings in bacterial endocarditis. *Circulation* 1976;53:474–482.
8. Erbel R, Rohmann S, Drexler M, et al. Improved diagnostic value of echocardiography in patients with infective endocarditis by transesophageal approach: a prospective study. *Eur Heart J* 1988;9:43–53.
9. Mügge A, Daniel WG, Frank G, Lichtlen PR. Echocardiography in infective endocarditis: reassessment of prognostic implications of vegetation size determined by the transthoracic and the transesophageal approach. *J Am Coll Cardiol* 1989;14:631–638.
10. Shively BK, Gurule FT, Roldan CA, Leggett JH, Schiller NB. Diagnostic value of transesophageal compared with transthoracic echocardiography in infective endocarditis. *J Am Coll Cardiol* 1991;18:391–397.
11. Taams MA, Gussenhoven EJ, Bos E, et al. Enhanced morphological diagnosis in infective endocarditis by transoesophageal echocardiography. *Br Heart J* 1990;63:109–113.
12. San Roman JA, Vilacosta I, Zamorano JL, Almeria C, Sanchez-Harguindey L. Transesophageal echocardiography in right-sided endocarditis. *J Am Coll Cardiol* 1993;21:1226–1230.
13. Vuille C, Nidorf M, Weyman AE, Picard MH. Natural history of vegetations during successful medical treatment of endocarditis. *Am Heart J* 1994;128:1200–1209.
14. Sanfilippo AJ, Picard MH, Newell JB, et al. Echocardiographic assessment of patients with infective endocarditis: prediction of risk for complications. *J Am Coll Cardiol* 1991;18:1191–1199.
15. Mullany CJ, Chua YL, Schaff HV, et al. Early and late survival after surgical treatment of culture-positive active endocarditis. *Mayo Clin Proc* 1995;70:517–525.
16. Daniel WG, Mügge A, Martin RP, et al. Improvement in the diagnosis of abscesses associated with endocarditis by transesophageal echocardiography. *N Engl J Med* 1991;324:795–800.
17. Bansal RC, Graham BM, Jutzy KR, Shakudo M, Shah PM. Left ventricular outflow tract to left atrial communication secondary to rupture of mitral-aortic intervalvular fibrosa in infective endocarditis: diagnosis by transesophageal echocardiography and color flow imaging. *J Am Coll Cardiol* 1990;15:499–504.
18. Karalis DG, Bansal RC, Hauck AJ, et al. Transesophageal echocardiographic recognition of subaortic complications in aortic valve endocarditis: clinical and surgical implications. *Circulation* 1992;86:353–362.
19. Lindner JR, Case RA, Dent JM, Abbott RD, Scheld WM, Kaul S. Diagnostic value of echocardiography in suspected endocarditis. An evaluation based on the pretest probability of disease. *Circulation* 1996;93:730–736.
20. Khandheria BK. Suspected bacterial endocarditis: to TEE or not to TEE. *J Am Coll Cardiol* 1993;21:222–224.
21. Libman E, Sacks B. A hitherto undescribed form of valvular and mitral endocarditis. *Arch Intern Med* 1924;33:701–737.
22. Skyrme-Jones RA, Wardrop CA, Wiles CM, Fraser AG. Transesophageal echocardiographic demonstration of resolution of mitral vegetations after warfarin in a patient with the primary antiphospholipid syndrome. *J Am Soc Echocardiogr* 1995;8:251–256.

CHAPTER 12

Cardiomyopathies

In 1995, the World Health Organization/International Society and Federation of Cardiology Task Force (1) on the definition and classification of cardiomyopathies redefined cardiomyopathy as "disease of the myocardium associated with cardiac dysfunction." Previously, it was defined as "heart muscle disease of unknown cause." The Task Force recommended that cardiomyopathies be classified by the dominant pathophysiologic mechanism or etiologic/pathogenic factor (Table 12-1), thus the following classification: (a) *dilated cardiomyopathy,* (b) *hypertrophic cardiomyopathy,* (c) *restrictive cardiomyopathy,* and (d) *arrhythmogenic right ventricular* (RV) *cardiomyopathy.* Each of these four classes of cardiomyopathy has distinctive morphologic and functional characteristics, with salient echocardiographic features.

1. Dilated cardiomyopathy is characterized by dilatation and impaired contraction of the left ventricle (LV) or both the LV and RV.

2. Hypertrophic cardiomyopathy is characterized by hypertrophy of the LV or RV (or both); the hypertrophy usually is asymmetric and involves the ventricular septum. LV cavity size usually is normal or decreased; a subset of the patients has LV outflow tract (LVOT) obstruction.

3. Restrictive cardiomyopathy is characterized by restrictive filling and decreased diastolic volume of either or both ventricles, with normal or near-normal systolic function and wall thickness. The atria are dilated because the stiff ventricles cause restrictive diastolic filling.

4. Arrhythmogenic RV cardiomyopathy (RV dysplasia) is caused by progressive fibrofatty replacement of the RV myocardium; occasionally, the LV is involved, with relative sparing of the septum.

Although cardiomyopathy can be classified in most patients on the basis of the clinical features and echocardiographic findings, the morphologic and functional features overlap, especially in patients with cardiomyopathy of advanced stage. Diastolic function becomes "restrictive" (grade 3 to 4 diastolic dysfunction) during the decompensation or end stage of any cardiomyopathy, regardless of the underlying lesion or classification. The unusual as well as the typical echocardiographic features of the four classes of cardiomyopathy are described in this chapter.

The Task Force also recommended that specific cardiomyopathies be used to describe heart muscle diseases that are associated with specific cardiac or systemic disorders (see Table 12-1). Echocardiographic findings in systemic illnesses are described in Chapter 13.

DILATED CARDIOMYOPATHY

Two-Dimensional Echocardiography

Dilated cardiomyopathy is the primary indication for cardiac transplantation, and the prevalence in Olmsted County, Minnesota, was 37 per 100,000 (from 1975 to 1984) (2). It is characterized by a dilated LV cavity and decreased global systolic function (Fig. 12-1). Both end-diastolic and end-systolic dimensions and volumes are moderately to markedly increased, and the variables of systolic function [ejec-

TABLE 12-1. *Classification of cardiomyopathies*

Cardiomyopathies	Specific cardiomyopathies
Dilated cardiomyopathy	Ischemic cardiomyopathy
Hypertrophic cardiomyopathy	Valvular cardiomyopathy
	Hypertensive cardiomyopathy
Restrictive cardiomyopathy	Inflammatory cardiomyopathy
Arrhythmogenic right ventricular cardiomyopathy	Metabolic cardiomyopathy
	General system disease
Unclassified cardiomyopathies	Muscular dystrophy
	Neuromuscular disorders
	Sensitivity and toxic reaction
	Peripartum cardiomyopathy

From ref. 1, with permission.

153

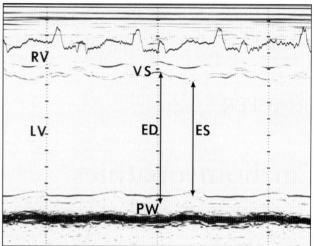

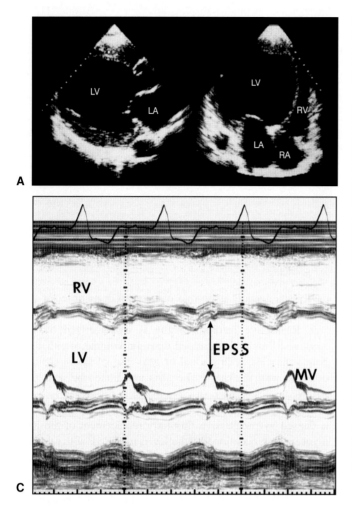

FIG. 12-1. A: Typical two-dimensional echocardiogram of dilated cardiomyopathy; systolic frame from parasternal long-axis **(left)** and apical four-chamber views **(right)**. The left ventricular (*LV*) cavity is markedly dilated, wall thickness is normal, and function is severely reduced. **B:** Typical M-mode echocardiogram of dilated cardiomyopathy at the mid-ventricular (or papillary muscle) level. Both end-diastolic (*ED*) and end-systolic (*ES*) dimensions are increased (78 mm and 68 mm, respectively). Ejection fraction calculated from these dimensions: $(ED^2 - ES^2)/ED^2 \times 100\% = 24\%$. Wall thickening is globally reduced. *PW*, posterior wall; *VS*, ventricular septum. **C:** At the mitral valve (*MV*) level, valve opening is reduced because of low cardiac output, and increased E-point septal separation (*EPSS*) of 30 mm indicates decreased systolic function.

tion fraction (EF), fractional shortening, stroke volume, and cardiac output] are uniformly decreased (3). Wall thickness varies but typically is within normal limits; however, LV mass is uniformly increased. Usually, contractility is reduced globally, but superimposed regional wall motion abnormalities can also be present. Similar findings occur in patients with extensive myocardial ischemia, myocarditis, alcoholic cardiomyopathy, hemochromatosis, sarcoidosis, acute catecholamine crisis, or doxorubicin (Adriamycin) toxicity.

Secondary features in dilated cardiomyopathy include dilated mitral annulus and incomplete coaptation of the mitral leaflets responsible for the associated functional mitral regurgitation, evidence of low cardiac output (decreased excursion of mitral leaflets), enlarged atrial cavities, RV enlargement, and apical mural thrombus.

It is recommended that echocardiographic screening of immediate family members of a patient with dilated cardiomyopathy be performed because of the high incidence (24.2%) of familial dilated cardiomyopathy (4). Clinical attributes of this familial disease have not been identified.

Doppler (Pulsed-Wave, Continuous-Wave) and Color-Flow Imaging

Doppler echocardiography is useful for determining cardiac output, pulmonary artery pressure, and mitral inflow filling pattern (i.e., diastolic function). Cardiac output is routinely measured using the LVOT time velocity integral (TVI) and diameter (see Chapter 6). Mitral inflow filling patterns provide insight into LV filling pressures as well as into diastolic function.

Although patients with dilated cardiomyopathy have similar global systolic dysfunction, their clinical symptoms and hemodynamic status can differ markedly. One group of these patients may be minimally symptomatic, whereas another group may have chronic heart failure symptoms. Doppler and color-flow imaging provide important hemodynamic information that is helpful in assessing LV filling pressures, management strategy, and prognosis.

Patients who are compensated have near-normal stroke volume and cardiac output and impaired relaxation pattern

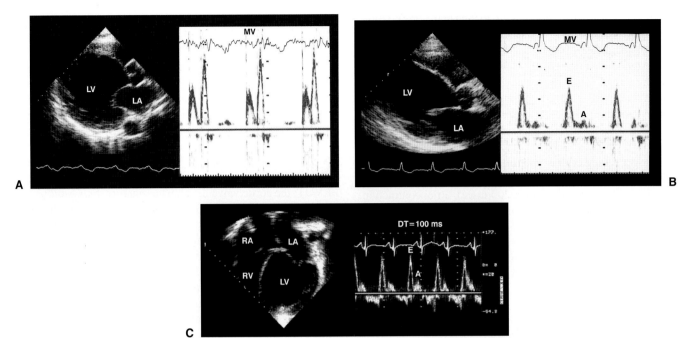

FIG. 12-2. A: Two-dimensional parasternal long-axis view of typical dilated cardiomyopathy **(left)** and pulsed-wave Doppler velocity recording **(right)** of mitral valve (*MV*) inflow showing a relaxation abnormality pattern with increased A velocity. Patients with this type of diastolic filling pattern usually have minimal to mild symptoms, despite severe left ventricular (*LV*) systolic dysfunction. Two-dimensional parasternal long-axis view **(B)**, and apical view **(C)** of typical dilated cardiomyopathy **(left)** and MV inflow velocity pattern **(right)** of restrictive physiology, with a markedly decreased A velocity and an increased E/A ratio. Deceleration time (*DT*) of mitral E velocity is shortened. Patients with this type of diastolic filling have increased filling pressure and symptomatic congestive heart failure.

as the diastolic filling abnormality (Fig. 12-2). Patients who have more advanced and decompensated dilated cardiomyopathy have a decreased stroke volume (LVOT TVI is decreased) and a restrictive diastolic filling pattern because of decreased compliance and increased LV filling pressures (5). The evolution of diastolic dysfunction from an impaired relaxation pattern to a restrictive filling pattern was demonstrated elegantly in an animal model with tachycardia-induced dilated cardiomyopathy (6). Of the various diastolic filling variables, deceleration time (DT) has the most

prognostic value. The shorter the DT (i.e., more restrictive diastolic filling), the worse the prognosis (7,8). As a patient's heart failure is treated, diastolic filling becomes less restrictive and deceleration time increases. The persistence of the restrictive filling after therapy is associated with a high mortality and transplantation rate. Patients with reversible restrictive filling have a high probability of improvement and excellent survival (Fig. 12-3) (9,10). The status of pulmonary artery pressure estimated from tricuspid regurgitation velocity is also prognostic in dilated car-

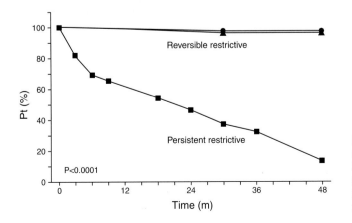

FIG. 12-3. Survival curves—free from heart transplantation—of patients with dilated cardiomyopathy. Mortality plus heart transplantation was significantly higher in patients with a persistent restrictive filling pattern than in patients with reversed restrictive filling to nonrestrictive filling after treatment. *m*, months. (Modified from ref. 9, with permission.)

diomyopathy (11). Patients with a tricuspid regurgitation velocity greater than 3 m/sec have a higher mortality, a higher incidence of heart failure, and more frequent hospitalization than those with a lower velocity. High tricuspid regurgitation velocities usually are seen in patients who have a restrictive diastolic filling pattern (12). Therefore, a restrictive diastolic filling pattern and high tricuspid regurgitation velocity identify patients who are at increased risk for death and heart failure.

Proper timing of diastolic filling may be important in optimizing cardiac output (Fig. 12-4). If the PR interval becomes prolonged (longer than 200 msec), atrial contraction may occur before early diastolic filling is completed. If the PR interval is too short (60 to 100 msec), the atrium may contract at the same time the ventricle contracts. Therefore, optimizing the PR interval with the guidance of Doppler, mitral inflow may increase cardiac output and the patient's symptoms may improve (13).

HYPERTROPHIC CARDIOMYOPATHY

Two-Dimensional/M-Mode Echocardiography

Although asymmetric septal hypertrophy is the most common type of morphologic pattern, hypertrophic car-

diomyopathy (Fig. 12-5) can present with concentric, apical, or free wall LV hypertrophy (14–17). When the basal septum is hypertrophied and bulging, the LVOT becomes narrowed, providing a substrate for dynamic obstruction. The velocity of blood flow across the narrowed LVOT increases and produces the *Venturi effect*. Consequently, the mitral leaflets and support apparatus are drawn toward the septum [i.e., *systolic anterior motion* (SAM)], obstructing the LVOT (Fig. 12-6). This obstruction is dynamic and depends on the loading conditions and LV size and contractility. When aortic flow is interrupted by obstruction of the LVOT, the aortic valve develops *premature midsystolic closure*. SAM of the mitral valve distorts the configuration of the mitral valve, resulting in mitral regurgitation. Therefore, varying degrees of mitral regurgitation almost invariably accompany the obstructive form of hypertrophic cardiomyopathy.

M-mode echocardiography is useful in documenting asymmetric septal hypertrophy, SAM of the mitral valve, and midsystolic aortic valve closure (18–20) (Fig. 12-7); however, the M-mode findings are not specific for hypertrophic cardiomyopathy. Asymmetric septal hypertrophy is also seen in RV hypertrophy, hypertension, and inferior wall myocardial infarction with preceding LV hypertrophy. SAM of the mitral valve also can be seen in other hyper-

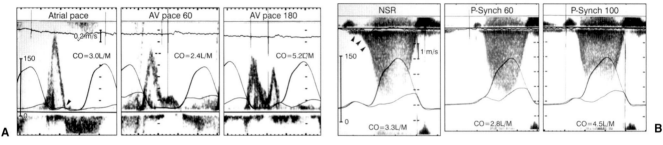

FIG. 12-4. A: Mitral flow velocity curve and simultaneous left atrial (LA) and left ventricular (LV) pressure curves in a 76-year-old man with long PR interval and severe LV dysfunction (ejection fraction, 25%) due to severe coronary artery disease. He has severe New York Heart Association functional class IV symptoms. **Left:** Atrial pacing with anterograde native conduction and a long atrioventricular (*AV*) delay. There is an increase in LV pressure above LA pressure during atrial relaxation in mid-diastole (*arrowhead*), culminating in a shortening of diastolic filling time and onset of diastolic regurgitation. The baseline cardiac output (*CO*) is 3.0 L/min. **Center:** AV pacing at a short AV interval of 60 msec. Diastolic filling occurs through all of diastole. Atrial contraction now occurs simultaneously with LV contraction, resulting in a lower CO than on the left. Note that mean LA pressure increased from 31 mm Hg **(left)** to 42 mm Hg **(center)**. **Right:** AV pacing at the optimal AV interval of 180 msec. The relation of atrial contraction to the onset of ventricular contraction is now optimal (see text), resulting in diastolic filling throughout the entire diastolic filling period. An appropriate relation exists between mechanical LA and LV contraction, so that mean LA pressure is maintained at a low level (34 mm Hg), with LA contraction occurring just before LV contraction. This causes an increase in LV end-diastolic pressure to 43 mm Hg. CO has increased to 5.2 L/min. **B:** Continuous-wave Doppler image of mitral regurgitation signal and simultaneous LA and LV pressure curves in a patient with long PR interval. **Left:** Normal sinus rhythm (*NSR*) with a long intrinsic PR interval. Diastolic mitral regurgitation (*arrowheads*) is due to an increase in LV pressure above LA pressure before ventricular contraction. **Center:** P-synchronous pacing (*P-Synch*) with a short AV interval of 60 msec. Diastolic mitral regurgitation is no longer present, but there is a decrease in CO from that on the left due to an atrial contraction that is ineffective because it occurs during ventricular contraction. **Right:** P-synchronous pacing at the optimal AV interval (100 msec). Diastolic mitral regurgitation is no longer present. LV diastolic pressure increases appropriately at the onset of ventricular contraction. LV pressure has increased from 30 mm Hg **(left)** to 43 mm Hg **(right)**. (From ref. 13, with permission.)

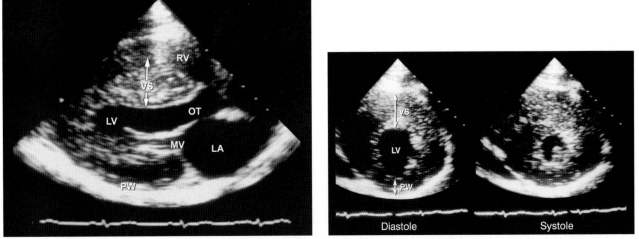

FIG. 12-5. A: Parasternal long-axis view of hypertrophic cardiomyopathy (nonobstructive variant). The ventricular septum (*VS*) is asymmetrically hypertrophied compared with the posterior wall (*PW*). Left atrium (*LA*) is mildly enlarged. *MV*, mitral valve; *OT*, outflow tract. **B:** Diastolic and systolic frames of the parasternal short-axis view. The entire VS is uniformly and markedly thickened, as is the anterolateral left ventricular (*LV*) free wall. Note that the posteroinferior wall is of normal thickness. Also note the abnormal texture of the involved myocardium. The principal difference from another form of hypertrophic cardiomyopathy is that there is no resting LV outflow track obstruction.

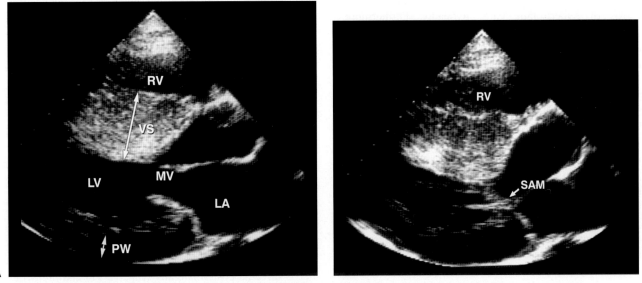

FIG. 12-6. Two-dimensional echocardiogram of hypertrophic obstructive cardiomyopathy. **A:** Diastolic frame. The ventricular septum (*VS*) is markedly thickened (34 mm) and has abnormal myocardial texture. *MV*, mitral valve; *PW*, posterior wall. **B:** Systolic frame. Systolic anterior motion (*SAM*) of the anterior mitral leaflet is shown, contributing to the obstruction of the LV outflow tract.

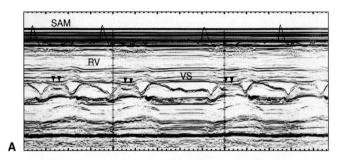

FIG. 12-7. A: M-mode echocardiogram showing systolic anterior motion (*SAM, double arrowheads*) of the anterior mitral leaflet. *VS*, ventricular septum. **B:** M-mode echocardiogram showing midsystolic aortic valve notching (*arrow*), from the same patient as in A. The aortic valve (*AV*) partially closes when obstruction to left ventricle (*LV*) ejection occurs. **C:** M-mode TEE echocardiogram of the aortic valve before (*baseline*) and after (*post*) myectomy in a patient with hypertrophic obstructive cardiomyopathy. Midsystolic aortic notching (*arrows*) disappeared after relief of the LV outflow obstruction by myectomy. *Ao*, aorta.

dynamic cardiac conditions. Two-dimensional (2D) echocardiography is the method of choice to establish the diagnosis of hypertrophic cardiomyopathy. Furthermore, detailed morphologic characterization also is provided by 2D echocardiographic imaging (14,21). The most frequent morphologic variety of hypertrophic cardiomyopathy consists of diffuse hypertrophy of the ventricular septum and anterolateral free wall (70% to 75%), followed by basal septal hypertrophy (10% to 15%), concentric hypertrophy (5%), apical hypertrophy (<5%), and hypertrophy of the lateral wall (1% to 2%). Apical hypertrophic cardiomyopathy may be missed by 2D echocardiography unless an apical examination is performed carefully. Parasternal examination may not provide the diagnosis, because the hypertrophy is usually confined to the apex (Fig. 12-8A and C). Because of massive apical hypertrophy, epicardial motion may suggest a dyskinetic apex (which suggests the false diagnosis of apical aneurysm), but endocardial motion shows nearly complete obliteration of the apical cavity. This condition typically is associated with giant T-wave inversion in the precordial leads (15) (see Fig. 12-8D). The presence of asymmetric septal hypertrophy and severe SAM of the mitral valve predicts a good outcome after septal myectomy (22).

Doppler (Pulsed-Wave, Continuous-Wave) and Color-Flow Imaging

LVOT Obstruction

The degree of LV obstruction is readily assessed by continuous-wave Doppler echocardiography. Increased flow velocity across the LVOT typically is detected from the apical transducer position, but other transducer positions also should be tried. The resulting Doppler spectrum has a characteristic late-peaking *dagger-shaped* appearance (Fig. 12-9). With the simplified Bernoulli equation, the peak velocity can be converted to the pressure gradient across the LVOT. The correlation between Doppler-derived and catheter-derived pressure gradients is good (23) (Fig. 12-10). The dynamic nature of LVOT obstruction can be documented by continuous-wave Doppler during the Valsalva maneuver or amyl nitrite inhalation (Fig. 12-9). LVOT velocity also increases after a meal or ingestion of alcohol (24,25).

Mitral Regurgitation

Mitral regurgitation frequently accompanies the obstructive form of hypertrophic cardiomyopathy. Typically, the jet is directed posterolaterally (Fig. 12-11) and temporally occurs after the onset of LVOT obstruction: ejection→obstruction→leak (26). It produces a high-velocity jet away from the apex, which can be confused with the LVOT velocity. Flow duration and Doppler spectral configuration help to differentiate mitral regurgitation from LVOT obstruction (Fig. 12-12). Color-flow imaging helps to separate the mitral regurgitation from LVOT flow and to guide the continuous-wave Doppler beam. Color-flow imaging is also the best means to assess the severity of mitral regurgitation. The peak velocity of the mitral regurgitant jet also can be used to determine the magnitude of LVOT obstruction, for example,

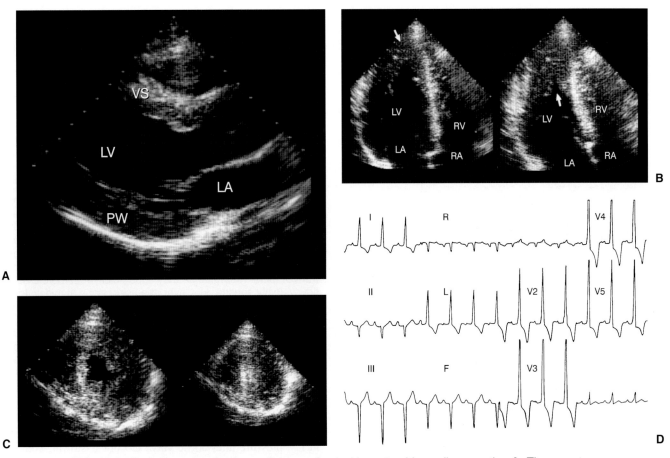

FIG. 12-8. Two-dimensional echocardiogram of apical hypertrophic cardiomyopathy. **A:** The parasternal long-axis view is unremarkable. Thickness of the ventricular septum (*VS*) and posterior wall (*PW*) is normal. **B:** Apical four-chamber view during diastole **(left)** and systole **(right)**. The apical wall thickness during diastole is markedly increased (18 mm, *arrow* on left) and the apical cavity is nearly obliterated except for a small slit during systole (*arrow* on right). **C:** Apical short-axis view during diastole **(left)** and systole **(right)** demonstrating apical hypertrophy and apical cavity obliteration. **D:** Typical electrocardiogram of apical hypertrophic cardiomyopathy, with a marked increase in QRS voltage and giant negative T waves in the precordial (V2-V5), I, and aVL leads.

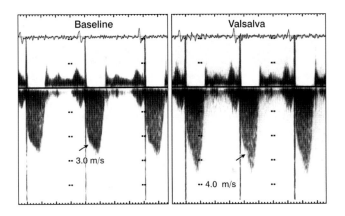

FIG. 12-9. Continuous-wave Doppler spectra obtained from the apex demonstrating dynamic left ventricular (LV) outflow tract obstruction. Note the typical late-peaking configuration resembling a dagger or ski slope (*arrow*). The baseline **(left)** velocity is 2.8 m/sec, corresponding to the peak LV outflow tract gradient of 31 mm Hg ($= 4 \times 2.8^2$). With the Valsalva maneuver **(right)**, the velocity increased to 3.5 m/sec, corresponding to the gradient of 50 mm Hg.

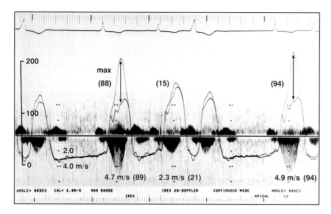

FIG. 12-10. Simultaneous continuous-wave Doppler and cardiac catheterization study. Left ventricular (LV) apex and outflow pressures are recorded to determine the severity of outflow obstruction. Doppler velocities are converted to pressure gradients with the simplified Bernoulli equation and correlate well with maximal (*max*) catheter-derived gradients. The resting gradient is 15 to 20 mm Hg, and it is markedly accentuated in the postextrasystolic contractions (second and fifth beats), with resultant gradients derived by catheter of 88 and 94 mm Hg and by Doppler of 89 and 94 mm Hg, respectively. Note that the LV pressure tracing has a late-peaking appearance corresponding to the late-peaking Doppler profile.

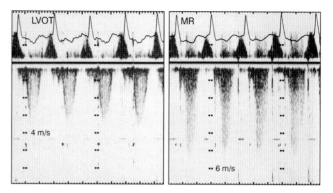

FIG. 12-12. Continuous-wave Doppler spectra from left ventricular outflow tract (*LVOT*) obstruction and mitral regurgitation (*MR*) obtained from the apex. It may be difficult to distinguish between them. MR in hypertrophic cardiomyopathy usually begins at midsystole when there is systolic anterior motion of the mitral valve. Therefore, the Doppler spectrum of mitral regurgitation may superficially resemble LVOT flow velocity spectra. However, the rising slope at midsystole is usually perpendicular to the baseline in MR, whereas it is curvilinear until it reaches the highest velocity in the LVOT signal. Furthermore, the MR velocity signal extends beyond ejection and culminates in mitral forward flow during onset of diastole. Remember that MR velocity will always be higher than LVOT jet velocity.

$$\textit{Mitral regurgitant jet velocity} = 7 \text{ m/sec}$$

$$\textit{LV–LA gradient} = 4 \times 7^2 = 196 \text{ mm Hg}$$

$$\textit{LV pressure} = 196 + 20 \ (\textit{LA pressure}) = 216 \text{ mm Hg}$$

If the blood pressure is 120/80 mm Hg, LVOT gradient = 216 − 120 = 96 mm Hg.

Diastolic Filling Pattern

The predominant diastolic abnormality in hypertrophic cardiomyopathy is markedly impaired myocardial relaxation due to the hypertrophic myocardium (27). The decline in LV pressure after aortic valve closure is slower; consequently, isovolumic relaxation time (IVRT) is prolonged, early rapid filling (E) is reduced, DT is prolonged, and atrial filling (A) is increased (Fig. 12-13). Atrial contraction contributes significantly to LV filling. If atrial contraction is compromised because of tachycardia or atrial fibrillation, cardiac output decreases and pulmonary venous congestion occurs. As the LV becomes less compliant and LA pressure

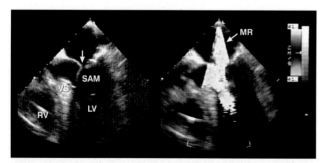

FIG. 12-11. Transverse transesophageal view of the ventricular septum (*VS*) and mitral valve in hypertrophic obstructive cardiomyopathy **(left)**. The dimension of the VS is increased, and systolic anterior motion (*SAM*) of the mitral valve obstructs the LV outflow tract **(right)**. Because of the distortion of the mitral valve (*arrow*), mitral regurgitation (*MR*) is directed posterolaterally.

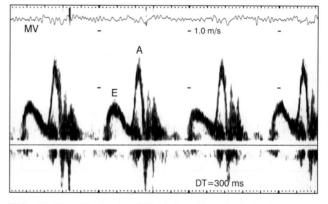

FIG. 12-13. Mitral valve (*MV*) inflow Doppler velocity pattern of abnormal relaxation in a patient with hypertrophic cardiomyopathy. The typical features include reduced E velocity (0.3 m/sec), increased A velocity (0.75 m/sec), decreased E/A ratio (0.4), and prolonged deceleration time (DT, 300 msec).

increases, early filling gradually increases and DT decreases; however, the same degree of increase in LA pressure does not produce similar shortening of DT in patients with hypertrophic cardiomyopathy as it does in those with dilated cardiomyopathy, because DT is markedly prolonged at baseline. Hence, there is no significant correlation between DT and LV filling pressures in patients with hypertrophic cardiomyopathy (28).

Because of asynchronous myocardial relaxation, redistri-

bution of intracavitary flow may occur during the isovolumic relaxation period in patients with hypertrophic cardiomyopathy (Figs. 12-14 and 12-15). This has no significant clinical or hemodynamic implication, but it may cause an erroneous interpretation of mitral inflow velocities and diastolic filling pattern. Also, this pattern should be differentiated from the triphasic diastolic filling pattern that shows a marked relaxation abnormality in combination with initial restrictive filling (Fig. 12-16).

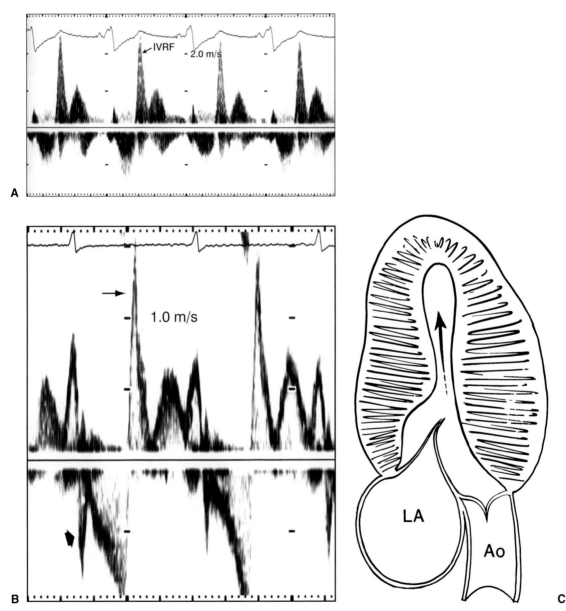

FIG. 12-14. A: Continuous-wave Doppler from the apex demonstrating accentuated isovolumic relaxation flow (*IVRF*). Note the isovolumic velocity is higher than the mitral E velocity. **B:** Pulsed-wave Doppler from the apex with the sample volume in the LV midcavity **(right)**. IVRF (*arrow*) is recorded best at midcavity because the flow is directed from the base of the heart to the apex across the narrowest portion of the left ventricle (*LV*) at the papillary muscle level. Note the peak IVRF velocity is 1.4 m/sec, markedly exceeding the mitral E velocity of 0.6 m/sec. **C:** IVRF (*arrow*) velocity is toward the apex. An intracavitary gradient is produced by relaxation of the apex, which lowers the pressure in the region. The aortic and mitral valves are both closed. *Ao,* aorta.

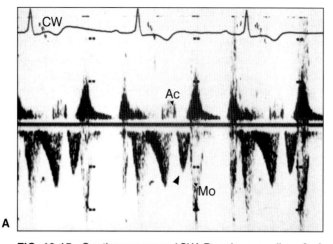

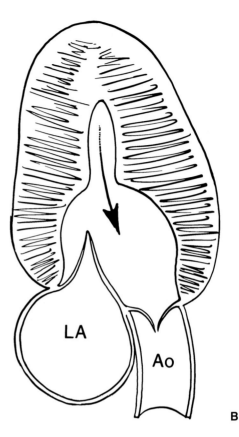

FIG. 12-15. Continuous-wave (*CW*) Doppler recording. **A:** A different isovolumic relaxation flow pattern (*arrowhead*) is noted in patients with apical hypertrophy and midcavity or apical obliteration. The isovolumic relaxation flow is directed away from the involved apex. The left ventricular (LV) apical pressure remains higher than that at the basal portion of the LV during isovolumic relaxation. *Ac*, aortic valve closure; *Mo*, mitral valve opening. **B:** Isovolumic relaxation flow (*arrow*) is directed away from the apex in the midcavitary or apical hypertrophic variant. LV pressure at the apex is higher than at the basal area, and there is a transient intracavitary gradient from the apex to the base during isovolumic relaxation. The aortic and mitral valves are both closed. *Ao*, aorta.

Dynamic LVOT Obstruction in Other Diseases

Not all dynamic LVOT obstruction is due to hypertrophic cardiomyopathy. If ventricular systolic function becomes hyperdynamic (because of medication or other factors) in a patient with basal septal hypertrophy, the LVOT becomes obstructed in a dynamic fashion and, hemodynamically, it behaves exactly the same as hypertrophic obstructive cardiomyopathy. This tends to happen in elderly patients who have a history of hypertension, although hypertension is not a prerequisite (29). These patients can be symptomatic, with dyspnea, chest pain, or hypotension (or a combination of these), which are exacerbated by treatment with vasodilators, diuretics, or digoxin. Although this has been called *hypertensive hypertrophic cardiomyopathy,* it clearly is different from true hypertrophic cardiomyopathy. Another frequent clinical setting associated with dynamic LVOT obstruction is the postoperative period when intravascular volume is depleted and the patient is receiving treatment with an inotropic agent. Patients with aortic stenosis are especially vulnerable to this acute life-threatening LVOT obstruction after aortic valve replacement. Myectomy of the basal septum prevents this hemodynamic complication.

Dynamic LVOT obstruction may be an initial presentation of cardiac amyloidosis. Acute LVOT obstruction can occur in a patient with acute anterior-apical myocardial infarction, especially when there is preexisting basal septal hypertrophy (see Fig. 7-11). Compensatory hyperdynamic motion of the inferobasal myocardium results in SAM of the mitral valve, which may cause an extreme hemodynamic compromise that requires prompt treatment with fluid, a β-blocker or even a pure α-agonist (phenylephrine). Discrete subaortic stenosis can mimic hypertrophic obstructive cardiomyopathy. LV hypertrophy associated with discrete subaortic stenosis produces many similar features.

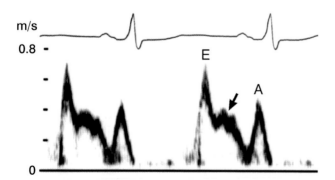

FIG. 12-16. Pulsed-wave Doppler recording of triphasic mitral inflow in a patient with left ventricular (*LV*) hypertrophy. The first wave is E velocity (not isovolumic relaxation flow), and the second wave (*arrow*) is due to marked delayed myocardial relaxation. This triphasic mitral inflow pattern can be differentiated from isovolumic relaxation flow by paying attention to the timing of velocities in reference to that of mitral regurgitation or LV outflow velocity.

Transesophageal Echocardiography

There are several clinical situations in which transesophageal echocardiography (TEE) is useful in evaluating patients with hypertrophic obstructive cardiomyopathy, for example, in assisting and evaluating intraoperatively the result of myectomy (see Chapter 19) and in evaluating the mitral leaflets and chordal apparatus in a patient with hypertrophic obstructive cardiomyopathy and sudden hemodynamic deterioration. Chordal rupture develops in a subgroup of patients with hypertrophic obstructive cardiomyopathy and results in severe mitral regurgitation (30) (Fig. 12-17). These patients require mitral valve repair or replacement in addition to myectomy. TEE is also indicated in the delineation of the anatomy of the LVOT and in the assessment of hemodynamics in a patient in whom a surface (transthoracic) study is not adequate. TEE is also useful in differentiating discrete subaortic stenosis from dynamic obstruction. The flow velocity and pressure gradient across the LVOT can be obtained by multiplane TEE from a transgastric view, with the transducer array rotated to about 130 degrees.

Limitations and Pitfalls

The 2D echocardiographic features of hypertrophic cardiomyopathy can be mimicked by chronic hypertension (especially in combination with renal failure), cardiac amyloidosis, pheochromocytoma, and Friedreich ataxia. Therefore, the echocardiographic finding of markedly increased LV wall thickness should be interpreted in its clinical context. Even dynamic LVOT obstruction can be present in these clinical conditions. Apical hypertrophic cardiomyopathy occasionally escapes echocardiographic detection, because LV wall thickness is not significantly increased at the basal and papillary muscle levels, so that the parasternal long- and short-axis views may appear normal (see Fig. 12-8A). Apical hypertrophy is best visualized from apical short-axis and four-chamber views with good endocardial definition, demonstrating thickened apical walls and obliteration of the apical cavity during systole. Because of the massive apical hypertrophy, the epicardial motion of the apex may appear to be dyskinetic. Apical hypertrophy should be differentiated from apical cavity obliteration due to hypereosinophilic syndrome (see Chapter 13). In apical hypertrophic cardiomyopathy, a small apical cavity is present during diastole, but this cavity is usually obliterated in hypereosinophilic syndrome. Eosinophilic thrombotic material also has a different echocardiographic density from that of the underlying myocardium. Occasionally, a false-positive diagnosis of asymmetric septal hypertrophy is made because of RV papillary muscle and prominent trabeculations that overlie the ventricular septum (Fig. 12-18).

RESTRICTIVE CARDIOMYOPATHY

Primary restrictive cardiomyopathy is characterized by restricted ventricular filling resulting from an idiopathic myocardial abnormality (stiffening fibrosis or decreased compliance or both) (31). Ventricular systolic function usually is well preserved in the initial stage, but diastolic pressure is elevated, which in turn results in increased atrial

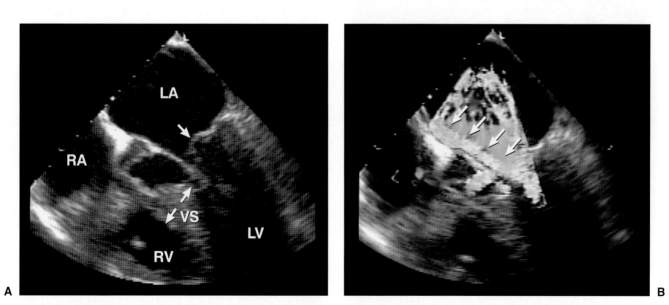

FIG. 12-17. A: Transesophageal echocardiography shows rupture of chordae tendineae (*arrow*) of the mitral valve, resulting in a flail segment in a patient with hypertrophic obstructive cardiomyopathy. The ventricular septum (*VS; double-headed arrow*) is markedly thickened. **B:** Color-flow imaging shows severe mitral regurgitation, with the jet directed medially (*arrows*) instead of posterolaterally as in mitral regurgitation due to systolic anterior motion of the mitral valve (see Fig. 12-11).

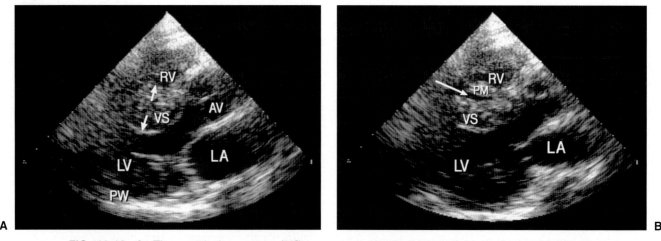

FIG. 12-18. A: The ventricular septum (*VS*) appears markedly thickened (*arrows*), consistent with hypertrophic cardiomyopathy. **B:** However, the asymmetric septal hypertrophy was mimicked by right ventricle (*RV*) muscle bands and papillary muscle (*PM*) overlying the VS. With a slight tilt and rotation, an echo-free space (*arrow*) between these two structures could be demonstrated, hence avoiding misdiagnosis. *AV*, aortic valve; *PW*, posterior wall.

pressures and marked biatrial enlargement. Therefore, the characteristic morphologic features of primary restrictive cardiomyopathy on 2D echocardiography include ventricular cavities of normal size, normal wall thicknesses, with relatively preserved global systolic function, and biatrial en-

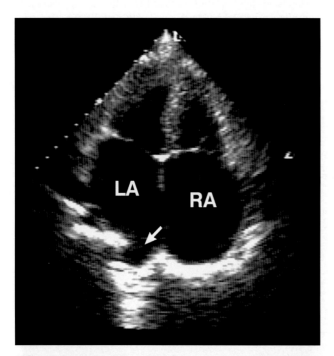

FIG. 12-19. Apical four-chamber view in a young patient shows marked biatrial enlargement typical of restrictive cardiomyopathy. Atrial size is considerably larger than ventricular size. Ventricular systolic function (i.e., ejection fraction) was normal in spite of the patient being in congestive failure. Pulmonary vein was also dilated (*arrow*), indicative of high diastolic filling pressures.

largement (Fig. 12-19). Also, restrictive cardiomyopathy is accompanied by restrictive diastolic filling (the reverse is not true; restrictive diastolic filling pattern, grade III–IV diastolic dysfunction, can be present in all cardiac diseases). The typical hemodynamic feature of restrictive cardiomyopathy is the *dip-and-plateau,* or "√" configuration in the ventricular diastolic pressure tracing (Fig. 12-20). This hemodynamic feature produces shortened DT of early rapid filling (E) in the mitral inflow velocity (Fig. 12-21). With the increase in left atrial (LA) pressure, the mitral valve opens at a higher pressure, resulting in a decrease in IVRT. High atrial pressure also results in an increased transmitral pressure gradient, an increased E mitral velocity, and decreased systolic pulmonary venous flow velocity (Fig. 12-21). Because of high ventricular pressure at end diastole, atrial contraction does not contribute significantly to ven-

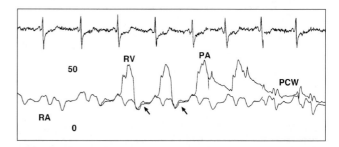

FIG. 12-20. Pressure tracing from catheterization of the right side of the heart of a patient with restrictive cardiomyopathy. There is a dip-and-plateau, or square root (√), configuration (*arrows*) of early right ventricular (*RV*) diastolic filling pressure. Right atrial (*RA*) pressure = 23 mm Hg; RV pressure = 62/18 mm Hg; pulmonary artery (*PA*) pressure = 62/30 mm Hg; pulmonary capillary wedge (*PCW*) pressure = 23 mm Hg.

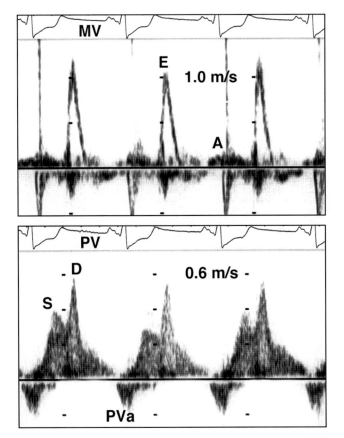

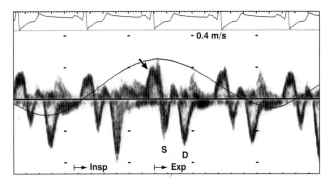

FIG. 12-22. Hepatic vein pulsed-wave Doppler recording together with respirometer recording from the same patient in Figs. 12-20 and 12-21, consistent with restrictive physiology. Note the higher diastolic velocity (*D*) than systolic velocity (*S*) and greater reversal of diastolic flow during inspiration (*Insp*) (*arrow*). *Exp*, expiration.

FIG. 12-21. Mitral valve (*MV*) and pulmonary vein (*PV*) pulsed-wave Doppler recordings from the same patient in Fig. 12-20. E velocity is high with shortened deceleration time. The mitral A velocity is markedly decreased. Short deceleration time corresponds to rapid rise of LV diastolic pressure during early filling. PV flow velocity **(bottom)** has a dominant diastolic component with rapid deceleration. Pulmonary vein atrial flow reversal velocity (*PVa*) is not increased, suggesting decreased atrial contractile force.

tricular filling, and A velocity is usually decreased. As a result, the E/A ratio is increased markedly (>2.0). Because of the increase in atrial pressure, venous flow velocity decreases during systole and increases with diastole (Fig.12-21 and 12-22). In contrast to constrictive pericarditis, hepatic vein diastolic flow reversal is greater during inspiration (Fig. 12-22).

Typical Doppler features in restrictive cardiomyopathy are as follows:

Mitral (*M*) and tricuspid (*T*) inflow
  Increased E velocity (*M* >1 m/sec; *T* > 0.7 m/sec)
  Decreased A velocity (*M* <0.5 m/sec; *T* < 0.3 m/sec)
  Increased E/A ratio (≥ 2.0)
  Decreased IVRT (<70 msec)
  Decreased A duration
Pulmonary and hepatic vein flow
  Systolic velocity much smaller than diastolic velocity
  Increased diastolic flow reversal in the hepatic vein during inspiration

  Increased atrial flow reversal velocity and duration in pulmonary vein

Restrictive cardiomyopathy should be distinguished from restrictive hemodynamics or physiology (32,33). The latter indicates the hemodynamic abnormality of impaired ventricular filling and the rapid increase in ventricular diastolic pressure from decreased compliance or increased LA pressure (or both), regardless of the underlying pathologic condition, whereas restrictive cardiomyopathy indicates an inherent myocardial process that produces the typical morphologic as well as the hemodynamic features described in this chapter.

Prognosis of primary restrictive cardiomyopathy is poor, especially in children (34). Medical treatment is for relief of systemic and pulmonary venous congestion. The underlying myocardial abnormality usually is not reversible. In addition to symptoms of heart failure, patients with restrictive cardiomyopathy may experience an embolic event or sudden death. Cardiac transplantation should be considered before significant pulmonary congestion or severe pulmonary hypertension develops.

Arrhythmogenic Right Ventricular Cardiomyopathy

Arrhythmogenic RV cardiomyopathy is commonly referred to as *RV dysplasia*. RV dysplasia is caused primarily by progressive replacement of the RV myocardium with fatty and fibrous tissue. Patients present with ventricular arrhythmia, congestive heart failure, heart murmur, or sudden death. In the Mayo Clinic experience with 20 patients (from 1978 to 1993), a familial association was noted in 30%, with first-order relatives being affected (35). In certain areas of Europe, RV dysplasia is the most common cause of cardiac death in young patients (36). Echocardiographically, the RV is predominantly dilated, with poor contractility. In some patients, LV dilatation and dysfunction also occur. RV systolic pressure is typically in the low

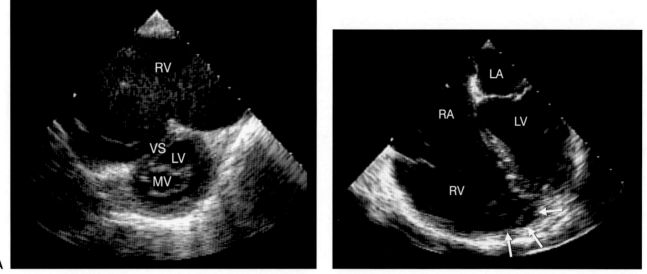

FIG. 12-23. Echocardiogram showing right ventricular (*RV*) dysplasia. **A:** Short-axis view at the mitral valve (*MV*) level. Note marked RV enlargement. Left ventricular (*LV*) size and function were normal. *VS*, ventricular septum. **B:** Apical view demonstrating RV dysplasia associated with small aneurysm formation (*arrows*). Right atrium (*RA*) and RV are dilated, but LV and left atrium (*LA*) are normal.

normal range because of RV pump failure; hence, tricuspid regurgitation velocity usually is <2 m/sec. Typical echocardiographic findings are shown in Fig. 12-23. Although the echocardiographic features are quite typical, the disease may actually present before the development of overt morphological change. Magnetic resonance imaging for fat in the RV myocardium has been helpful in some patients.

REFERENCES

1. Richardson P, McKenna W, Bristow M, et al. Report of the 1995 World Health Organization/International Society and Federation of Cardiology Task Force on the definition and classification of cardiomyopathies. *Circulation* 1996;93:841–842.
2. Codd MB, Sugrue DD, Gersh BJ, Melton LJ III. Epidemiology of idiopathic dilated and hypertrophic cardiomyopathy: a population-based study in Olmsted County, Minnesota, 1975–1984. *Circulation* 1989;80:564–572.
3. Corya B, Feigenbaum H, Rasmussen S, Black MJ. Echocardiographic features of congestive cardiomyopathy compared with normal subjects and patients with coronary artery disease. *Circulation* 1974;49:1153–1159.
4. Goerss JB, Michels VV, Burnett J, et al. Frequency of familial dilated cardiomyopathy. *Eur Heart J* 1995;16(Suppl):2–4.
5. St. Goar FG, Masuyama T, Alderman EL, Popp RL. Left ventricular diastolic dysfunction in end-stage dilated cardiomyopathy: simultaneous Doppler echocardiography and hemodynamic evaluation. *J Am Soc Echocardiogr* 1991;4:349–360.
6. Ohno M, Cheng CP, Little WC. Mechanism of altered patterns of left ventricular filling during the development of congestive heart failure. *Circulation* 1994;89:2241–2250.
7. Xie GY, Berk MR, Smith MD, Gurley JC, DeMaria AN. Prognostic value of Doppler transmitral flow patterns in patients with congestive heart failure. *J Am Coll Cardiol* 1994;24:132–139.
8. Rihal CS, Nishimura RA, Hatle LK, Bailey KR, Tajik AJ. Systolic and diastolic dysfunction in patients with clinical diagnosis of dilated cardiomyopathy. Relation to symptoms and prognosis. *Circulation* 1994;90:2772–2779.
9. Pinamonti B, Zecchin M, Di Lenarda A, Gregori D, Sinagra G, Camerini F. Persistence of restrictive left ventricular filling pattern in dilated cardiomyopathy: an ominous prognostic sign. *J Am Coll Cardiol* 1997;29:604–612.
10. Lee D-C, Oh JK, Osborn SL, Mahoney DW, Seward JB. Repeat evaluation of diastolic filling pattern after treatment of congestive heart failure in patients with restrictive diastolic filling: Implication for long-term prognosis. *J Am Soc Echocardiogr* 1997;10:431(abst).
11. Abramson SV, Burke JF, Kelly JJ Jr, et al. Pulmonary hypertension predicts mortality and morbidity in patients with dilated cardiomyopathy. *Ann Intern Med* 1992;116:888–895.
12. Hurrell DG, Nishimura RA, Higano ST, et al. Value of dynamic respiratory changes in left and right ventricular pressures for the diagnosis of constrictive pericarditis. *Circulation* 1996;93:2007–2013.
13. Nishimura RA, Hayes DL, Holmes DR Jr, Tajik AJ. Mechanism of hemodynamic improvement by dual-chamber pacing for severe left ventricular dysfunction: an acute Doppler and catheterization hemodynamic study. *J Am Coll Cardiol* 1995;25:281–288.
14. Maron BJ, Gottdiener JS, Epstein SE. Patterns and significance of distribution of left ventricular hypertrophy in hypertrophic cardiomyopathy: a wide angle, two dimensional echocardiographic study of 125 patients. *Am J Cardiol* 1981;48:418–428.
15. Yamaguchi H, Ishimura T, Nishiyama S, et al. Hypertrophic nonobstructive cardiomyopathy with giant negative T waves (apical hypertrophy): ventriculographic and echocardiographic features in 30 patients. *Am J Cardiol* 1979;44:401–412.
16. Keren G, Belhassen B, Sherez J, et al. Apical hypertrophic cardiomyopathy: evaluation by noninvasive and invasive techniques in 23 patients. *Circulation* 1985;71:45–56.
17. Wigle ED, Rakowski H, Kimball BP, Williams WG. Hypertrophic cardiomyopathy: clinical spectrum and treatment. *Circulation* 1995;92:1680–1692.
18. Shah PM, Gramiak R, Kramer DH. Ultrasound localization of left ventricular outflow obstruction in hypertrophic obstructive cardiomyopathy. *Circulation* 1969;40:3–11.
19. Tajik AJ, Giuliani ER. Echocardiographic observations in idiopathic hypertrophic subaortic stenosis. *Mayo Clin Proc* 1974;49:89–97.
20. Popp RL, Harrison DC. Ultrasound in the diagnosis and evaluation of therapy of idiopathic hypertrophic subaortic stenosis. *Circulation* 1969;40:905–914.
21. Tajik AJ, Seward JB, Hagler DJ. Detailed analysis of hypertrophic obstructive cardiomyopathy by wide-angle two-dimensional sector echocardiography. *Am J Cardiol* 1979;43:348 (abst).
22. McCully RB, Nishimura RA, Bailey KR, Schaff HV, Danielson GK, Tajik AJ. Hypertrophic obstructive cardiomyopathy: preoperative echo-

cardiographic predictors of outcome after septal myectomy. *J Am Coll Cardiol* 1996;27:1491–1496.

23. Sasson Z, Yock PG, Hatle LK, Alderman EL, Popp RL. Doppler echocardiographic determination of the pressure gradient in hypertrophic cardiomyopathy. *J Am Coll Cardiol* 1988;11:752–756.

24. Gilligan DM, Marsonis A, Joshi J, et al. Cardiovascular and hormonal responses to a meal in hypertrophic cardiomyopathy: a comparison of patients with and without postprandial exacerbation of symptoms. *Clin Cardiol* 1996;19:129–135.

25. Paz R, Jortner R, Tunick PA, et al. The effect of the ingestion of ethanol on obstruction of the left ventricular outflow tract in hypertrophic cardiomyopathy. *N Engl J Med* 1996;335:938–941.

26. Nishimura RA, Tajik AJ, Reeder GS, Seward JB. Evaluation of hypertrophic cardiomyopathy by Doppler color flow imaging: initial observations. *Mayo Clin Proc* 1986;61:631–639.

27. Maron BJ, Spirito P, Green KJ, Wesley YE, Bonow RO, Arce J. Noninvasive assessment of left ventricular diastolic function by pulsed Doppler echocardiography in patients with hypertrophic cardiomyopathy. *J Am Coll Cardiol* 1987;10:733–742.

28. Nishimura RA, Appleton CP, Redfield MM, Ilstrup DM, Holmes DR Jr, Tajik AJ. Noninvasive Doppler echocardiographic evaluation of left ventricular filling pressures in patients with cardiomyopathies: a simultaneous Doppler echocardiographic and cardiac catheterization study. *J Am Coll Cardiol* 1996;28:1226–1233.

29. Topol EJ, Traill TA, Fortuin NJ. Hypertensive hypertrophic cardiomyopathy of the elderly. *N Engl J Med* 1985;312:277–283.

30. Zhu WX, Oh JK, Kopecky SL, Schaff HV, Tajik AJ. Mitral regurgitation due to ruptured chordae tendineae in patients with hypertrophic obstructive cardiomyopathy. *J Am Coll Cardiol* 1992;20:242–247.

31. Seward J, Tajik AJ. Restrictive cardiomyopathy. *Curr Opin Cardiol* 1987;2:499–501.

32. Appleton CP, Hatle LK, Popp RL. Demonstration of restrictive ventricular physiology by Doppler echocardiography. *J Am Coll Cardiol* 1988;11:757–768.

33. Little WC, Ohno M, Kitzman DW, Thomas JD, Cheng CP. Determination of left ventricular chamber stiffness from the time for deceleration of early left ventricular filling. *Circulation* 1995;92:1933–1939.

34. Cetta F, O'Leary PW, Seward JB, Driscoll DJ. Idiopathic restrictive cardiomyopathy in childhood: diagnostic features and clinical course. *Mayo Clin Proc* 1995;70:634–640.

35. Kullo IJ, Edwards WD, Seward JB. Right ventricular dysplasia: the Mayo Clinic experience. *Mayo Clin Proc* 1995;70:541–548.

36. Thiene G, Nava A, Corrado D, Rossi L, Pennelli N. Right ventricular cardiomyopathy and sudden death in young people. *N Engl J Med* 1988;318:129–133.

CHAPTER 13

Cardiac Diseases Due to Systemic Illness, Medication, or Infection

Various systemic illnesses, chemicals, medications, or sepsis can cause morphologic, functional, and hemodynamic abnormalities of the heart. Cardiac abnormalities include secondary forms of cardiomyopathies (dilated, infiltrative, or restrictive), valvular disease, carcinoid, hypereosinophilia, pericardial diseases (pericardial effusion, tamponade, or constriction), intracardiac mass, and marantic or Libman-Sacks endocarditis. Infective endocarditis is discussed separately in Chapter 11. Echocardiography is the method of choice for the detection and evaluation of these cardiac abnormalities. Two-dimensional (2D) echocardiographic studies provide morphologic and functional information; Doppler and color-flow studies provide information about intracardiac pressures, severity of valvular stenosis and regurgitation, and diastolic filling pattern. Not uncommonly, the echocardiographic detection of a particular cardiac abnormality may be the first diagnostic clue, for example, the typical tricuspid and pulmonary valve involvement and appearance in carcinoid or increased ventricular wall thickness and granular appearance in cardiac amyloidosis. Table 13-1 lists various cardiac manifestations of systemic illnesses frequently seen in the echocardiography laboratory. The typical echocardiographic findings in these cardiac abnormalities are described in more detail in this chapter, and illustrative examples are given.

AMYLOIDOSIS

Amyloidosis is due to the deposition of amyloid fibrils in various organs. It may involve the myocardium and result in infiltrative cardiomyopathy (Fig. 13-1). Contrary to the general perception, not all infiltrative cardiomyopathies produce restrictive cardiac morphology or hemodynamics. Myocardial *infiltration is primarily interstitial in amyloidosis,* and the predominant morphologic feature is an increase in myocardial wall thickness without dilatation of the left ventricular (LV) cavity (1) (Fig. 13-2). Ventricular

systolic function is not reduced until cardiac amyloidosis reaches the advanced stage with a marked increase in wall thickness (>15 mm). Although increased wall thickness seen on 2D echocardiography is the hallmark of cardiac amyloidosis, the diagnosis cannot be excluded when wall thickness is not increased (2). Amyloid deposits in the heart are diffuse, involving the valves, myocardium, interatrial septum, and pericardium (3). It is common to detect multivalvular regurgitation due to diffuse amyloid deposits in the cardiac valves. Amyloid deposits make the myocardium sparkle on 2D echocardiography, which produces a beautiful image, but the sparkling appearance alone is not diagnostic of cardiac amyloidosis. Other conditions may produce similar echocardiographic features, for example, hypertensive disease (especially in patients with renal failure), glycogen storage disease (4), and hypertrophic cardiomyopathy. Patients with cardiac amyloidosis usually have a *low QRS voltage* or a pseudoinfarct pattern on the electrocardiogram (Fig. 13-3), whereas those with LV hypertrophy, hypertrophic cardiomyopathy, or glycogen storage disease have increased QRS voltages of the LV hypertrophy pattern. During an early stage of cardiac amyloidosis, systolic function can be hyperdynamic, and it is not uncommon to see systolic anterior motion of the mitral valve and intracavitary obstruction, as in hypertrophic cardiomyopathy (5). As the disease progresses, however, systolic function gradually deteriorates.

Pulsed-wave Doppler echocardiography has been helpful in evaluation of the diastolic abnormalities of cardiac amyloidosis. The initial diastolic abnormality is abnormal relaxation (grade 1 diastolic dysfunction) resulting from increased ventricular wall thickness; the pattern becomes restrictive (grade 3–4 diastolic dysfunction) when progressive amyloid infiltration decreases LV compliance and increases LA pressure (6) (Fig. 13-4). The filling pattern may even normalize temporarily ("pseudonormalized"; grade 2 diastolic dysfunction) as a result of combined relaxation

TABLE 13-1. *Echocardiographic features of cardiac manifestations of systemic illnesses*

Amyloidosis
  Increased LV and RV wall thickness (moderate to marked)
  Normal LV cavity size
  Gradual deterioration of ventricular systolic function
  Granular appearance of myocardium (abnormal texture)
  Pericardial effusion
  Spectrum of diastolic dysfunction
  Thickening of the valves and multivalvular regurgitation
Ankylosing spondylitis
  Dilatation of the aortic annulus
  Dilatation of sinuses of Valsalva
  Thickened aortic valve with aortic regurgitation
Carcinoid
  Thickening and retraction of tricuspid valve with severe tricuspid regurgitation
  Tricuspid stenosis, usually mild
  Pulmonary valve thickening and retraction with pulmonic stenosis
  RV volume overload
  Thickening of valves on left side (<15%)
Friedreich ataxia
  LV hypertrophy, usually concentric (68%), resembling hypertrophic cardiomyopathy
  Dilated LV with systolic dysfunction (7%)
Hemochromatosis
  Appearance of dilated cardiomyopathy, dilated LV with decreased systolic function
  Normal ventricular wall thickness
  Restrictive diastolic filling characteristic at advanced stage
HIV infection or AIDS
  Pericardial effusion
  Dilated cardiomyopathy
  Pulmonary hypertension
Hypereosinophilic syndrome
  Posterior mitral leaflet thickening and tethering
  Ventricular apical thrombus with cavity obliteration
  Rarely, diffuse myocarditis with LV cavity increased in size with systolic dysfunction

Hyperthyroidism or hypothyroidism
  Pericardial effusion
  LV systolic dysfunction
Marfan syndrome
  Dilatation of the ascending aorta
  Dilatation of the aortic annulus and the sinus of Valsalva
  Aortic dissection
  Mitral valve prolapse
Muscular dystrophy (Duchenne)
  Posterior basal and lateral wall fibrosis
Pheochromocytoma
  Concentric LV hypertrophy (20%)
  Myocarditis (acute) with catecholamine crisis
Rheumatoid arthritis
  Pericardial effusion
  Constrictive pericarditis
  Cardiac granuloma
Sarcoidosis
  Regional wall motion abnormalities
  Thinning of the basal and posterolateral walls
  Posterobasal aneurysm
  Restrictive morphology
Scleroderma
  Pericardial effusion
  Pulmonary hypertension
  Valvular sclerosis
Systemic lupus erythematosus
  Pericarditis
  Tamponade
  Myocarditis
  Endocarditis, Libman-Sacks
Tuberous sclerosis
  Rhabdomyoma
  Cardiomyopathy

AIDS, acquired immunodeficiency syndrome; HIV, human immunodeficiency virus; LV, left ventricle; RV, right ventricle.

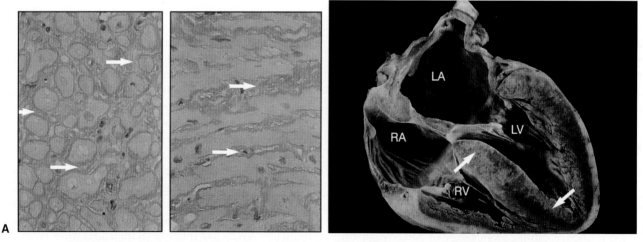

FIG. 13-1. Amyloidosis. **A:** Histologic sections of myocardial biopsy stained with sulfated alcian blue. Amyloid (*arrows*) occurs around and between myocardial cells. **B:** Gross cardiac specimen showing amyloid infiltration (*white arrows*) and thickened left ventricular (*LV*) walls. (From Click RL, Olson LJ, Edwards WD, et al. Echocardiography and systemic diseases. *J Am Soc Echocardiogr* 1994;7:201–216, with permission.)

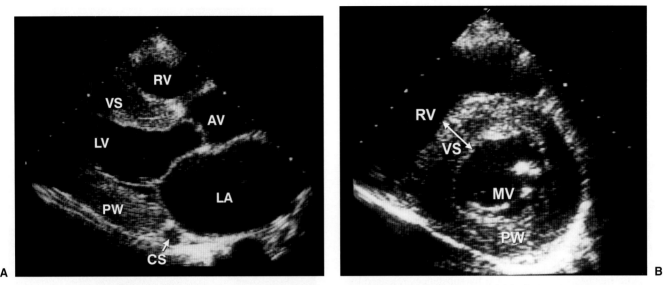

FIG. 13-2. A: Parasternal long-axis view showing typical findings of cardiac amyloidosis: concentric increase in left ventricular (*LV*) wall thickness, sparkling granular appearance of the myocardium, and thickened valve leaflets. The coronary sinus (*CS, arrow*) is enlarged because of increased right atrial pressure. **B:** Parasternal short-axis view showing marked concentric increase in LV wall thickness. *Double-headed arrow* indicates the thickness (18 mm) of the ventricular septum (*VS*). *AV*, aortic valve; *MV*, mitral valve; *PW*, posterior wall.

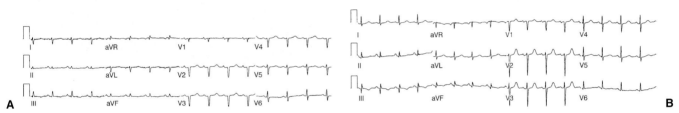

FIG. 13-3. A: Electrocardiogram (ECG) from a 78-year-old woman with dyspnea. Echocardiography was performed because of concern about anterior myocardial infarction. ECG shows low QRS voltage in the limb leads and suggests anterior wall myocardial infarction. Echocardiography showed typical features of cardiac amyloidosis, which was confirmed by biopsy. **B:** ECG from the same patient 2 years earlier. There is a Q wave in lead III, but QRS voltages are not decreased.

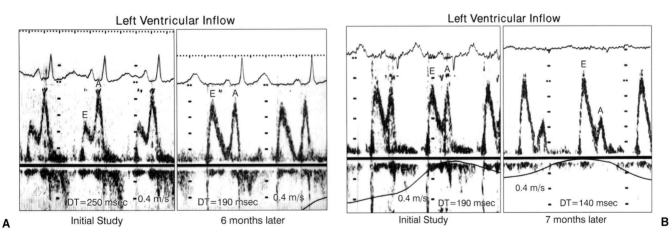

FIG. 13-4. Serial mitral inflow Doppler velocities from two patients with cardiac amyloidosis. **A:** The initial Doppler **(left)** showed a relaxation abnormality, with decreased E, increased A, and prolonged deceleration time (*DT*). Six months later **(right)**, it had become pseudonormalized, with progressive cardiac amyloidosis. **B:** In another patient, the initial study **(left)** showed a DT of 190 msec, with normal E and A. Seven months later **(right)**, the mitral inflow became typical of a restrictive pattern (increased E, decreased A, and decreased DT), indicating that the initial Doppler pattern was of a "pseudonormalized" inflow. (From ref. 6, with permission.)

abnormality and a moderate increase in LA filling pressure before becoming frankly restrictive. Deceleration time (DT) is one of the most important prognostic variables in cardiac amyloidosis (7). The shorter the DT, the poorer the prognosis. The average survival for patients with a DT of ≤150 msec is <1 year, compared with 3 years when DT is >150 msec (Fig. 13-5). In summary, the echocardiographic evaluation of cardiac amyloidosis provides comprehensive morphologic, functional (systolic and diastolic), and prognostic information.

CARCINOID

Carcinoid heart disease is caused by a slow-growing metastatic carcinoid tumor, which usually originates in the ileum. Cardiac involvement occurs almost exclusively with hepatic metastases and is caused by substances released by the tumor, such as serotonin and bradykinin. Because the tumor substances are inactivated by the lung, cardiac involvement is predominantly on the right side, but it may involve the left side (7% of cases), most likely because a patent foramen ovale allows the tumor substances to pass from the right atrium (RA) to the LA or because of pulmonary metastasis (8). The predominant lesion of cardiac carcinoid is fibrosis of the cardiac valves and endocardium, especially the tricuspid and pulmonary valves (9). These valvular abnormalities produce characteristic thickening (fibrosis) and restricted motion of the valves that are responsible for severe tricuspid regurgitation, usually mild tricuspid stenosis, and varying degrees of pulmonic stenosis (Figs. 13-6 and 13-7).

These morphologic changes of carcinoid valvular involvement are readily detected by 2D echocardiography. The tricuspid valve is thickened and retracted with limited

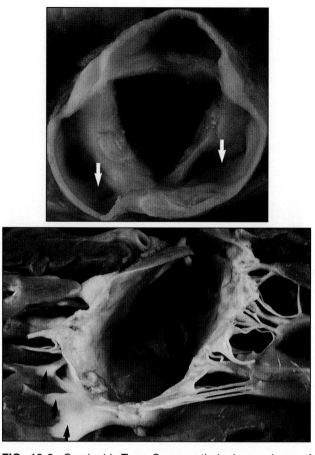

FIG. 13-6. Carcinoid. **Top:** Gross pathologic specimen of carcinoid heart disease. Pulmonic valve leaflets are thickened, retracted, and shortened, with a fixed opening. Note fibrous endocardial plaque (*arrows*). **Bottom:** Tricuspid valve leaflets and chordae are thickened and retracted. (From Click RL, Olson LJ, Edwards WD, et al. Echocardiography and systemic diseases. *J Am Soc Echocardiogr* 1994;7:201–216, with permission.)

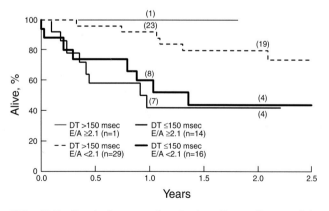

FIG. 13-5. Survival curve of patients with cardiac amyloidosis. Patients with deceleration time (*DT*) of ≤150 msec had a 1-year mortality rate of 50%, which was 90% when DT was >150 msec. (From ref. 7, with permission.)

mobility and coaptation is incomplete, resulting in severe tricuspid regurgitation. The severe tricuspid regurgitation produces a right ventricular (RV) volume overload pattern, with an enlarged RV and ventricular septal motion abnormalities. The pulmonary valve, whose increased thickness and retraction result in pulmonic stenosis, is occasionally difficult to image with the transthoracic approach. The transesophageal longitudinal-axis view of the RV outflow tract may be needed to visualize the pulmonary valve. Characteristically, the wall thickness of the ventricles is normal in carcinoid heart disease, and carcinoid plaque over the endocardial walls in the chambers on the right side may be seen by using transesophageal echocardiography (TEE). Carcinoid also may produce a metastatic tumor embedded in the myocardium (Fig. 13-8) (8). The 2D echocardiographic features of carcinoid heart disease are distinctive

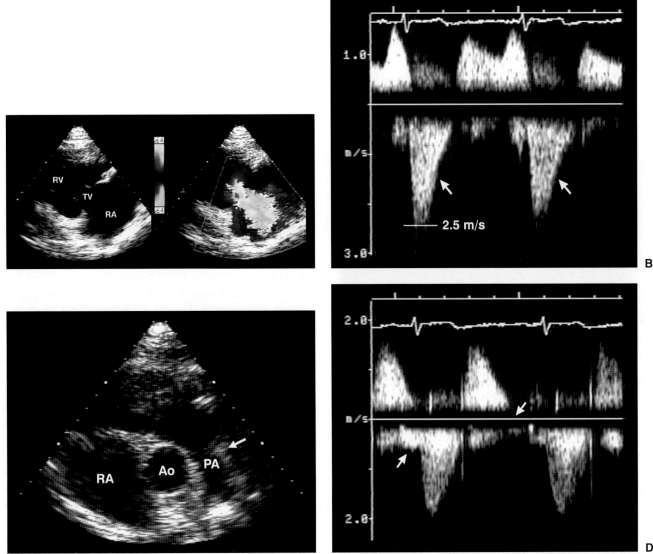

FIG. 13-7. A: Left: Two-dimensional systolic frame of right ventricular (*RV*) inflow view showing carcinoid involvement of the tricuspid valve (*TV*). Anterior and septal tricuspid leaflets do not coapt because of retraction and thickening, which results in severe tricuspid regurgitation. **Right:** Color-flow imaging shows severe tricuspid regurgitation. **B:** Continuous-wave Doppler signal of tricuspid flow in carcinoid heart disease. Systolic tricuspid regurgitation velocity is 2.5 m/sec, which is higher than expected for pure severe tricuspid regurgitation. If right atrial (*RA*) pressure is assumed to be 20 mm Hg, RV systolic pressure is 45 mm Hg, because of mild degree of pulmonary stenosis in carcinoid. Concavity (*arrows*) of downslope of tricuspid regurgitation corresponds to the "V" wave because of severe regurgitation. Diastolic inflow velocity is increased because of severe tricuspid regurgitation. **C:** Parasternal short-axis view at the level of the pulmonary valve showing carcinoid involvement of the pulmonary valve. The pulmonary valve annulus (*arrow*) is retracted and narrowed, and the valve is diminutive. *Ao*, aorta; *PA*, pulmonary artery. **D:** Continuous-wave Doppler signal from the narrowed pulmonary valve shows mild stenosis, with a peak systolic velocity of 2 m/sec and a regurgitant signal with a short deceleration time due to rapid equalization (*downward arrow*) of RV and pulmonary artery diastolic pressures before the onset of QRS. There is also diastolic flow (*upward arrow*) across the pulmonary valve due to rapid rise in RV diastolic pressure.

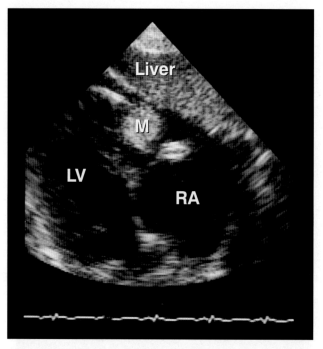

FIG. 13-8. Myocardial metastasis (*M*) in the left ventricular (*LV*) wall of a 61-year-old man who also had carcinoid involvement of the tricuspid and pulmonary valves. This was confirmed pathologically. (From ref. 8, with permission.)

and readily distinguishable from other lesions producing right-sided heart failure, such as Ebstein anomaly, RV contusion, RV infarct, tricuspid valve dysplasia, and severe tricuspid regurgitation due to intrinsic valvular abnormalities. Rarely, cardiac valvular lesions resembling carcinoid involvement may develop with excessive use of ergot or, more recently, a diet pill combination (''fen-phen'') (see the following).

DRUG-INDUCED CARDIAC DISEASES

Drugs have been identified as responsible agents for causing cardiomyopathy or valvulopathy. Doxorubicin (Adriamycin), a chemotherapy agent, is well known for producing LV dilatation and systolic dysfunction (10). Its cardiac toxicity is dose related and potentiated by concurrent or previous radiation therapy. Patients who need chemotherapy with doxorubicin should have a baseline 2D echocardiographic examination and follow-up studies at regular intervals thereafter. LV systolic dysfunction caused by doxorubicin may not be reversible and usually occurs after a dose greater than 450 g/m^2. A similar cardiomyopathy is produced by daunorubicin (>600 mg/m^2) and cyclophosphamide (>6.2 g/m^2) (11). In addition, pericardial effusion or tamponade may develop after cyclophosphamide treatment. Severe LV systolic dysfunction also has been

reported in bulimic patients who ingested ipecac (12). Emetine, the principal component of ipecac, causes mitochondrial damage by inhibiting oxidative phosphorylation. Chronic high-dose steroid therapy may result in LV systolic dysfunction. Cardiac function can be suppressed by phenothiazines and tricyclic antidepressants.

Cardiac valves may be affected by drug toxicity. Ergot alkaloids may produce valvular lesions similar to those of rheumatic or carcinoid (or both) valvular disease (13). The 2D echocardiographic findings are similar to those for the abnormalities already mentioned, but microscopic examination shows fibrous plaque stuck on relatively normal valve tissue in patients who have taken ergot alkaloids. Anorectic drugs have been implicated as causes of valvulopathy or pulmonary hypertension (or both). In the late 1960s and early 1970s in Europe, aminorex was found to cause pulmonary hypertension. More recently, Connolly et al. (14) at our institution reported 24 patients who took ''fen-phen'' and were found to have aortic, mitral, or tricuspid regurgitation (Fig. 13-9). Because four to six million people worldwide have been exposed to fenfluramine or dexfenfluramine with or without phentermine, the health implications of this finding are potentially huge. Subsequent studies have documented an 8% to 30% prevalence of valvular regurgitation in patients who took ''fen-phen'' for various lengths of time. Valvular regurgitation or pulmonary hypertension has been identified in patients who took the medication for less than 1 month. It is recommended that patients who did take fenfluramine or dexfenfluramine with or without phentermine undergo echocardiography if symptoms or signs of valvular regurgitation develop. Valvular regurgitation is considered to be associated with ''fen-phen'' when echocardiography demonstrates mild aortic regurgitation or a moderate degree of mitral regurgitation. Aortic regurgitation is more common than mitral regurgitation.

HEMOCHROMATOSIS

Idiopathic hemochromatosis is an autosomal recessive disease, with an incidence of two to three per 1,000 population. It is characterized by large deposits of iron in various organs, including the heart, liver, testes, and pancreas. When the heart is involved, the disease is usually in an advanced stage, with multiorgan involvement. The severity of myocardial dysfunction is proportional to the amount of iron deposited in the myocardium. Myocardial deposits of excessive iron interfere with myocardial cellular function and result in LV dilatation and systolic dysfunction, as in dilated cardiomyopathy (Fig. 13-10). Progressive congestive heart failure is the most frequent cause of death of patients with hemochromatosis. Therefore, in patients who present with heart failure and features of dilated cardiomyopathy of unknown cause, the iron level, iron-binding

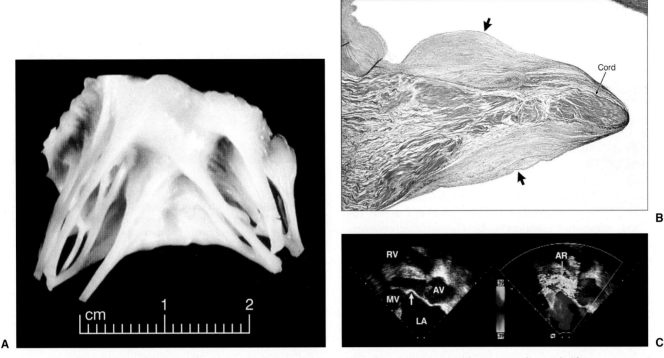

FIG. 13-9. A: Gross specimen of explanted mitral valve from a 45-year-old woman who took "fen-phen" for 11 months. Leaflets and chordae are glistening and thickened. **B:** Low-power view of section of resected mitral valve from a 44-year-old woman who took fen-phen for 12 months. Note the intact valve structure, with "stuck-on" plaques (*arrows*). (Elastic-van Gieson stain; ×36.) (From ref. 14, with permission.) **C:** Typical echocardiographic features of mitral valve associated with "fen-phen" treatment. Both the aortic (*AV*) and mitral valves (*MV*) are thickened. The anterior mitral leaflet (*arrow*) has a doming during diastole, resembling a rheumatic MV. Color-flow imaging shows severe aortic regurgitation (*AR*).

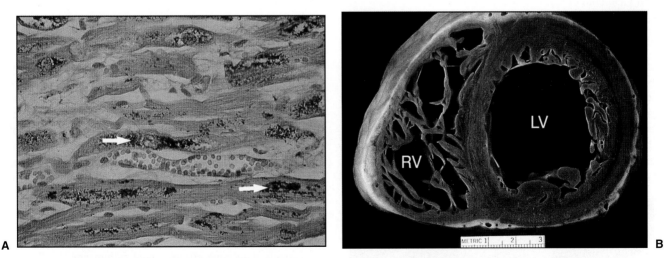

FIG. 13-10. Hemochromatosis. **A:** Histologic section of myocardial biopsy specimen showing iron (*black stain*) within the myocardial cells (*arrows*). **B:** Gross pathologic specimen with the reddish brown rust appearance and dilated cardiac chambers characteristic of cardiac hemochromatosis. (From Click RL, Olson LJ, Edwards WD, et al. Echocardiography and systemic diseases. *J Am Soc Echocardiogr* 1994;7:201–216, with permission.)

capacity, and ferritin level should be determined. Typical 2D echocardiographic findings of cardiac hemochromatosis include mild LV dilatation, LV systolic dysfunction, normal wall thickness, normal heart valves, and biatrial enlargement (Fig. 13-11) (15). Dilatation of heart chambers produces varying degrees of mitral and tricuspid valve regurgitation. When a patient presents with congestive heart failure, the LV diastolic filling pattern is usually restrictive and the morphologic features are those of dilated cardiomyopathy. These typical echocardiographic findings were found in 37% of patients with hemochromatosis seen at the Mayo Clinic (15). Most of the patients with these echocardiographic findings died within 6 months after the echocardiographic examination. LV dysfunction can be reversed, sometimes completely, by chronic phlebotomies. Serial echocardiographic examination is useful to monitor the response of LV function.

HUMAN IMMUNODEFICIENCY VIRUS INFECTION

Various cardiovascular abnormalities have been described in patients with human immunodeficiency virus infection, including pericardial effusion, tamponade, dilated cardiomyopathy, pulmonary hypertension, endocarditis, and intracardiac tumor (Fig. 13-12) (16,17). A prospective study with serial echocardiography showed that the incidence of pericardial effusion in surviving acquired immunodeficiency syndrome patients was 11% per year. Pericardial effusion is usually small and asymptomatic; however, survival was shorter for patients in whom pericardial effusion developed independently of albumin level and CD4 count (17).

HYPEREOSINOPHILIC SYNDROME

Hypereosinophilic syndrome is defined as a persistent eosinophilia with more than 1,500 eosinophils/mm^3 and evidence of organ involvement. Cardiac involvement in hypereosinophilic syndrome is very common and involves both the right and left sides of the heart, with endocardial thickening of the inflow areas and thrombotic-fibrotic obliteration of the ventricular apices. Typical echocardiographic

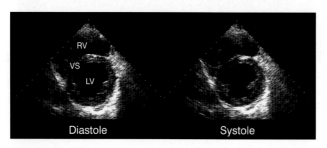

FIG. 13-11. Typical parasternal short-axis views of two-dimensional echocardiographic image of hemochromatosis, resembling dilated cardiomyopathy. *VS*, ventricular septum.

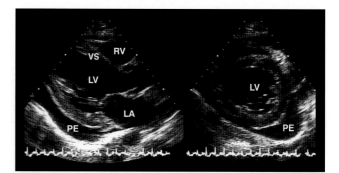

FIG. 13-12. Systolic frames of parasternal long- **(left)** and short-axis **(right)** views of transthoracic echocardiogram, demonstrating dilated cardiomyopathy and pericardial effusion (*PE*) in a young man with acquired immunodeficiency syndrome. *VS*, ventricular septum.

features include limited motion of the posterior mitral leaflet (resulting in mitral regurgitation of varying severity) together with thickening of the inferobasal LV wall, endocardial thrombotic-fibrotic lesion, and biventricular apical obliteration by thrombus (Fig. 13-13) (18). The obliteration of the apical cavity and eosinophilic involvement of the endocardium decrease ventricular compliance and limit ventricular diastolic filling, producing restrictive physiology on pulsed-wave Doppler echocardiography. Rarely, acute hypereosinophilic crisis produces diffuse myocarditis with ventricular cavity dilatation, with a marked decrease in systolic function. Patients usually die of severe heart failure or uncontrollable ventricular arrhythmias.

RADIATION-INDUCED CARDIAC DISEASES

Radiation to the mediastinum can damage the coronary arteries, pericardium, valves, or myocardium, resulting in proximal coronary stenosis, pericardial effusion, constrictive pericarditis, regurgitant valve, restrictive cardiomyopathy, or a combination of these. Radiation-induced valve damage is manifested as thickening and regurgitation of any valve, although the tricuspid valve is most frequently involved. A more severe cardiac manifestation is failure of the right side of the heart, from constrictive pericarditis or restrictive cardiomyopathy (or both). Echo-Doppler features of constriction and restriction are discussed in detail in Chapter 14.

RENAL FAILURE

Patients who have chronic renal failure are usually hypertensive, and the most prominent echocardiographic finding is increased LV wall thicknesses related to LV hypertrophy. The myocardial texture with LV hypertrophy appears similar to that of cardiac amyloidosis, but these two conditions can be distinguished. Chronic renal failure is associated with LV hypertrophy and cardiac amyloidosis, with decreased voltage on ECG. Although systolic function

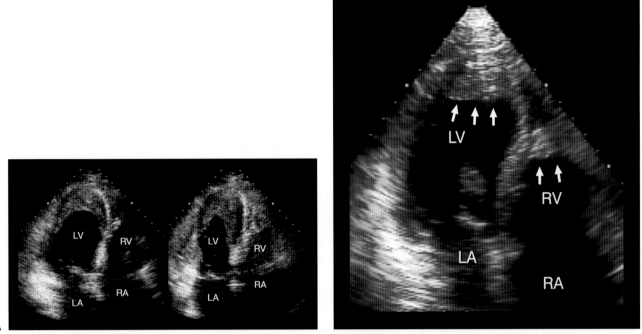

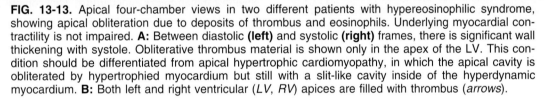

FIG. 13-13. Apical four-chamber views in two different patients with hypereosinophilic syndrome, showing apical obliteration due to deposits of thrombus and eosinophils. Underlying myocardial contractility is not impaired. **A:** Between diastolic **(left)** and systolic **(right)** frames, there is significant wall thickening with systole. Obliterative thrombus material is shown only in the apex of the LV. This condition should be differentiated from apical hypertrophic cardiomyopathy, in which the apical cavity is obliterated by hypertrophied myocardium but still with a slit-like cavity inside of the hyperdynamic myocardium. **B:** Both left and right ventricular (*LV, RV*) apices are filled with thrombus (*arrows*).

is normal in the early stage of chronic renal failure, diastolic function is abnormal, with decreased myocardial relaxation. As the disease progresses with decreased compliance of the myocardium, LV filling pressure increases and the diastolic filling pattern may become pseudonormalized or even restrictive. LV systolic function also may decrease with long-standing hypertension. Also, small amounts of pericardial effusion are common, especially in patients undergoing chronic hemodialysis. Chronic renal failure commonly causes valvular sclerosis with calcification; the mitral annulus is also calcified.

SARCOIDOSIS

Sarcoidosis is a granulomatous disease of unknown cause involving multiple organs. Its most important manifestation is caused by pulmonary involvement, resulting in diffuse pulmonary fibrosis, right-sided heart failure, and pulmonary hypertension (19). Cardiac involvement is uncommon and occurs in fewer than 20% of patients. The myocardium is involved by noncaseating granulomas, producing myocardial fibrosis and regional wall motion abnormalities. The fibrosis occurs predominantly at the mid and basal levels of the LV, although global involvement may occur. Thinning and aneurysmal formation occur, mainly at the basal inferior and lateral portions of the LV. Therefore, the 2D

echocardiographic features include a dilated LV with regional wall motion abnormalities, especially at the mid and basal levels of the LV (20). Posterior basal aneurysm may be seen. These echocardiographic features were found in 14% of the patients with sarcoidosis examined at the Mayo Clinic, and the symptoms of congestive heart failure were more common in these patients (20). Although the angiotensin-converting enzyme (ACE) level is commonly used to diagnose sarcoidosis, most patients who had the echocardiographic features of cardiac involvement had normal ACE levels and noncaseating granulomas in the endomyocardial biopsy specimen. Therefore, normal ACE levels do not exclude active cardiac sarcoidosis and should not deter one from obtaining endomyocardial biopsy specimens to make the diagnosis.

SCLERODERMA

The most common cardiac abnormality associated with scleroderma is a pericardial lesion, which occurs in up to 78% of patients (21). Cardiac tamponade that requires pericardiocentesis rarely develops, although pericardial effusion is common. Pulmonary hypertension is a prominent feature of scleroderma and the cause of a patient's shortness of breath. Tricuspid regurgitation velocity should be reported in all patients with scleroderma. The myocardium may be involved with fibrosis or sclerosis, resulting in systolic and diastolic dysfunction. Therefore, global systolic and diastolic function evaluation should be an essential part of the echocardiographic examination of patients with scleroderma.

SEPSIS

LV dilatation and decreased ejection fraction (EF) frequently are observed in patients with sepsis and septic shock (22). Patients who survive the septic shock have a lower left ventricular ejection fraction (LVEF) than those who did not (23). In patients who survive, the LV dilatation and systolic dysfunction are reversible. The cause of myocardial dysfunction and sepsis is not clear. It may be related to a circulating myocardial depressant, such as an endotoxin, tumor necrosis factor, or interleukin. Therefore, echocardiography frequently shows a dilated LV with a decreased EF in patients with sepsis. Stroke volume is maintained (normal LV outflow tract time velocity integral and velocity), however, because of a decrease in systemic vascular resistance. Certain infections result in characteristic cardiac and echocardiographic abnormalities: an intracardiac mass in echinococcosis or tuberculosis (Chapter 16); pericarditis in viral, bacterial, or tuberculosis infection; and ventricular aneurysm in Chagas disease.

Chagas disease (American trypanosomiasis) is little known in North America but is endemic in all Latin American countries. In infected patients, heart muscle is invaded by the protozoan parasite *Trypanosoma cruzi,* resulting in characteristic abnormalities: biventricular enlargement, ventricular aneurysms, thinning of the ventricular wall, and mural thrombi (24). The conduction system is also affected, producing conduction abnormalities. With an increasing number of persons infected with *T. cruzi* immigrating to North America, it is important for physicians and sonographers to be familiar with the echocardiographic manifestations of this infection.

SPONDYLOARTHROPATHIES

Spondyloarthropathies with cardiac involvement include ankylosing spondylitis and Reiter syndrome. Cardiac manifestations of ankylosing spondylitis include aortic regurgitation, pericardial effusion, and conduction abnormalities. Aortic regurgitation results from thickening of the aortic valve cusps, displacement of the cusps by the fibrous tissue bump, and dilatation of the aortic root. Patients with ankylosing spondylitis may need aortic valve replacement because of severe aortic valve regurgitation. Aortic regurgitation with the dilatation of the aorta is also seen in patients with Reiter syndrome or psoriatic arthritis.

SYSTEMIC LUPUS ERYTHEMATOSUS

Lupus is a systemic disease characterized by the presence of antinuclear antibodies, which produce immune complexes that cause inflammation of various organs. The most common cardiac involvement is pericarditis, found in more than two-thirds of patients. Thus, detection of pericardial effusion by echocardiography is one of the diagnostic criteria for systemic lupus erythematosus. Despite the frequent presence of pericardial effusion, tamponade and constrictive pericarditis are uncommon. The myocardium may be involved by vasculitis, resulting in myocarditis, but significant LV diastolic dysfunction is rare. Another characteristic cardiac lesion is *Libman-Sacks endocarditis*, with a verrucous valvular lesion usually involving the mitral valve (25). It is found most commonly on the basal portion of the mitral valve but can extend to the chordal structure or papillary muscles (Fig. 13-14). Aortic valve involvement in Libman-Sacks endocarditis is uncommon. These lesions are difficult to see on transthoracic echocardiograms, but detection is enhanced with TEE. Metastatic tumors also involve cardiac valves, producing lesions similar to those seen in Libman-Sacks endocarditis. This condition is called *marantic endocarditis,* which occurs most commonly with Hodgkin disease and adenocarcinoma of the lung, pancreas, stomach, and colon.

OTHER CONDITIONS

The heart is affected by many other systemic, rheumatic, endocrine, genetic, and infectious diseases. Pheochromocytoma and Friedreich ataxia produce a concentric increase in LV wall thickness (26,27). Friedreich ataxia is an auto-

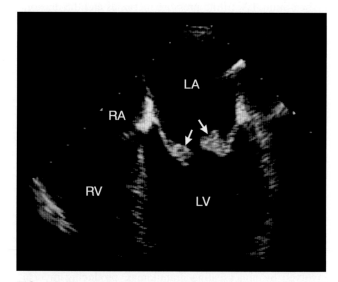

FIG. 13-14. Libman-Sacks endocarditis in a 36-year-old woman with systemic lupus erythematosus and no clinical evidence of bacterial endocarditis. Diastolic frame of the horizontal transesophageal echocardiographic view of the mitral valve shows large verrucous vegetations (*arrows*).

somal recessive disease that produces spinal cerebellar ataxia. Ninety percent of patients with this disease have cardiac involvement. The 2D echocardiographic findings are mostly similar to those of hypertrophic cardiomyopathy, although LV hypertrophy is more often concentric. Asymmetric septal hypertrophy is unusual and LV outflow tract obstruction is not common. In a small proportion of patients (7%), the LV may be dilated, with decreased systolic function due to diffuse interstitial fibrosis (15). Most patients with pheochromocytoma have normal echocardiographic findings except for hyperdynamic systolic function, but occasionally concentric LV hypertrophy occurs (26). When a catecholamine crisis develops in a patient with pheochromocytoma, acute myocarditis may result with LV dilatation, with decreased systolic function that may be reversible with treatment of the pheochromocytoma.

Certain neuromuscular diseases also involve the myocardial segment, especially Duchenne dystrophy, which involves the inferobasal area with myocardial fibrosis. The 2D echocardiographic findings in Duchenne dystrophy are similar to those of inferior myocardial infarction. Patients with hypothyroidism, or rarely hyperthyroidism, may develop dilated cardiomyopathy, which resolves when the underlying endocrine abnormalities are corrected.

REFERENCES

1. Siqueira-Filho AG, Cunha CL, Tajik AJ, Seward JB, Schattenberg TT, Giuliani ER. M-mode and two-dimensional echocardiographic features in cardiac amyloidosis. *Circulation* 1981;63:188–196.
2. Gertz MA, Grogan M, Kyle RA, Tajik AJ. Endomyocardial biopsy-proven light chain amyloidosis (AL) without echocardiographic features of infiltrative cardiomyopathy. *Am J Cardiol* 1997;80:93–95.
3. Roberts WC, Waller BF. Cardiac amyloidosis causing cardiac dysfunction: analysis of 54 necropsy patients. *Am J Cardiol* 1983;52:137–146.
4. Olson LJ, Reeder GS, Noller KL, Edwards WD, Howell RR, Michels VV. Cardiac involvement in glycogen storage disease III: Morphologic and biochemical characterization with endomyocardial biopsy. *Am J Cardiol* 1984;53:980–981.
5. Oh JK, Tajik AJ, Edwards WD, Bresnahan JF, Kyle RA. Dynamic left ventricular outflow tract obstruction in cardiac amyloidosis detected by continuous-wave Doppler echocardiography. *Am J Cardiol* 1987;59:1008–1010.
6. Klein AL, Hatle LK, Taliercio CP, et al. Serial Doppler echocardiographic follow-up of left ventricular diastolic function in cardiac amyloidosis. *J Am Coll Cardiol* 1990;16:1135–1141.
7. Klein AL, Hatle LK, Taliercio CP, et al. Prognostic significance of Doppler measures of diastolic function in cardiac amyloidosis: a Doppler echocardiography study. *Circulation* 1991;83:808–816.
8. Pellikka PA, Tajik AJ, Khandheria BK, et al. Carcinoid heart disease: clinical and echocardiographic spectrum in 74 patients. *Circulation* 1993;87:1188–1196.
9. Callahan JA, Wroblewski EM, Reeder GS, Edwards WD, Seward JB, Tajik AJ. Echocardiographic features of carcinoid heart disease. *Am J Cardiol* 1982;50:762–768.
10. Bristow MR, Mason JW, Billingham ME, Daniels JR. Doxorubicin cardiomyopathy: evaluation by phonocardiography, endomyocardial biopsy, and cardiac catheterization. *Ann Intern Med* 1978;88:168–175.
11. Gottdiener JS, Appelbaum FR, Ferrans VJ, Deisseroth A, Ziegler J. Cardiotoxicity associated with high-dose cyclophosphamide therapy. *Arch Intern Med* 1981;141:758–763.
12. Schiff RJ, Wurzel CL, Brunson SC, Kasloff I, Nussbaum MP, Frank SD. Death due to chronic syrup of ipecac use in a patient with bulimia. *Pediatrics* 1986;78:412–416.
13. Redfield MM, Nicholson WJ, Edwards WD, Tajik AJ. Valve disease associated with ergot alkaloid use: echocardiographic and pathologic correlations. *Ann Intern Med* 1992;117:50–52.
14. Connolly HM, Crary JL, McGoon MD, et al. Valvular heart disease associated with fenfluramine-phentermine. *N Engl J Med* 1997;337:581–588.
15. Olson LJ, Baldus WP, Tajik AJ. Echocardiographic features of idiopathic hemochromatosis. *Am J Cardiol* 1987;60:885–889.
16. Hoit BD, Ramrakhyani K. Pulmonary venous flow in cardiac tamponade: Influence of left ventricular dysfunction and the relation to pulsus paradoxus. *J Am Soc Echocardiogr* 1991;4:559–570.
17. Heidenreich PA, Eisenberg MJ, Kee LL, et al. Pericardial effusion in AIDS: incidence and survival. *Circulation* 1995;92:3229–3234.
18. Gottdiener JS, Maron BJ, Schooley RT, Harley JB, Roberts WC, Fauci AS. Two-dimensional echocardiographic assessment of the idiopathic hypereosinophilic syndrome: anatomic basis of mitral regurgitation and peripheral embolization. *Circulation* 1983;67:572–578.
19. Newman LS, Rose CS, Maier LA. Sarcoidosis. *N Engl J Med* 1997;336:1224–1234.
20. Burstow DJ, Tajik AJ, Bailey KR, DeRemee RA, Taliercio CP. Two-dimensional echocardiographic findings in systemic sarcoidosis. *Am J Cardiol* 1989;63:478–482.
21. Byers RJ, Marshall DA, Freemont AJ. Pericardial involvement in systemic sclerosis. *Ann Rheum Dis* 1997;56:393–394.
22. Bunnell E, Parrillo JE. Cardiac dysfunction during septic shock. *Clin Chest Med* 1996;17:237–248.
23. Parker MM, Suffredini AF, Natanson C, et al. Responses of left ventricular function in survivors and nonsurvivors of septic shock. *J Crit Care* 1989;4:19–25.
24. Kirchhoff LV. American trypanosomiasis (Chagas disease)—a tropical disease now in the United States. *N Engl J Med* 1993;329:639–644.
25. Libman E, Sacks B. A hitherto undescribed form of valvular and mural endocarditis. *Arch Intern Med* 1924;33:701–738.
26. Shub C, Williamson MD, Tajik AJ, Eubanks DR. Dynamic left ventricular outflow tract obstruction associated with pheochromocytoma. *Am Heart J* 1981;102:286–290.
27. Alboliras ET, Shub C, Gomez MR, et al. Spectrum of cardiac involvement in Friedreich's ataxia: clinical, electrocardiographic and echocardiographic observations. *Am J Cardiol* 1986;58:518–524.

CHAPTER 14

Pericardial Disease

The detection of pericardial effusion was one of the most exciting initial clinical applications of cardiac ultrasonography (1–4). Echocardiography continues to be essential in the diagnosis and management of pericardial disease. Pericardial effusion, tamponade, pericardial cyst, and absent pericardium are readily recognized on two-dimensional (2D) echocardiography. When a pericardial effusion needs to be drained, pericardiocentesis can be performed safely under the guidance of 2D echocardiography. Although it usually is difficult to establish the diagnosis of constrictive pericarditis with 2D echocardiography alone, the characteristic respiratory variation in flow velocities, as recorded on Doppler echocardiography, has added strength and confidence to the noninvasive diagnosis of constrictive pericarditis.

Transesophageal echocardiography (TEE) is helpful in measuring pericardial thickness, in evaluating diastolic function (for tamponade or constrictive physiology) from the pulmonary vein, and in detecting loculated pericardial effusion or other structural abnormalities of the pericardium. The various applications of echocardiography in the evaluation of pericardial diseases are discussed in this chapter.

CONGENITALLY ABSENT PERICARDIUM

The congenital absence of the pericardium usually involves the left side of the pericardium. Complete absence of the pericardium on the right side is uncommon. The defect is more frequent in males, and it rarely creates symptoms such as chest pain, dyspnea, or syncope. Because of the pericardial defect, cardiac motion is exaggerated, especially the posterior wall of the left ventricle (LV). The entire cardiac structure is shifted to the left; hence, the right ventricular (RV) cavity appears enlarged from the standard parasternal windows, mimicking the RV volume overload pattern on echocardiography (5,6). The absence of pericardium should be considered when the RV appears enlarged from the parasternal window and is at the center of the usual apical image (Fig. 14-1A). This condition is also associated with a high incidence of atrial septal defect, bi-

cuspid aortic valve, and bronchogenic cysts. It is readily recognized because of its typical 2D echocardiographic features, and the diagnosis can be confirmed with computed tomography or magnetic resonance imaging (Fig. 14-1B).

Pericardial Cyst

A pericardial cyst typically is a benign structural abnormality of the pericardium that usually is detected as an incidental mass lesion on chest radiographs (Fig. 14-2). Most frequently, pericardial cysts are located in the right costophrenic angle, but they also are found in the left costophrenic angle, hilum, and superior mediastinum. Pericardial cysts need to be differentiated from malignant tumors, cardiac chamber enlargement, and diaphragmatic hernia. Two-dimensional echocardiography is useful in differentiating a pericardial cyst from other solid structures, because a cyst is filled with clear fluid and appears as an echo-free structure (Fig. 14-3).

Pericardial Effusion/Tamponade

When the potential pericardial space is filled with fluid or blood, it is detected as an echo-free space. When the amount of effusion is greater than 25 mL, an echo-free space persists throughout the cardiac cycle. A smaller amount of pericardial effusion may be detected as a posterior echo-free space that is present only during the systolic phase. As pericardial effusion increases, movement of the parietal pericardium decreases. When the amount of pericardial effusion is massive, the heart may have a ''swinging'' motion in the pericardial cavity (Fig. 14-4), which is responsible for the electrocardiographic manifestation of cardiac tamponade, ''electrical alternans.'' The swinging motion is not always present in cardiac tamponade, however. Various M-mode and 2D echocardiographic signs have been reported in this life-threatening condition (7,8): early diastolic collapse of the RV, late diastolic right atrial (RA) inversion, abnormal ventricular septal motion, respiratory variation in ventricle chamber size (Fig. 14-5),

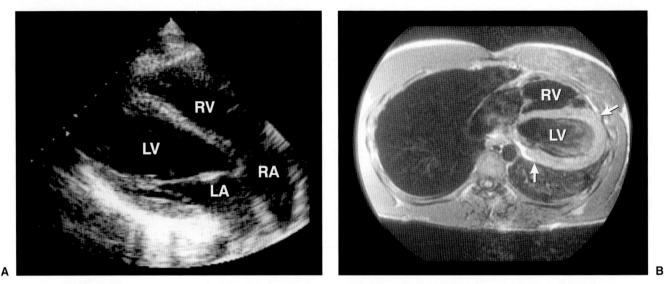

FIG. 14-1. **A:** Two-dimensional still-frame obtained from the normal apical position (left fifth intercostal space at the midclavicular line) in a patient with a congenitally absent pericardium. Because of the leftward shift of the heart, the right ventricle (*RV*) is at the center of the apical image rather than the left ventricular (*LV*) apex; this is often confused with RV volume overload. Cardiac catheterization was performed elsewhere to evaluate an atrial septal defect and showed no shunt prior to this evaluation. **B:** Magnetic resonance image of the chest showing a marked shift of the heart to the left side of the chest because of the partial absence of the pericardium on the left side. *Arrows* indicate area of absent pericardium.

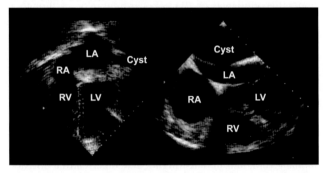

FIG. 14-3. Transthoracic and transesophageal echocardiographic images of a pericardial cyst. Apex-down apical four-chamber view **(left)** showing a large echo-free cyst structure next to the left atrium (*LA*) and left ventricle (*LV*). Transverse transesophageal four-chamber view **(right)** showing a large pericardial cyst compressing the LA posterior wall.

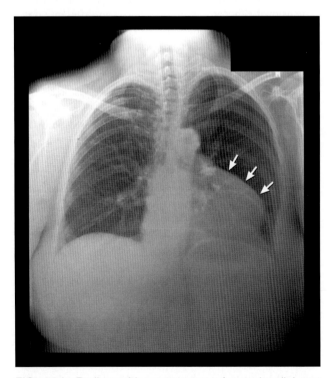

FIG. 14-2. Radiographic appearance of a pericardial cyst (*arrows*).

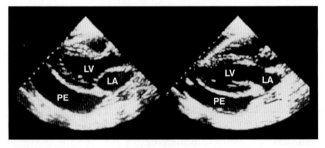

FIG. 14-4. With a large amount of pericardial effusion (*PE*), the heart has a swinging motion, which is an ominous sign of cardiac tamponade. When the left ventricular (*LV*) cavity is close to the surface **(left)**, the QRS voltage increases on the electrocardiogram, but it decreases when the LV swings away from the surface **(right)**, producing electrical alternans.

182

Effusion/Tamponade

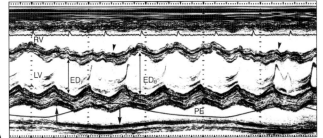

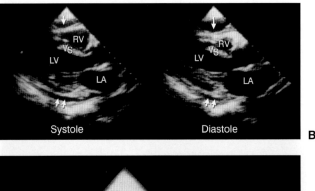

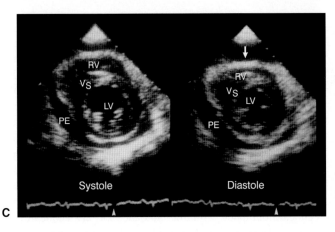

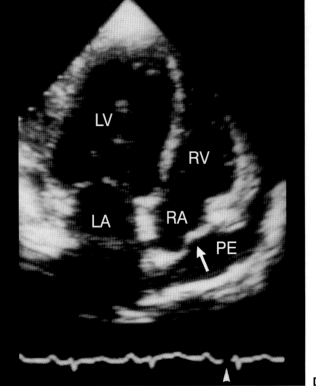

FIG. 14-5. A: M-mode echocardiogram from the parasternal window in a patient with cardiac tamponade and large circumferential pericardial effusion (*PE*). The M-mode was recorded simultaneously with the respirometer tracing at the bottom (*upward arrow* indicates onset of inspiration and *downward arrow* indicates onset of expiration). The left ventricular (*LV*) dimension during inspiration (*ED*ᵢ) becomes smaller than with expiration (*ED*ₑ). The opposite changes occur in the right ventricle (*RV*). The ventricular septum (*arrowheads*) moves toward the LV with inspiration and toward the RV with expiration, accounting for the abnormal ventricular septum in patients with cardiac tamponade. Parasternal long-axis (**B**) and short-axis (**C**) views of a patient with tamponade during systole and diastole. The pericardial effusion (*double arrows* in **B**; *PE* in **C**) appears small in the long axis and moderate in the short axis during systole, but during early diastole, the RV free wall collapses (*arrow* at top). *VS*, ventricular septum. **D:** Apical four-chamber view demonstrating late diastolic (*arrowhead* on electrocardiograph) collapse of right atrium (*RA*) wall (*arrow*). This sign is sensitive but not specific for tamponade. When RA inversion lasts longer than a third of the RR interval, it is specific for hemodynamically significant pericardial effusion.

and plethora of the inferior vena cava with blunted respiratory changes. In case of acute myocardial rupture or proximal aortic dissection, clotted blood may be seen in the pericardial sac; this finding is highly suggestive of hemopericardium (Fig. 14-6). When there is air in the pericardial sac (pneumopericardium) as a result of esophageal perforation, cardiac imaging [both transthoracic echocardiography (TTE) and TEE] is difficult because ultrasound does not penetrate air well.

Recently, the Doppler echocardiographic features of pericardial effusion/tamponade have been reported to be more sensitive than the features mentioned above (9,10). The Doppler findings of cardiac tamponade are based on the

following characteristic respiratory variations in intrathoracic and intracardiac hemodynamics (Fig. 14-7). Normally, intrapericardial pressure (hence, LV diastolic pressure) and intrathoracic pressure fall the same degree during inspiration, but in cardiac tamponade intrapericardial pressure falls substantially less than intrathoracic pressure. Therefore, the LV filling pressure gradient [from pulmonary wedge pressure to LV diastolic pressure (the shaded area in Fig. 14-7)] decreases with inspiration. With the decreased LA filling pressure, mitral valve opening is delayed, which lengthens the isovolumic relaxation time (IVRT) and decreases mitral E velocity. In cardiac tamponade, the ventricles are coupled because of the relatively fixed cardiac volume; thus, recip-

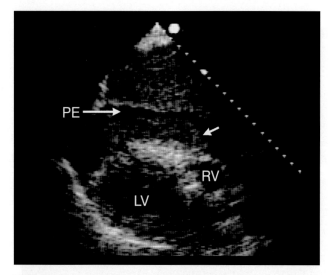

FIG. 14-6. Subcostal echocardiogram of a patient with cardiogenic shock after acute myocardial infarction. In addition to pericardial effusion (*PE*), there is an echo-dense structure (*small arrow*) along the ventricular walls that indicates clot formation. Urgent pericardiocentesis was performed to temporize the clinical situation, after which the patient underwent an emergency operation and survived. (Courtesy of S. Hayes, M.D.)

rocal changes occur in the cardiac chambers on the right side (Fig. 14-8).

The respiratory flow velocity changes across the mitral and tricuspid valves are reflected in the pulmonary and hepatic venous flow velocities, respectively: inspiratory decrease and expiratory increase in pulmonary vein diastolic forward flow and expiratory decrease in hepatic vein forward flow and increase in expiratory reversal flow (Fig. 14-9) (10).

Echocardiographically Guided Pericardiocentesis

The most effective treatment for cardiac tamponade is removal of the pericardial fluid. Although pericardiocentesis is lifesaving, a blind percutaneous attempt has a high rate of complications, including pneumothorax, puncture of the cardiac wall, or death. Two-dimensional echocardiography can guide pericardiocentesis by locating the optimal site of puncture, by determining the depth of the pericardial effusion and the distance from the puncture site to the effusion, and by monitoring the results of the pericardiocentesis (Fig. 14-10) (11–13). At the Mayo Clinic, most pericardiocentesis procedures are performed by an echocardiographer with the guidance of 2D echocardiography. Among more than 1,000 of these procedures, only one death has been related to the procedure.

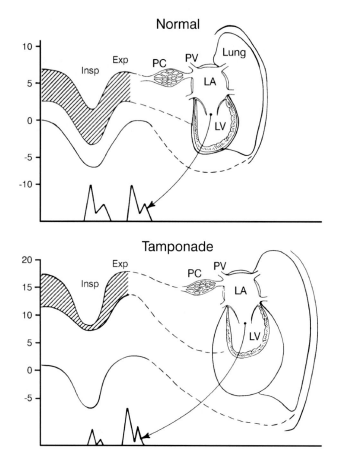

FIG. 14-7. Diagram of intrathoracic and intracardiac pressure changes with respiration in normal and tamponade physiology. The shaded area indicates left ventricle (*LV*) filling pressure gradients (difference between pulmonary capillary wedge pressure and LV diastolic pressure). At the bottom of each drawing is a schematic mitral inflow Doppler velocity profile reflecting LV diastolic filling. In tamponade, there is a decrease in LV filling after inspiration (*Insp*) because the pressure decrease in the pericardium and LV cavity is smaller than the pressure fall in the pulmonary capillaries (*PC*). LV filling is restored after expiration (*Exp*). *PV*, pulmonary vein. (Modified from Sharp JT, Bunnell IL, Holland JF, Griffith GT, Greene DG. Hemodynamics during induced cardiac tamponade in man. *Am J Med* 1960;29:640–646, with permission.)

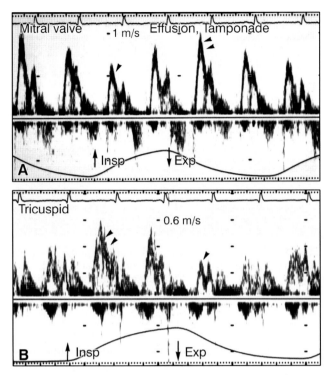

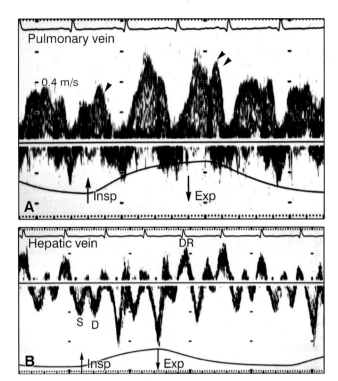

FIG. 14-8. Typical pulsed-wave Doppler pattern of tamponade recorded with a nasal respirometer. **A:** Mitral inflow velocity decreases (*single arrowhead*) after inspiration (*Insp*) and increases (*double arrowheads*) after expiration (*Exp*). **B:** Tricuspid inflow velocity has the opposite changes. E velocity increases (*double arrowheads*) after inspiration and decreases (*single arrowhead*) after expiration. (From Oh JK, Hatle LK, Mulvagh SL, Tajik AJ. Transient constrictive pericarditis: diagnosis by two-dimensional Doppler echocardiography. *Mayo Clin Proc* 1993;68:1158–1164, with permission.)

FIG. 14-9. Pulmonary vein and hepatic vein Doppler patterns of tamponade. **A:** Diastolic forward pulmonary venous flow decreases (*single arrowhead*) after inspiration (*Insp*) and increases (*double arrowheads*) after expiration (*Esp*). **B:** The hepatic vein has a significant reduction in diastolic forward flow and an increase in diastolic reversals (*DR*) after expiration. *D*, diastolic flow; *S*, systolic flow. (From Oh JK, Hatle LK, Mulvagh SL, Tajik AJ. Transient constrictive pericarditis: diagnosis by two-dimensional Doppler echocardiography. *Mayo Clin Proc* 1993;68:1158–1164, with permission.)

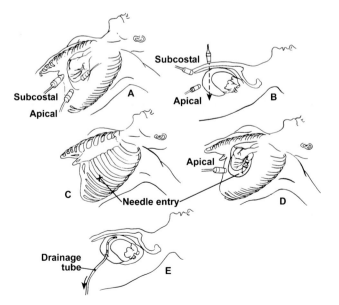

FIG. 14-10. Echocardiographically guided pericardiocentesis.

Step 1. Locate an area on the chest or subcostal region from which the largest amount of pericardial effusion can be visualized, and mark it **(A–C)**.

Step 2. Determine the depth of effusion from the marked position and the optimal angulation.

Step 3. After sterile preparation and local anesthesia, perform pericardiocentesis **(D)**.

Step 4. When in doubt about the location of the needle, inject saline solution through the needle and image it from a remote site to locate the bubbles.

Step 5. Monitor the completeness of the pericardiocentesis by repeat echocardiography.

Step 6. Place a 6F or 7F pigtail catheter in the pericardial space to minimize reaccumulation of fluid **(E)**.

Step 7. Drain any residual fluid or fluid that has reaccumulated via the pigtail catheter every 4 to 6 hours. If after 2 to 3 days pericardial fluid has not reaccumulated, as demonstrated echocardiographically, the pigtail catheter may be removed. Always have the pericardial fluid analyzed: cell counts, glucose and protein measurements, culture, and cytology. (Modified from Callahan JA, Seward JB, Tajik AJ, et al. Pericardiocentesis assisted by two-dimensional echocardiography. *J Thorac Cardiovasc Surg* 1983:85:877–879, with permission.)

Pericardial Effusion Versus Pleural Effusion

Pericardial effusion usually is located circumferentially. If there is an echo-free space anteriorly alone, it more likely is an epicardial fat pad than pericardial effusion. Posteriorly, pericardial effusion is located anterior to the descending thoracic aorta, whereas pleural effusion is present posterior to the aorta (Fig. 14-11). Two-dimensional ultrasonographic imaging of pleural effusion is also helpful in thoracentesis to locate the optimal puncture site. Pleural effusion on the left side allows cardiac imaging from the back (Fig.14-12).

Constrictive Pericarditis

The M-mode and 2D echocardiographic features of constrictive pericarditis include thickened pericardium, abnormal ventricular septal motion, flattening of the LV posterior wall during diastole, respiratory variation in ventricular size, and a dilated inferior vena cava (14–17) (Fig. 14-13), but these findings are not sensitive or specific. Hatle et al. (18) described the Doppler features typical of constriction, which are distinct from those of restrictive hemodynamics. Although the underlying pathologic mechanism is different from that of cardiac tamponade, the hemodynamic events of constriction in regard to respiratory variation in LV and RV filling are similar to those of tamponade.

The following two hemodynamic characteristics need to be demonstrated to establish the diagnosis of constrictive pericarditis:

1. Dissociation between intrathoracic and intracardiac pressures
2. Exaggerated ventricular interdependence in diastolic filling

A thickened or inflamed pericardium prevents full transmission of the intrathoracic pressure changes that occur with respiration to the pericardial and intracardiac cavities,

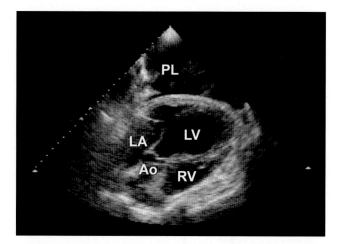

FIG. 14-12. Two-dimensional echocardiographic examination from the back through a pleural effusion (*PL*). This unique view may be the only available ultrasound window to the heart in some patients. *Ao*, aorta.

creating respiratory variations in the left-side filling pressure gradient [the pressure difference between the pulmonary vein and the left atrium (LA)]. With inspiration, intrathoracic pressure falls (5 to 7 mm Hg normally) and the pressure in other intrathoracic structures (pulmonary vein, pulmonary capillaries) falls to a similar degree. This inspiratory pressure change is not fully transmitted to the intrapericardial and intracardiac cavities. As a result, the driving pressure gradient for LV filling decreases immediately

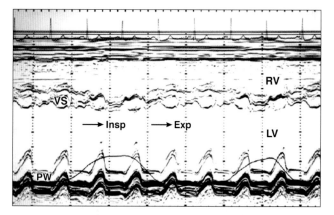

FIG. 14-13. M-mode echocardiogram from the parasternal window of a patient with constrictive pericarditis. It was recorded simultaneously with the respirometer tracing at the bottom. An upward deflection of the respirometer recording indicates the onset of inspiration (*Insp*). A downward deflection indicates the onset of expiration (*Exp*). The typical features of constrictive pericarditis include thickened pericardium, abnormal ventricular septal (*VS*) motion with septal shift toward the left ventricle (*LV*) on inspiration and toward the right ventricle (*RV*) on expiration (resulting in the respiratory variation in ventricular size), and flattening of the LV posterior wall (*PW*) due to limited diastolic filling.

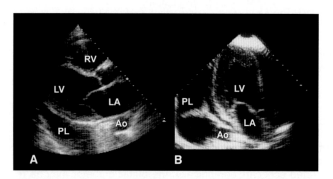

FIG. 14-11. Two-dimensional imaging of pleural effusion (*PL*) from the parasternal long-axis **(A)** and apical long-axis **(B)** views. Pericardial effusion is present between the descending thoracic aorta (*Ao*) and the posterior cardiac walls, whereas pleural effusion is present behind the descending thoracic aorta.

after inspiration and increases with expiration. This characteristic hemodynamic pattern is best illustrated by simultaneous pressure recordings from the LV and the pulmonary capillary wedge together with mitral inflow velocities (Fig. 14-14).

Diastolic filling (or distensibility) of the LV and RV relies on each other because the overall cardiac volume is relatively fixed within the thickened or noncompliant pericardium. Hence, reciprocal respiratory changes occur in the filling of the LV and RV. With inspiration, decreased LV filling allows increased filling in the RV. As a result, the ventricular septum shifts to the left, and tricuspid inflow E velocity and hepatic vein diastolic flow velocity increase (Fig. 14-15 and 14-16). With expiration, LV filling increases, causing the ventricular septum to shift to the right, which limits RV filling. Tricuspid inflow decreases and hepatic vein diastolic forward flow decreases, with significant flow reversals. Usually, diastolic forward flow velocity is higher than systolic forward flow velocity in the hepatic vein, which corresponds to the Y and X waves of systemic venous pressure, respectively.

Optimally, a respiratory variation of 25% or greater in the mitral inflow E velocity and increased diastolic flow reversal with expiration in the hepatic vein need to be demonstrated to establish the diagnosis of constrictive pericarditis (Fig. 14-17). Up to 20% of patients with constrictive pericarditis demonstrate less than 25% of respiratory variation in mitral E velocity (19,20), however, because of (a) mixed constriction and restriction or (b) marked increase of atrial pressures.

If LA pressure is markedly increased, mitral valve opening occurs at a steep portion of the LV pressure curve, when the respiratory change has little effect on the transmitral pressure gradient (Fig. 14-18). In this case, a Doppler echocardiographic examination should be repeated after an attempt to reduce preload (i.e., head-up tilt or sitting position) (Fig. 14-19).

Pitfalls and Caveats

Several other clinical entities can produce a similar respiratory variation in mitral inflow velocities: acute dilatation of the heart, pulmonary embolism, RV infarct, pleural effusion, and chronic obstructive lung disease. Most of these conditions do not present a significant diagnostic problem in the interpretation of Doppler findings because their clinical and 2D echocardiographic features are different from those of constrictive pericarditis. Patients with chronic obstructive lung disease, however, may have symptoms of right-sided heart failure similar to those of constrictive pericarditis.

Several features of Doppler echocardiographic studies can be used to distinguish between chronic obstructive lung disease and constrictive pericarditis (21).

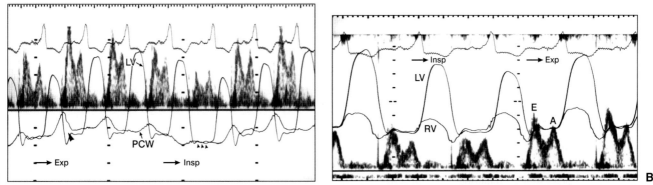

FIG. 14-14. A: Simultaneous pressure recordings from the left ventricle (*LV*) and pulmonary capillary wedge together with mitral inflow velocity on a Doppler echocardiogram. The onset of the respiratory phase is indicated at the bottom. *Exp*, expiration; *Insp*, inspiration. With the onset of expiration, pulmonary capillary wedge pressure (*PCW*) increases much more than LV diastolic pressure, creating a large driving pressure gradient (*large arrowhead*). With inspiration, however, PCW decreases much more than LV diastolic pressure, with a very small driving pressure gradient (*three small arrowheads*). These respiratory changes in the LV filling gradient are well reflected by the changes in the mitral inflow velocities recorded on Doppler echocardiography. **B:** Simultaneous pressure measurements from the LV and right ventricle (*RV*) together with mitral inflow velocities on Doppler echocardiography. The LV pressure decreases from the second to the third cardiac cycle toward the end of inspiration, but RV systolic pressure increases from the second to the third cardiac cycle. This represents discordant pressure changes with respiration. The increase in RV systolic pressure (third cardiac cycle) follows the decrease in the mitral inflow velocity (second complete mitral inflow velocity recording), indicating that the initial hemodynamic event responsible for respiratory variation in ventricular filling comes from the left side. The typical square root sign and the equalization of diastolic pressure between the LV and RV are well shown in the simultaneous LV and RV pressure tracings.

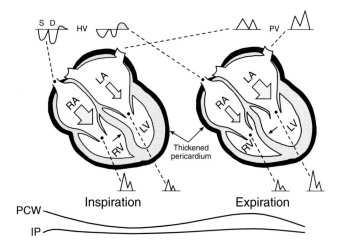

FIG. 14-15. Diagram of a heart with a thickened pericardium to illustrate the respiratory variation in ventricular filling and the corresponding Doppler features of the mitral valve, tricuspid valve, pulmonary vein (*PV*), and hepatic vein (*HV*). These changes are related to discordant pressure changes in the vessels in the thorax, such as pulmonary capillary wedge pressure (*PCW*) and intrapericardial (*IP*) and intracardiac pressures. *Hatched area under curve* indicates the reversal of flow. *Thicker arrows* indicate greater filling. *D*, diastolic flow; *S*, systolic flow.

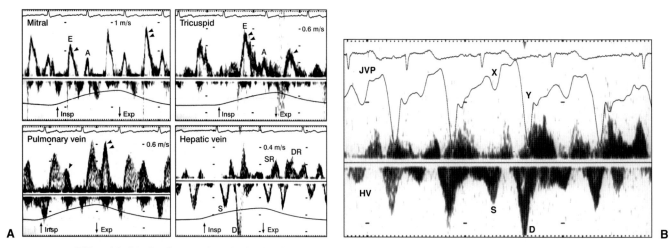

FIG. 14–16. A: Composite of mitral valve, tricuspid valve, pulmonary vein, and hepatic venous flow velocities typically seen in constrictive pericarditis (see text). *DR*, diastolic flow reversal; *Exp*, expiration; *Insp*, inspiration; *SR*, systolic flow reversal. **B:** Simultaneous jugular venous pressure (*JVP*) tracing and pulsed-wave Doppler recording of hepatic vein (*HV*) velocities. There is the characteristic Y descent. *D*, diastolic flow; *S*, systolic flow; *X* and *Y*, jugular venous pressure wave forms.

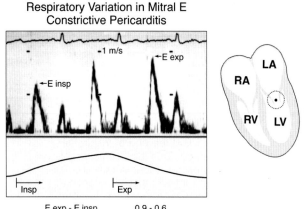

FIG. 14-17. Calculation of the extent of respiratory variation in mitral inflow E velocity is shown in the diagram and Doppler recording. Percent respiratory changes calculated as the difference between peak E velocity at expiration (*E exp*) and peak E velocity at inspiration (*E insp*) divided by E insp. In this example, E exp is 0.9 m/sec and E insp is 0.6 m/sec. Therefore, the difference in E velocity is 0.3 m/sec, or 50% of E insp.

% change = $\dfrac{E\ exp - E\ insp}{E\ Insp} \times 100 = \dfrac{0.9 - 0.6}{0.6} \times 100 = 50\%$

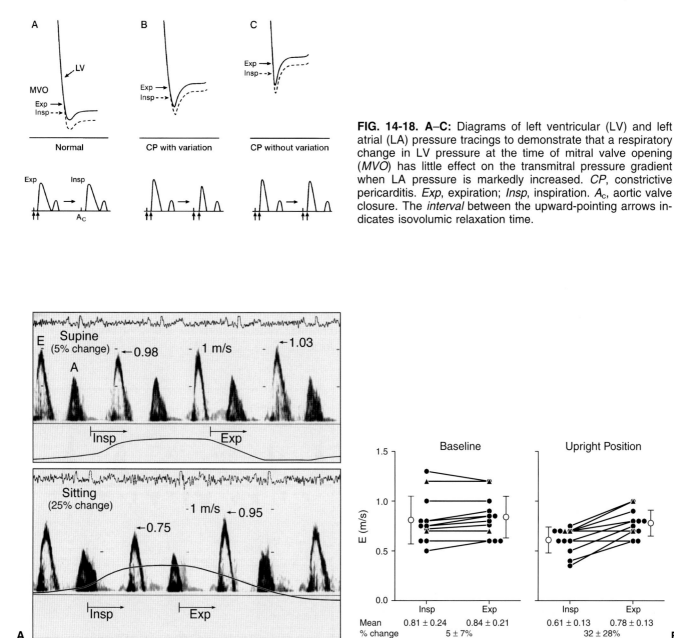

FIG. 14-18. A–C: Diagrams of left ventricular (LV) and left atrial (LA) pressure tracings to demonstrate that a respiratory change in LV pressure at the time of mitral valve opening (*MVO*) has little effect on the transmitral pressure gradient when LA pressure is markedly increased. *CP*, constrictive pericarditis. *Exp*, expiration; *Insp*, inspiration. *A*$_c$, aortic valve closure. The *interval* between the upward-pointing arrows indicates isovolumic relaxation time.

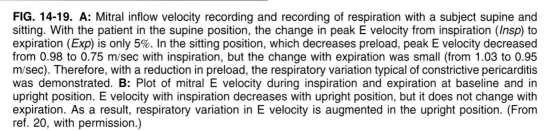

FIG. 14-19. A: Mitral inflow velocity recording and recording of respiration with a subject supine and sitting. With the patient in the supine position, the change in peak E velocity from inspiration (*Insp*) to expiration (*Exp*) is only 5%. In the sitting position, which decreases preload, peak E velocity decreased from 0.98 to 0.75 m/sec with inspiration, but the change with expiration was small (from 1.03 to 0.95 m/sec). Therefore, with a reduction in preload, the respiratory variation typical of constrictive pericarditis was demonstrated. **B:** Plot of mitral E velocity during inspiration and expiration at baseline and in upright position. E velocity with inspiration decreases with upright position, but it does not change with expiration. As a result, respiratory variation in E velocity is augmented in the upright position. (From ref. 20, with permission.)

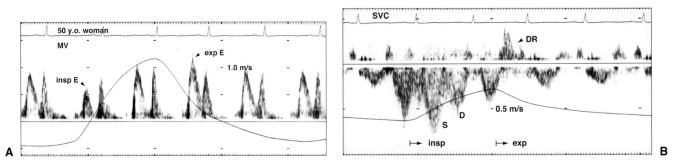

FIG. 14-20. A: Pulsed-wave Doppler recording of mitral inflow velocity (*MV*) showing respiratory variation in a 50-year-old woman with chronic obstructive lung disease. There is 100% change in E velocity (from 0.6 m/sec with inspiration to 1.2 m/sec with expiration. *insp*, inspiration; *exp*, expiration. **B:** Pulsed-wave Doppler recording from the superior vena cava (*SVC*) showing a marked increase in SVC flow velocity with inspiration and a marked diminution with expiration. *D*, diastolic flow; *DR*, diastolic flow reversal; *S*, systolic flow.

1. In chronic obstructive lung disease, individual mitral inflow velocities usually are not restrictive because the LV filling pressure is not increased (Fig. 14-20A).

2. In chronic obstructive lung disease, the highest mitral E velocity occurs toward the end of expiration, but it occurs immediately after the onset of expiration in constrictive pericarditis.

3. The Doppler finding that most reliably distinguishes between these two entities is superior vena cava flow velocities. In chronic obstructive lung disease, superior vena cava flow is markedly increased with inspiration (Fig. 14-20B), because the underlying mechanism for respiratory variation in chronic obstructive lung disease is a greater decrease in intrathoracic pressure with inspiration, which generates greater negative pressure changes in the thorax. This enhances flow to the RA from the superior vena cava with inspiration. In constrictive pericarditis, superior vena cava flow velocities do not change significantly with respiration (Fig. 14-21); the difference in systolic forward flow velocity between inspiration and expiration is rarely 20 cm/sec in constrictive pericarditis (21).

Atrial fibrillation makes the interpretation of respiratory variation in Doppler velocities difficult. Patients with constrictive pericarditis and atrial fibrillation still have typical 2D echocardiographic features and require longer observation of Doppler velocities to detect velocity variation with respiration, regardless of underlying cardiac cycle length. Hepatic vein diastolic flow reversal with expiration is an important Doppler finding to suggest constrictive pericarditis, even when mitral inflow velocity pattern is not diagnostic. Occasionally, it may be necessary to regularize the patient's rhythm with a temporary pacemaker to evaluate the respiratory variation of Doppler velocities. Respirometer recording may have a phase delay up to 1,000 msec, which may make the timing of velocity variation erroneous. A good rule of thumb is to remember that the lowest mitral inflow velocity usually occurs during inspiration. It also is important to instruct the patient to breathe smoothly during Doppler recording. An erratic breathing pattern distorts the timing of Doppler flow velocities.

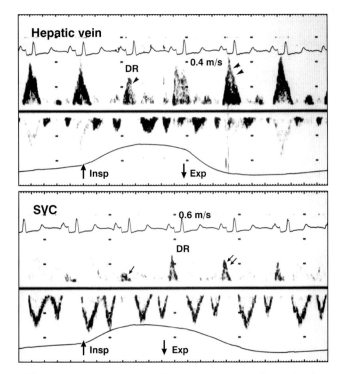

FIG. 14-21. Pulsed-wave Doppler recording from the hepatic vein and superior vena cava (*SVC*) in a patient with constrictive pericarditis. Diastolic flow reversal (*DR*) increases (*double arrowheads*) in the hepatic vein with expiration (*Exp*) compared with DR with inspiration (*Insp*) (*single arrowhead*). However, there is a smaller diastolic flow reversal (*double arrows*) in the SVC during expiration compared with that in the hepatic vein. Diastolic flow reversal during inspiration is minimal (*single arrow*). Also, there was no significant change in the SVC forward flow velocity during inspiration and expiration, compared with SVC flow in chronic obstructive lung disease.

RESTRICTION VERSUS CONSTRICTION

The clinical and hemodynamic profiles of restriction and constriction are similar, although their pathophysiologic mechanisms are distinctly different. Both are caused by diastolic filling abnormalities, with relatively preserved global systolic function. Diastolic dysfunction in restrictive cardiomyopathy is the result of a stiff and noncompliant ventricular myocardium, but in constrictive pericarditis, it is related to a thickened noncompliant pericardium. Both disease processes limit diastolic filling and result in diastolic heart failure. Restrictive cardiomyopathy resulting from infiltrative cardiomyopathy is the abnormality easiest to diagnose because it has typical 2D echocardiographic and biochemical features. A noninfiltrative type of restrictive cardiomyopathy is more difficult to diagnose. The myocardium becomes noncompliant because of fibrosis and scarring, and systolic function is usually maintained. Because of limited diastolic filling and increased diastolic pressure, the atria become enlarged. In contrast, myocardial compliance usually is not decreased in constrictive pericarditis. The thickened and sometimes calcific pericardium limits diastolic filling, resulting in hemodynamic features that are similar to but distinctly different from those of restrictive cardiomyopathy. Atrial enlargement is less prominent in constriction than in restrictive cardiomyopathy, but it can be as large. When restrictive cardiomyopathy affects both ventricles, clinical signs due to abnormalities of right-sided heart failure are apparent, with increased jugular venous pressure and peripheral edema. An early diastolic gallop sound (S_3) is a rule in restriction, but it often is difficult to differentiate it from pericardial knock.

Electrocardiographic and chest radiographic findings are nonspecific, although a calcified pericardium should point to constrictive pericarditis and low voltage of QRS on the electrocardiogram suggests cardiac amyloidosis. Echocardiographically, it is difficult to distinguish between restriction and constriction only on the basis of M-mode and 2D findings, although diagnostic abnormalities may be detected with careful observation. In constrictive pericarditis, the most striking finding is ventricular septal motion abnormalities, which can be explained on the basis of respiratory variation in ventricular filling (discussed subsequently). The pericardium usually is thickened, but this may not be obvious on TTE. Recent data suggest that TEE measurements of pericardial thickness correlate well with those of electron-beam computed tomography (22); however, 2D echocardiographic findings alone usually are not sufficient to differentiate restriction from constriction, and additional hemodynamic information supplied by Doppler echocardiography is necessary.

The main characteristic hemodynamic feature of constriction is respiratory variation of ventricular filling and ventricular interdependence (18,19), as discussed. These hemodynamic characteristics are not present in restrictive cardiomyopathy. Therefore, the demonstration of respiratory variation in left-side and right-side diastolic filling is essential for diagnosing (invasively or noninvasively) constrictive pericarditis. These changes may not be present in a subgroup of patients with constrictive pericarditis, however, if the filling pressure is markedly increased; thus, an attempt should be made to decrease preload to augment the respiratory changes (20). A corollary to this is that although the typical respiratory variation is diagnostic for constrictive pericarditis, the lack of respiratory variation does not exclude constrictive pericarditis, and additional studies are required. It should be noted, however, that the individual ventricular filling pattern in constriction is usually restrictive.

Despite the significant difference in the pathophysiologic mechanisms of restriction and constriction, there is significant overlap between these two entities. Increased atrial pressures, equalization of end-diastolic pressures, and dip-and-plateau or square root sign of the ventricular diastolic pressure recording have been advocated as hemodynamic features typical of constrictive pericarditis (23). Hemodynamic pressure tracings with characteristics almost identical to these can be obtained in patients with either constriction or restrictive cardiomyopathy (24). Therefore, in addition to these hemodynamic features, a respiratory variation in ventricular filling should be demonstrated to diagnose constriction, either invasively or noninvasively. The dissociation between intrathoracic and intracardiac pressure changes with inspiration are well seen in simultaneous recordings of LV and pulmonary capillary wedge pressures. In constrictive pericarditis, the fluctuation in the pulmonary capillary wedge pressure is more marked in parallel with intrathoracic pressure changes than with changes in LV diastolic pressure. Ventricular interdependence also is observed in simultaneous recordings of LV and RV pressures. With inspiration, which induces less filling of the LV, LV pressure decreases; the opposite changes occur in the RV so that RV pressure increases with inspiration. This discor-

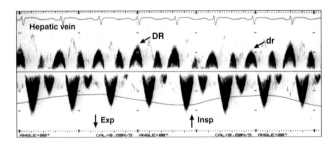

FIG. 14-22. Pulsed-wave Doppler recording from the hepatic vein of a patient with advanced constrictive pericarditis who was referred for cardiac transplantation with the diagnosis of restrictive cardiomyopathy. The hepatic vein has flow reversal during both inspiration (*Insp*) and expiration (*Exp*). However, this reversal becomes more prominent after the onset of expiration (*DR*) with decreased forward flow during diastole as compared with the flow velocities on inspiration (*dr*).

TABLE 14-1. *Doppler variables of mitral inflow, tricuspid inflow, and hepatic venous flow velocities in normal subjects and those with constriction or restriction*[a]

Normal
  Mitral inflow
    No (≤ 10%) respiratory variation in E
    DT, ≥ 160 msec
  Tricuspid inflow
    Mild (≤ 15%) respiratory variation in E
    DT, ≥ 160 msec
  Hepatic vein
    Systolic forward (S) flow greater than diastolic forward (D) flow (in sinus rhythm)
    Systolic forward flow less than diastolic forward flow (in atrial fibrillation)
    Slight increase in systolic (SR) and diastolic reversals (DR) with expiration
Constriction
  Mitral inflow
    Inspiratory E less than expiratory E (≥ 25% change)
    DT, not always, but usually shortened (≤ 160 msec)
  Tricuspid inflow
    Inspiratory E greater than expiratory E (≥ 40% change)
    DT usually shortened (≤ 160 msec)
  Hepatic vein
    Decreased diastolic forward flow with expiration
    Marked decrease in diastolic forward flow and increase in diastolic flow reversals with expiration
    Constriction is usually diagnosed on the basis of changes in mitral inflow and hepatic vein flow velocity with respiration
    When mitral inflow is difficult to obtain, pulmonary vein diastolic forward flow velocity changes of 25% or more with respiration are used to represent respiratory variation in LV filling. Pulmonary vein Doppler recording may be obtained with TEE
Restriction
  Mitral inflow
    No respiratory variation of E velocity
    Increased E velocity (usually ≥ 1.0 m/sec)
    Decreased A velocity (usually ≤ 0.5 m/sec)
    Increased E/A ratio (≥ 2.0)
    Shortened DT of E (< 160 ms)
  Tricuspid inflow
    Mild respiratory variation (≤ 15%) in E velocity
    Increased E/A ratio (≥ 2.0)
    Shortened DT of E (≤ 160 m/sec)
  Hepatic vein
    Systolic forward flow (S) less than diastolic forward flow (D)
    Increase in systolic and diastolic flow reversals with inspiration

A, filling wave due to atrial contraction; DT, deceleration time; E, early rapid filling wave; TEE, transesophageal echocardiography.
[a] See Fig. 14-23.
From ref. 19, with permission.

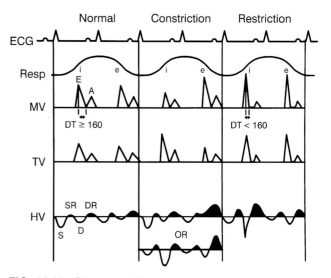

FIG. 14-23. Diagram of Doppler velocities from mitral inflow (*MV*), tricuspid inflow (*TV*), and hepatic vein (*HV*) and the electrocardiographic (*ECG*) and respirometer recordings (*Resp*) indicating inspiration (*i*) and expiration (*e*). D, diastolic flow; *DR*, diastolic flow reversal; *DT*, deceleration time; *S*, systolic flow; *SR*, systolic flow reversal; *Blackened areas under curve*, flow reversal. (Modified from ref. 19, with permission.)

dant pressure change between the LV and RV in constrictive pericarditis does not occur in restrictive cardiomyopathy.

In restrictive cardiomyopathy, mitral inflow velocity rarely shows respiratory variation (unless the patient also has chronic obstructive lung disease), although each velocity pattern appears similar to that of constriction, with increased E velocity, an E/A ratio usually greater than 2.0 and a short deceleration time (DT). Hepatic vein flow reversals are more prominent with inspiration in restrictive cardiomyopathy, although it is not unusual to see significant diastolic flow reversals in the hepatic vein during both inspiration and expiration in patients with advanced constriction or with constriction and restriction combined (Fig. 14-22). The Doppler features of constriction and restriction are summarized in Table 14-1 and Fig. 14-23. Therefore, invasively or noninvasively, the diagnostic criteria of restriction and constriction should be based on the respiratory changes of ventricular filling and hemodynamic features in-

TABLE 14-2. *Traditional hemodynamic criteria for constriction versus restriction*

Criterion	Constriction	Restriction
LVEDP-RVEDP (mm Hg)	≤5	>5
RV systolic pressure (mm Hg)	≤50	>50
RVEDP/RVSP	≥0.33	<0.3

LVEDP, left ventricular end-diastolic pressure; RVEDP, right ventricular end-diastolic pressure; RVSP, right ventricular systolic pressure.

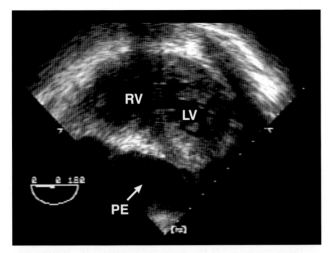

FIG. 14-24. Transesophageal echocardiographic (TEE) imaging from the transgastric view in a patient with hypotension after cardiac surgery. Transthoracic echocardiography was not adequate for imaging pericardial effusion. The study shows posteriorly loculated pericardial effusion (*PE*). Left ventricular (*LV*) and right ventricular (*RV*) size was small (underfill). On the basis of this TEE finding, the patient was returned to the operating room for evacuation of hemopericardium.

stead of previously proposed criteria using the level of systolic RV pressure or equalization of ventricular end-diastolic pressures (Table 14-2), because there is significant overlap of the hemodynamic values between constriction and restriction (25). Instead, during cardiac catheterization for evaluation of constrictive pericarditis, discordant respiratory change between RV and LV pressures during inspiration should be looked for as a sign of interdependence of ventricular filling (26). Another promising technique to differentiate constrictive pericarditis from restrictive cardiomyopathy is the measurement of mitral annular velocity by Doppler tissue imaging. Mitral annular velocity is markedly decreased in restrictive cardiomyopathy, whereas it is well preserved in constrictive pericarditis (27).

TRANSESOPHAGEAL ECHOCARDIOGRAPHY

When TTE is not adequate for obtaining satisfactory imaging of the pericardium and hemodynamic assessment of ventricular filling, TEE should be considered. A hemodynamically compromising loculated pericardial effusion may be difficult to detect on TTE, and TEE has been especially helpful in postoperative patients with tamponade due to loculated hemopericardium (Fig. 14-24). TEE also is useful in obtaining pulmonary venous flow pulsed-wave Doppler velocity with simultaneous respirometer recording in the evaluation of constrictive pericarditis. Furthermore, TEE is helpful in measuring the thickness of the pericardium (the correlation between these measurements and those of electron-beam computed tomography is good) and in evaluating abnormal structures near the pericardium (e.g., pericardial cyst, metastatic tumor) (Fig. 14-25).

CLINICAL IMPACT

Echocardiography is usually one of the first diagnostic procedures used in patients in whom a pericardial abnormality is suspected. This method is capable of providing a complete assessment of pericardial effusion (how much and how significant), identifying the best site for pericardiocentesis if necessary, and helping to establish or suggest the diagnosis of constrictive pericarditis. In some patients, constrictive pericarditis is transient, usually after acute pericarditis. The development and resolution of transient constrictive hemodynamics are readily assessed with serial 2D Doppler echocardiography (28). Detection of respiratory variation in mitral flow and central venous flow velocities may be the initial diagnostic clue to constrictive pericarditis, even in patients without any clinical suspicion of pericardial abnormality. Comprehensive 2D and Doppler echo-

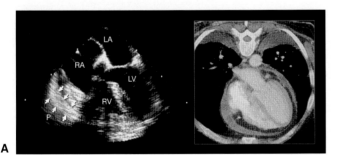

A

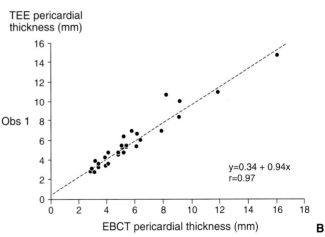

B

FIG. 14-25. A: Transesophageal echocardiographic (TEE) imaging of thickened pericardium (*arrows*, *P*) **(left)** and electron-beam computed tomographic (EBCT) scan **(right)** of the pericardium of the same patient. **B:** The correlation between the measurements of pericardial thickness by TEE and EBCT is good.

cardiography with simultaneous recording of respiration should be able to distinguish constriction from restriction in nearly all patients.

REFERENCES

1. Feigenbaum H, Waldhausen JA, Hyde LP. Ultrasound diagnosis of pericardial effusion. *JAMA* 1965;191:711–714.
2. Feigenbaum H, Zaky A, Waldhausen JA. Use of ultrasound in the diagnosis of pericardial effusion. *Ann Intern Med* 1966;65:443–452.
3. Tajik AJ. Echocardiography in pericardial effusion. *Am J Med* 1977;63:29–40.
4. Lemire F, Tajik AJ, Giuliani ER, Gau GT, Schattenberg TT. Further echocardiographic observations in pericardial effusion. *Mayo Clin Proc* 1976;51:13–18.
5. Nasser WK, Helmen C, Tavel ME, Feigenbaum H, Fisch C. Congenital absence of the left pericardium: clinical, electrocardiographic, radiographic, hemodynamic, and angiographic findings in six cases. *Circulation* 1970;41:469–478.
6. Connolly HM, Click RL, Schattenberg TT, Seward JB, Tajik AJ. Congenital absence of the pericardium: echocardiography as a diagnostic tool. *J Am Soc Echocardiogr* 1995;8:87–92.
7. Armstrong WF, Schilt BF, Helper DJ, Dillon JC, Feigenbaum H. Diastolic collapse of the right ventricle with cardiac tamponade: an echocardiographic study. *Circulation* 1982;65:1491–1496.
8. Gillam LD, Guyer DE, Gibson TC, King ME, Marshall JE, Weyman AE. Hydrodynamic compression of the right atrium: a new echocardiographic sign of cardiac tamponade. *Circulation* 1983;68:294–301.
9. Appleton CP, Hatle LK, Popp RL. Cardiac tamponade and pericardial effusion: respiratory variation in transvalvular flow velocities studied by Doppler echocardiography. *J Am Coll Cardiol* 1988;11:1020–1030.
10. Burstow DJ, Oh JK, Bailey KR, Seward JB, Tajik AJ. Cardiac tamponade: Characteristic Doppler observations. *Mayo Clin Proc* 1989;64:312–324.
11. Callahan JA, Seward JB, Tajik AJ. Cardiac tamponade: pericardiocentesis directed by two-dimensional echocardiography. *Mayo Clin Proc* 1985;60:344–347.
12. Callahan JA, Seward JB. Pericardiocentesis guided by two-dimensional echocardiography. *Echocardiography* 1997;14:497–504.
13. Kopecky SL, Callahan JA, Tajik AJ, Seward JB. Percutaneous pericardial catheter drainage: report of 42 consecutive cases. *Am J Cardiol* 1986;58:633–635.
14. Engel PJ, Fowler NO, Tei CW, et al. M-mode echocardiography in constrictive pericarditis. *J Am Coll Cardiol* 1985;6:471–474.
15. Gibson TC, Grossman W, McLaurin LP, Moos S, Craige E. An echocardiographic study of the interventricular septum in constrictive pericarditis. *Br Heart J* 1976;38:738–743.
16. Pandian NG, Skorton DJ, Kieso RA, Kerber RE. Diagnosis of constrictive pericarditis by two-dimensional echocardiography: studies in a new experimental model and in patients. *J Am Coll Cardiol* 1984;4:1164–1173.
17. Candell-Riera J, Garcia del Castillo H, Permanyer-Miralda G, Soler-Soler J. Echocardiographic features of the interventricular septum in chronic constrictive pericarditis. *Circulation* 1978;57:1154–1158.
18. Hatle LK, Appleton CP, Popp RL. Differentiation of constrictive pericarditis and restrictive cardiomyopathy by Doppler echocardiography. *Circulation* 1989;79:357–370.
19. Oh JK, Hatle LK, Seward JB, et al. Diagnostic role of Doppler echocardiography in constrictive pericarditis. *J Am Coll Cardiol* 1994;23:154–162.
20. Oh JK, Tajik AJ, Appleton CP, Hatle LK, Nishimura RA, Seward JB. Preload reduction to unmask the characteristic Doppler features of constrictive pericarditis: a new observation. *Circulation* 1997;95:796–799.
21. Boonyaratavej S, Oh JK, Appleton CP, Seward JB. Superior vena cava Doppler can distinguish chronic obstructive lung disease from constrictive pericarditis despite similar respiratory variation in mitral flow velocity. *J Am Coll Cardiol* (*in press*).
22. Ling LH, Oh JK, Tei C, et al. Pericardial thickness measured with transesophageal echocardiography: feasibility and potential clinical usefulness. *J Am Coll Cardiol* 1997;29:1317–1323.
23. Bloomfield RA, Lauson HD, Cournand A, Breed ES, Richards DW Jr. Recording of right heart pressures in normal subjects and in patients with chronic pulmonary disease and various types of cardiocirculatory disease. *J Clin Invest* 1946;25:639–664.
24. Meaney E, Shabetai R, Bhargava V, et al. Cardiac amyloidosis, constrictive pericarditis and restrictive cardiomyopathy. *Am J Cardiol* 1976;38:547–556.
25. Vaitkus PT, Kussmaul WG. Constrictive pericarditis versus restrictive cardiomyopathy: a reappraisal and update of diagnostic criteria. *Am Heart J* 1991;122:1431–1441.
26. Hurrell DG, Nishimura RA, Higano ST, et al. Value of dynamic respiratory changes in left and right ventricular pressures for the diagnosis of constrictive pericarditis. *Circulation* 1996;93:2007–2013.
27. Garcia MJ, Rodriguez L, Ares M, Griffin BP, Thomas JD, Klein AL. Differentiation of constrictive pericarditis from restrictive cardiomyopathy: assessment of left ventricular diastolic velocities in longitudinal axis by Doppler tissue imaging. *J Am Coll Cardiol* 1996;27:108–114.
28. Oh JK, Hatle LK, Mulvagh SL, Tajik AJ. Transient constrictive pericarditis: diagnosis by two-dimensional Doppler echocardiography. *Mayo Clin Proc* 1993;68:1158–1164.

CHAPTER 15

Diseases of the Aorta

With the use of multiple transthoracic (TTE) and transesophageal echocardiographic (TEE) imaging windows, the entire thoracic aorta can be visualized by echocardiography (1–5). The aortic arch and proximal portion of the descending thoracic aorta are seen well on a suprasternal notch examination, which should be a routine part of the TTE examination in all patients (Fig. 15-1). The ascending aorta is visualized best from the parasternal long-axis view on TTE and from a 120-degree to 140-degree multiplane TEE view. With monoplane TEE, there is a blind spot from the midascending aorta to the proximal portion of the arch (4), but biplane or multiplane TEE imaging usually allows visualization of the entire thoracic aorta (5–7). Diseases involving the aorta include aortic aneurysm, aortic dissection, coronary sinus aneurysm with or without rupture into the

surrounding cardiac chambers (most commonly the right cardiac chambers), aortic ulcer or intramural hematoma, aortic rupture, atheromatous debris, aortic abscess, and coarctation of the aorta. With TTE, the dimensions of the ascending aorta and arch usually are measured best from the parasternal long-axis and suprasternal views, respectively. The dimension of the aorta should be measured at the same location for follow-up in cases of aortic aneurysm and Marfan syndrome.

AORTIC DISSECTION

Aortic dissection is a potentially life-threatening disease that requires prompt diagnosis and treatment (8). The location of aortic dissection dictates the treatment modality. The classification of aortic dissections according to the location of the tear and the extent of involvement is shown in Fig. 15-2 (9). Proximal aortic dissection (DeBakey type I and II or Stanford type A) requires immediate surgical repair, whereas distal dissection (DeBakey type III or Stanford type B) is usually managed medically, unless there is persistent pain or a clinically significant compromise to vital organs. Therefore, not only diagnosis but also determination of the location and extent of an aortic dissection are important for optimal management.

Transthoracic Echocardiography

TTE is a good initial imaging modality for proximal aortic dissection (the ascending aorta and arch). The positive predictive value is good, but it may be difficult to exclude aortic dissection in patients with negative findings. Review of the 6-year experience at the Mayo Clinic in 67 patients with aortic dissection demonstrated that the sensitivity of TTE was 79% and the positive predictive accuracy was 91% (2). Although all patients with aortic dissection had a dilated aorta on two-dimensional (2D) echocardiography, an intimal flap was seen in only 79% of the patients (Fig. 15-3). Five patients (7%) had a false-positive diagnosis,

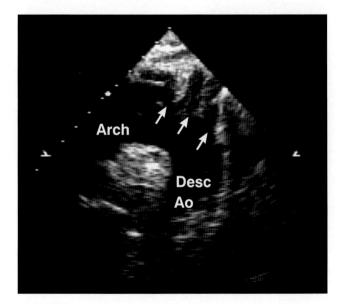

FIG. 15-1. Long-axis view of the thoracic aorta from the suprasternal notch window. The arch and descending thoracic aorta (*Desc Ao*) are clearly seen. The innominate, left carotid, and left subclavian arteries are also visualized (*arrows*).

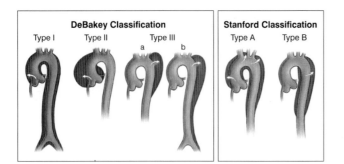

FIG. 15-2. The two most widely used classifications of aortic dissection. The DeBakey classification includes three types. In *type I* the intimal tear usually originates in the proximal ascending aorta and the dissection involves the ascending aorta, the arch, and variable lengths of the descending and abdominal aorta. In *type II* the dissection is confined to the ascending aorta. In *type III* the dissection may be confined to the descending thoracic aorta (*type IIIa*), or it may extend into the abdominal aorta and iliac arteries (*type IIIb*). The dissection may extend proximally to involve the arch and the ascending aorta. The Stanford classification has two types. *Type A* includes all cases in which the ascending aorta is involved by the dissection, with or without involvement of the arch or the descending aorta. *Type B* includes cases in which the descending thoracic aorta is involved, with or without proximal (retrograde) or distal (anterograde) extension. (From ref. 9, with permission.)

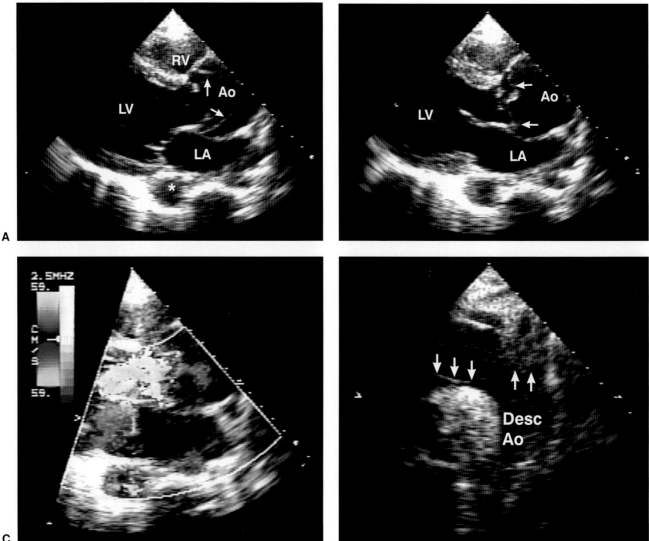

FIG. 15-3. Transthoracic parasternal long-axis view showing a dilated ascending aorta and an undulating intimal flap in proximal aortic dissection. These images were obtained in a 37-year-old woman with Marfan syndrome and chest pain. She underwent urgent surgical repair on the basis of these echocardiographic findings. **A:** Systolic frame shows an intimal flap (*arrows*) in the aorta (*Ao*), which is dilated. The *asterisk* indicates the descending thoracic aorta, which is not dilated. **B:** Diastolic frame shows movement of the flap (*arrows*) toward the aortic valve. **C:** Color-flow imaging showing severe aortic regurgitation. **D:** Suprasternal notch view of an intimal flap (*downward arrows*) in the arch. The takeoff of the left carotid and subclavian arteries is also visualized (*upward arrows*). *Desc Ao*, descending aorta.

usually because the membranous wall of a thrombus in the lumen of an aneurysmal descending thoracic aorta was misinterpreted as an intimal flap. Another limitation of TTE is the inability to visualize the descending thoracic aorta. Therefore, TTE is an inexpensive and rapid screening tool for aortic dissection, but negative findings or a suboptimal examination requires further diagnostic evaluation.

Transesophageal Echocardiography

Because of the intimate anatomic relationship between the esophagus and the thoracic aorta, TEE allows visualization of the entire thoracic aorta using biplane or multiplane transducers (5–7) (Fig. 15-4). It should be noted that the esophagus is anterior to the aorta at the level of the diaphragm, but they are intertwined in the thorax, and the esophagus is posterior to the aorta at the level of the arch. In a horizontal transesophageal view (0 degree in multi-

plane TEE), the distal portion of the ascending aorta and the proximal portion of the transverse aorta may not be well visualized because of the interposed trachea. This blind area on the horizontal plane can now be visualized with the longitudinal view (90-degree multiplane view). With a clearer and more complete view of the entire aorta, TEE has changed the role of echocardiography in the diagnosis and management of aortic dissection. TEE images of aortic dissection are shown in Figs. 15-5 through 15-8.

The multicenter European cooperative study (10) was the first to demonstrate that TEE was at least equal to or even superior to computed tomography (CT) and aortography in the diagnosis of aortic dissection (sensitivity of 99%). Aortic dissection was not detected in one of two patients studied with monoplane TEE (it was a localized type II dissection). Subsequent studies validated the highly accurate diagnostic capability of TEE in aortic dissection (11,12). Bansal and colleagues (6) also reported false-negative re-

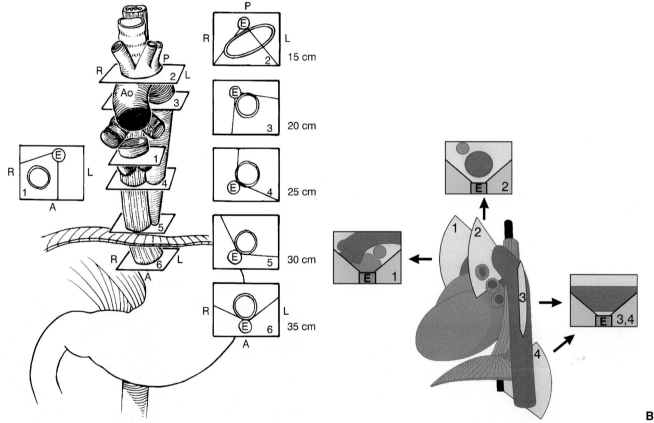

A

B

FIG. 15-4. **A:** Diagram of the anatomic relationship of the aorta (*Ao*), trachea, and esophagus (*E*) at various levels of horizontal scan planes of the thoracic aorta. *1*, level of the aortic root; *2*, arch; *3*, upper descending aorta; *4* to *5*, thoracic aorta; and *6*, upper abdominal aorta. Note that the esophagus is anterior to the aorta at the level of the diaphragm and posterior to the aorta at the level of the arch. A portion of the distal ascending aorta directly anterior to the trachea is a blind area for horizontal transesophageal echocardiography. *A*, anterior; *L*, left; *P*, posterior; *R*, right. (From ref. 4, with permission.) **B:** Transesophageal imaging of the thoracic aorta in the longitudinal plane. The aortic valve, aortic root, and the ascending aorta are visualized with transducer position at 110 to 135 degrees (*1*), whereas the arch is viewed in short axis (*2*), and the descending aorta in long axis (*3* and *4*). (From Freeman WK. Diseases of the thoracic aorta: assessment by transesophageal echocardiography. In: Freeman WK, Seward JB, Khandheria BK, Tajik AJ, eds. Transesophageal echocardiography. Boston: Little, Brown and Company, 1994:425–467, with permission.)

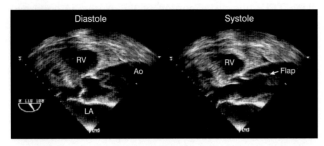

FIG. 15-5. Long-axis view of the heart with the multiplane transducer array rotated to 118 degrees showing a dilated ascending aorta (*Ao*) and intimal flap. It has a typical undulating motion from diastole to systole. On the basis of this transesophageal echocardiographic finding, the patient underwent repair of the proximal aortic dissection.

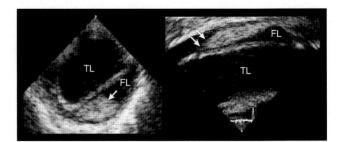

FIG. 15-7. Biplane transesophageal imaging of a type III dissection. The transverse plane image **(left)** shows a true lumen (*TL*) and a false lumen (*FL*). The false lumen is partially thrombosed (*arrow*). The longitudinal plane image **(right)** shows the descending thoracic aorta with a partially thrombosed false lumen (*arrows*).

sults in two of 65 patients examined with biplane TEE. Both patients had localized DeBakey type II aortic dissections. In the same study, aortography yielded a sensitivity of 77%, including a false-negative result in a type I dissection, mainly related to a completely thrombosed false lumen or intramural hematoma.

Intramural hematoma is a precursor for aortic dissection (usually in elderly patients with hypertension) and should be treated like an aortic dissection. From 15% to 20% of patients with aortic dissection may present with intramural hematoma (6,13). An intramural hematoma appears as an increased echodensity along the wall of the aorta, corresponding to thrombus formation between the intima and the adventitia (Fig. 15-9). This should be differentiated from atheromatous plaque in the aorta, which tends to have an irregular edge (Fig. 15-10). Also, it is easily seen on CT and magnetic resonance imaging (MRI) as an increased density along the aortic wall. A fresh hematoma has an even higher density on CT. Aortography is least valuable in the diagnosis of intramural hematoma (13). Currently, TEE or CT with contrast agent is the initial diagnostic procedure of choice for suspected aortic dissection. Although the diagnostic accuracy of MRI is superb, its clinical role

is limited by the distant location of the imaging facility from the emergency department and by difficulties in monitoring patients during the procedure.

As experience increases with TEE, the surgical repair of aortic dissections may be carried out on the basis of TEE findings (14). Mortality of patients with aortic dissection increases 1% for every hour after onset (15), especially in those with a DeBakey type I dissection. The advantages of echocardiography are that it is portable and can be performed quickly (about 10 to 30 minutes for each examination). If aortic dissection is suspected clinically, it would be prudent to sedate patients before passage of the transesophageal probe because TEE can produce an increase in heart rate and blood pressure. Another advantage is that echocardiography can be used to evaluate the potential complications of aortic dissection, including hemopericardium, coronary involvement, aortic regurgitation, and left ventricular (LV) systolic dysfunction. Patients with aortic dissection can be followed up with TEE after surgical or medical treatment (16). The

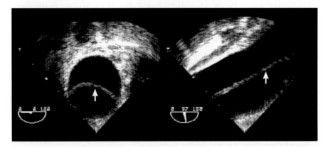

FIG. 15-6. Transverse **(left)** and longitudinal **(right)** views of the descending thoracic aorta with multiplane transesophageal echocardiography. The transverse view was obtained with the transducer at 0 degree, and the longitudinal view, with the transducer at 97 degrees. True and false lumina are separated by an intimal flap (*arrow*). This is the typical appearance of a dissection of the descending thoracic aorta.

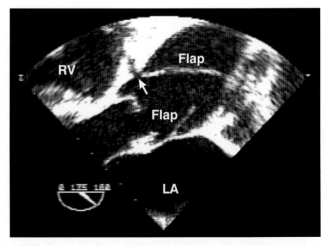

FIG. 15-8. Multiplane transesophageal echocardiogram with the transducer at the 135-degree position showing proximal aortic dissection, with an intimal flap originating from the ostium of the right coronary artery (*arrow*).

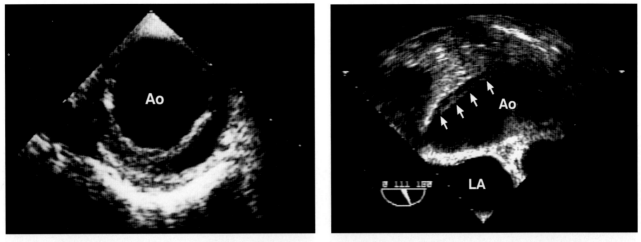

FIG. 15-9. A: Transverse transesophageal view of the descending thoracic aorta (*Ao*) showing an intramural hematoma in a patient with hypertension and severe back pain. The soft-tissue mass with a smooth surface appears different from aortic debris. During the next 6 months, the intramural hematoma disappeared while the patient was taking antihypertensive medications, including a β-blocker. **B:** Long-axis transesophageal view showing intramural hematoma in the ascending aorta (*arrows*).

morphological and flow characteristics of an aortic dissection and the status of thrombosis in the false lumen during follow-up may be important factors in a patient's prognosis. A subgroup of the patients with clinical symptoms identical to those of aortic dissection may have an aortic penetrating ulcer as well as an intramural hematoma, which can be detected with TEE.

Pitfalls

Several pitfalls exist in the echocardiographic diagnosis of aortic dissection, including (a) inadequate visualization of a portion of the aorta, (b) difficulty in differentiating an

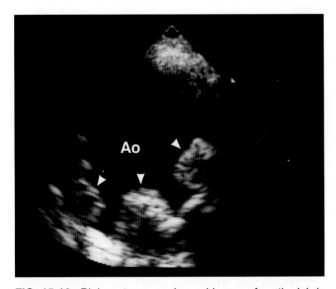

FIG. 15-10. Biplane transesophageal image of aortic debris in the descending thoracic aorta. Horizontal view showing mobile irregular masses (in real time) (*arrowheads*) attached to the aortic wall. This appearance is typical of an atherosclerotic plaque in the aorta (*Ao*).

artifact from an intimal flap, (c) misinterpreting a normal structure or nonaortic structure as an intimal flap or false lumen (innominate vein or azygous vein), and (d) localized aortic dissection or intramural hematoma.

It is recommended that additional imaging studies be performed to clarify a less-than-certain diagnosis of aortic dissection by echocardiography. We have encountered several cases of dilated azygous vein masquerading aortic dissection in patients with chronic obstruction of the superior vena cava. Contrast echocardiography (agitated saline injected into an arm vein opacifies azygous vein) is helpful in recognizing this entity (Fig. 15-11).

AORTIC RUPTURE

Aortic rupture is one of the most life-threatening complications of deceleration injury caused by a motor vehicle accident. Patient survival depends on prompt diagnosis and surgical treatment. Traditionally, aortography, CT, or MRI is used to diagnose aortic rupture. Because TEE is able to visualize the entire thoracic aorta, it may be well suited as the initial diagnostic procedure for patients with suspected ruptured thoracic aorta. Smith and colleagues (17) evaluated the role of TEE in 101 patients admitted to the emergency department with the diagnosis of possible traumatic rupture of the aorta. Echocardiography and aortography were performed in all patients. TEE was performed successfully in 93 patients, and the reason it failed in the others was related to lack of patient cooperation or significant facial trauma. No complications were noted with TEE, and the average time required for the examination was 20.9 ± 12 minutes. Echocardiography had a sensitivity of 100% and a specificity of 98%, with one false-positive result. The diagnosis of aortic rupture should be distinguished from aortic debris or

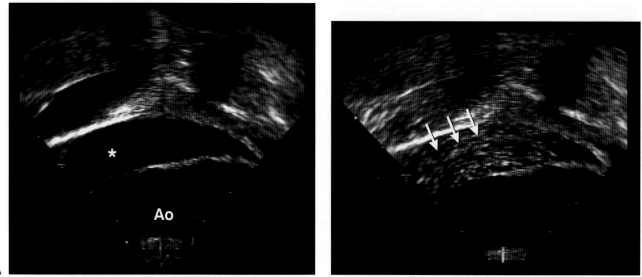

A   B

FIG. 15-11. A: A longitudinal transesophageal view (or 90-degree multiplane) of the thoracic aorta showing two lumens (*Ao* and *asterisk*) separated by a linear structure. The image initially was interpreted as aortic dissection. The lumen indicated by the *asterisk* is an enlarged azygous vein due to obstruction of the superior vena cava. (Venous drainage occurs from the upper extremity to the right atrium (*RA*) through the azygous veins and inferior vena cava.) **B:** Injection of 10 mL of agitated saline opacified the azygous vein (*arrows*).

atheromatous plaque along the aortic wall (Fig. 15-12). On the basis of their experience, Smith et al. (17) recommended that TEE be used as the primary imaging mo-

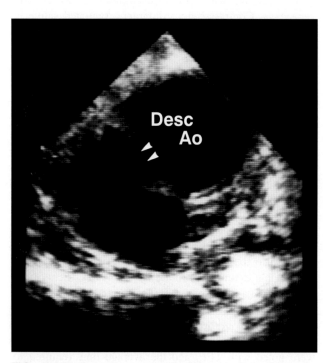

FIG. 15-12. Transverse transesophageal view of the descending thoracic aorta in a hypotensive patient after a motor vehicle accident. The aorta has a tear (*arrowheads*), with a large cavity communicating with the descending thoracic aorta (*Desc Ao*).

dality to evaluate aortic rupture. Aortography may be required if the TEE results are not diagnostic.

Trauma or infection may cause pseudoaneurysm to develop in the aorta. Pseudoaneurysm results from a tear or perforation in the aortic wall and from leakage of blood from the aorta into a contained aneurysmal cavity. Because pseudoaneurysms tend to rupture, repair is usually recommended. Pseudoaneurysm has a different appearance from true aneurysm, with a sharply demarcated rupture site where communication occurs between the aorta and the pseudoaneurysm (Fig. 15-12; see also Fig. 21-2).

AORTIC ANEURYSM

Aortic dilatation is detected easily with TTE and TEE. When the aneurysm reaches a diameter of 5.5 to 6 cm, the incidence of rupture increases. Smaller aneurysms require serial follow-up studies, in which the dimensions of the aorta are measured at specific locations. Patients with Marfan syndrome have a high prevalence of cardiovascular abnormalities, including aortic dilatation and mitral valve prolapse (Fig. 15-13 and 15-14) (18,19). In a study of 40 patients with Marfan syndrome, 78% had aortic root dilatation and 65% had mitral valve prolapse. In follow-up examination, the mean rate of aortic root dilatation was 1.9 mm per year. Aortic dissection is the most serious complication of Marfan syndrome, and prophylactic therapy with β-blockers appears to be effective in slowing the rate of aortic dilatation and reducing the development of aortic complications in the syndrome (20).

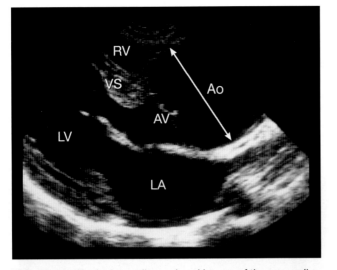

FIG. 15-13. Typical two-dimensional image of the ascending aorta in Marfan syndrome (annuloaortic ectasia). The proximal portion of the aorta (*Ao*) (aortic annulus and the sinuses of Valsalva) is diffusely enlarged (*double-headed arrow*). Annulus dilatation results in chronic aortic regurgitation. Progressive aortic dilatation predisposes to aortic rupture, and it is advised to perform prophylactic surgery (Bentall procedure) when the aortic diameter reaches 5.5 to 6 cm. Aortic dissection is also frequent. Cardiac complications (heart failure, aortic rupture, and aortic dissection) are common causes of death in patients with Marfan syndrome, accounting for more than 90% of deaths. Mitral valve prolapse also is frequently present in patients with Marfan syndrome. *AV*, aortic valve; *VS*, ventricular septum.

AORTIC DEBRIS

Because imaging of the aorta is a routine part of TEE examinations, new morphologic abnormalities of the aorta have been described. Atherosclerotic plaques and debris are common findings in elderly patients, and their clinical significance has been investigated. Unlike intramural hematoma, aortic plaques are usually irregularly shaped and frequently mobile (Fig. 15-10). The incidence of aortic debris is higher in patients who have had an embolic event (21–24). The prevalence of ulcerated plaques in the aortic arch

was studied by Amarenco and colleagues (22) in stroke patients. Ulcerated plaques were present in 26% of 239 patients who had a cerebrovascular accident but in only 5% of the 261 patients without a neurologic disease. Subsequently, the French stroke study group determined that atheromatous plaques 4 mm or more thick are more likely to cause an embolic event (24). Although preliminary data suggest that chronic anticoagulation with warfarin may be beneficial in patients with atheromatous plaque to decrease embolic events, surgical removal is indicated if embolism recurs during anticoagulation (25). An aortic plaque can be hemodynamically compromising or flow-limiting and result in acquired coarctation of the aorta (26) or ischemia of the lower extremity (or both), especially in the setting of low cardiac output (Fig. 15-15).

COARCTATION OF THE AORTA

Coarctation of the aorta is a narrowing of the descending thoracic aorta, usually immediately distal to the left subclavian artery. It is important to consider coarctation in patients with hypertension because it is surgically treatable. Coarctation is associated with Turner syndrome and other congenital anomalies such as bicuspid aortic valve, patent ductus arteriosus, ventricular septal defect, and aneurysm of the circle of Willis. Echocardiographically, coarctation is diagnosed by showing narrowing of the descending thoracic aorta and increased Doppler flow velocity across the narrowing (Fig. 15-16). Therefore, suprasternal notch 2D and continuous-wave Doppler examinations should be performed routinely in patients with hypertension. MRI is also a useful modality to demonstrate coarctation (see Chapter 18, Fig. 18–17).

ANEURYSM OF THE SINUS OF VALSALVA

The absence of the media in the sinus aortic wall results in aneurysmal dilatation of the sinus of Valsalva. Bulging of the sinus usually does not create symptoms, but it can cause compression of adjacent structures. It also can rupture

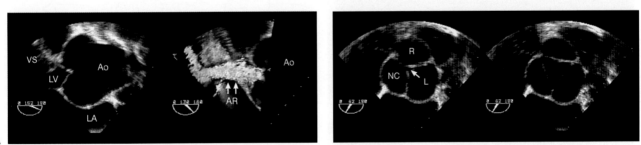

A **B**

FIG. 15-14. Multiplane transesophageal view of the aorta in a patient with Marfan syndrome. **A:** Long-axis view of the aorta (*Ao*) with a transducer at 130 to 150 degrees showing the dilated sinus of Valsalva and color-flow imaging (*arrows*) of severe aortic regurgitation (*AR*). *VS*, ventricular septum. **B:** Short-axis view of the aortic valve with the transducer at 62 degrees, demonstrating dilated sinus of Valsalva, with inadequate coaptation (*arrow*) of the right (*R*) and left (*L*) aortic cusps resulting in severe aortic regurgitation. *NC*, noncoronary cusp.

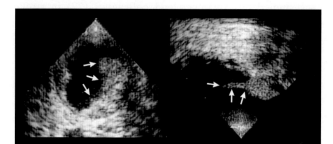

FIG. 15-15. Biplane transesophageal images of aortic debris (*arrows*) partially obstructing the descending thoracic aorta in a patient with ischemic cardiomyopathy and livedo below the umbilicus. The combination of low cardiac output and significant obstruction of the descending aorta resulted in a low flow state in the lower extremities. The livedo disappeared when cardiac output increased after administration of dopamine.

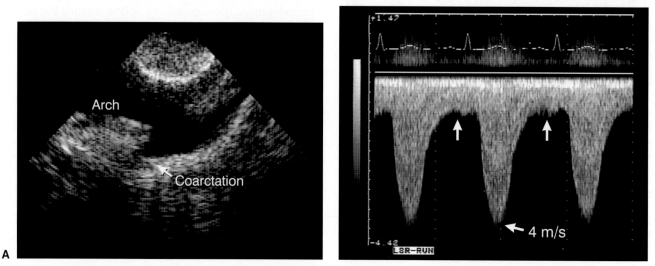

FIG. 15-16. Suprasternal two-dimensional and continuous-wave Doppler studies of coarctation of the aorta. **A:** Two-dimensional image showing narrowing of the descending thoracic aorta at the usual location. **B:** Continuous-wave Doppler spectrum of coarctation. Peak velocity is 4 m/sec, corresponding to a peak pressure gradient of 64 mm Hg. Continuous diastolic flow (*upward arrows*) is typical in severe coarctation because aortic pressure to coarctation remains high during diastole.

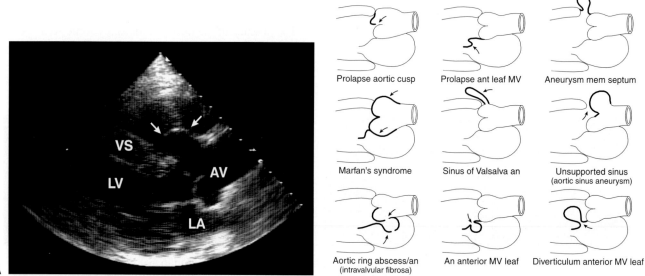

FIG. 15-17. A: Parasternal long-axis view of a transthoracic echocardiogram demonstrating aneurysm (*arrows*) of the sinus of Valsalva. *AV*, aortic valve; *VS*, ventricular septum. **B:** Drawings of various aneurysms found in the region of the left ventricular outflow tract. *an*, aneurysm; *ant*, anterior; *mem*, membranous; *MV*, mitral valve. (From ref. 30, with permission.)

into the cardiac chambers (most commonly, the right atrium or right ventricle) or ventricular septum (27,28). Parasternal long-axis and short-axis views should be able to demonstrate this aneurysm and associated structural abnormalities (Fig. 15-17). The apical view is helpful in distinguishing this from an aneurysm of a membranous ventricular septum. There are several other morphologically distinct aneurysms within the region of the LV outflow tract. Morphologic features of various aneurysms are shown schematically in Fig. 15-17B. These aneurysms can be distinguished confidently with comprehensive TTE and TEE examinations [29,30].

REFERENCES

1. Victor MF, Mintz GS, Kotler MN, Wilson AR, Segal BL. Two dimensional echocardiographic diagnosis of aortic dissection. *Am J Cardiol* 1981;48:1155–1159.
2. Khandheria BK, Tajik AJ, Taylor CL, et al. Aortic dissection: review of value and limitations of two-dimensional echocardiography in a six-year experience. *J Am Soc Echocardiogr* 1989;2:17–24.
3. Erbel R, Borner N, Steller D, et al. Detection of aortic dissection by transoesophageal echocardiography. *Br Heart J* 1987;58:45–51.
4. Seward JB, Khandheria BK, Oh JK, et al. Transesophageal echocardiography: technique, anatomic correlations, implementation, and clinical applications. *Mayo Clin Proc* 1988;63:649–680.
5. Seward JB, Khandheria BK, Freeman WK, et al. Multiplane transesophageal echocardiography: Image orientation, examination technique, anatomic correlations, and clinical applications. *Mayo Clin Proc* 1993;68:523–551.
6. Bansal RC, Chandrasekaran K, Ayala K, Smith DC. Frequency and explanation of false negative diagnosis of aortic dissection by aortography and transesophageal echocardiography. *J Am Coll Cardiol* 1995;25:1393–1401.
7. Keren A, Kim CB, Hu BS, et al. Accuracy of biplane and multiplane transesophageal echocardiography in diagnosis of typical acute aortic dissection and intramural hematoma. *J Am Coll Cardiol* 1996;28:627–636.
8. Spittell PC, Spittell JA Jr, Joyce JW, et al. Clinical features and differential diagnosis of aortic dissection: experience with 236 cases (1980 through 1990). *Mayo Clin Proc* 1993;68:642–651.
9. Kouchoukos NT, Dougenis D. Surgery of the thoracic aorta. *N Engl J Med* 1997;336:1876–1888.
10. Erbel R, Engberding R, Daniel W, Roelandt J, Visser C, Rennollet H, and the European Cooperative Study Group for Echocardiography. Echocardiography in diagnosis of aortic dissection. *Lancet* 1989;1:457–461.
11. Ballal RS, Nanda NC, Gatewood R, et al. Usefulness of transesophageal echocardiography in assessment of aortic dissection. *Circulation* 1991;84:1903–1914.
12. Sommer T, Fehske W, Holzknecht N, et al. Aortic dissection: a comparative study of diagnosis with spiral CT, multiplanar transesophageal echocardiography, and MR imaging. *Radiology* 1996;199:347–352.
13. Nienaber CA, von Kodolitsch Y, Petersen B, et al. Intramural hemorrhage of the thoracic aorta: diagnostic and therapeutic implications. *Circulation* 1995;92:1465–1472.
14. O'Gara PT, DeSanctis RW. Acute aortic dissection and its variants: toward a common diagnostic and therapeutic approach [Editorial]. *Circulation* 1995;92:1376–1378.
15. Jamieson WR, Munro AI, Miyagishima RT, Allen P, Tyers GF, Gerein AN. Aortic dissection: early diagnosis and surgical management are the keys to survival. *Can J Surg* 1982;25:145–149.
16. Mohr-Kahaly S, Erbel R, Rennollet H, et al. Ambulatory follow-up of aortic dissection by transesophageal two-dimensional and color-coded Doppler echocardiography. *Circulation* 1989;80:24–33.
17. Smith MD, Cassidy JM, Souther S, et al. Transesophageal echocardiography in the diagnosis of traumatic rupture of the aorta. *N Engl J Med* 1995;332:356–362.
18. Simpson IA, de Belder MA, Treasure T, Camm AJ, Pumphrey CW. Cardiovascular manifestations of Marfan's syndrome: improved evaluation by transoesophageal echocardiography. *Br Heart J* 1993;69:104–108.
19. Hwa J, Richards JG, Huang H, et al. The natural history of aortic dilatation in Marfan syndrome. *Med J Aust* 1993;158:558–562.
20. Shores J, Berger KR, Murphy EA, Pyeritz RE. Progression of aortic dilatation and the benefit of long-term (β-adrenergic blockade in Marfan's syndrome. *N Engl J Med* 1994;330:1335–1341.
21. Karalis DG, Chandrasekaran K, Victor MF, Ross JJ Jr, Mintz GS. Recognition and embolic potential of intraaortic atherosclerotic debris. *J Am Coll Cardiol* 1991;17:73–78.
22. Amarenco P, Duyckaerts C, Tzourio C, Henin D, Bousser MG, Hauw JJ. The prevalence of ulcerated plaques in the aortic arch in patients with stroke. *N Engl J Med* 1992;326:221–225.
23. Katz ES, Tunick PA, Rusinek H, Ribakove G, Spencer FC, Kronzon I. Protruding aortic atheromas predict stroke in elderly patients undergoing cardiopulmonary bypass: experience with intraoperative transesophageal echocardiography. *J Am Coll Cardiol* 1992;230:70–77.
24. The French Study of Aortic Plaques in Stroke Group. Atherosclerotic disease of the aortic arch as a risk factor for recurrent ischemic stroke. *N Engl J Med* 1996;334:1216–1221.
25. Laperche T, Laurian C, Roudaut R, Steg PG, for the Filiale Echocardiographie de la Société Française de Cardiologie. Mobile thromboses of the aortic arch without aortic debris: a transesophageal echocardiographic finding associated with unexplained arterial embolism. *Circulation* 1997;96:288–294.
26. Higano ST, Harris WO, Tajik AJ, Freeman WK, Joyce JW, Hayes DL. Calcified obstructive disease of the descending thoracic aorta. *Mayo Clin Proc* 1994;69:371–372.
27. van Son JAM, Danielson GK, Schaff HV, Orszulak TA, Edwards WD, Seward JB. Long-term outcome of surgical repair of ruptured sinus of Valsalva aneurysm. *Circulation* 1994;90(Suppl 2):II20–II29.
28. Katz ES, Cziner DG, Rosenzweig BP, Attubato M, Feit F, Kronzon I. Multifaceted echocardiographic approach to the diagnosis of a ruptured sinus of Valsalva aneurysm. *J Am Soc Echocardiogr* 1991;4:494–498.
29. Blackshear JL, Safford RE, Lane GE, Freeman WK, Schaff HV. Unruptured noncoronary sinus of Valsalva aneurysm: preoperative characterization by transesophageal echocardiography. *J Am Soc Echocardiogr* 1991;4:485–490.
30. Meier JH, Seward JB, Miller FA Jr, Oh JK, Enriquez-Sarano M. Aneurysms in the left ventricular outflow tract: clinical presentation, causes and echocardiographic features. *J Am Soc Echocardiogr* 1998;11:729–745.

CHAPTER 16

Cardiac Tumors and Masses

Echocardiography is the diagnostic procedure of choice for detecting and characterizing cardiac masses. Its diagnostic accuracy has been enhanced by the use of transesophageal echocardiography (TEE). The first publication from the Mayo Clinic on echocardiography was about an intracardiac tumor and was entitled "Echocardiographic diagnosis of left atrial myxoma," by T. T. Schattenberg in the *Mayo Clinic Proceedings* in 1968 (1). Cardiac masses can be classified as (a) cardiac tumor, (b) thrombus, (c) vegetation, (d) iatrogenic material, (e) normal variant, and (f) extracardiac structure. The size, shape, location, mobility, and attachment site of a cardiac mass as well as the clinical presentation usually can differentiate these masses. Accurate diagnosis is crucial because misinterpretation may result in an incorrect management strategy, including an unnecessary surgical procedure. This chapter discusses the echocardiographic and relevant clinical features of cardiac tumors and masses.

BENIGN TUMORS

Cardiac tumors are *primary* (originate from the heart) or *secondary* to metastases from other malignancies. Although primary cardiac tumors are usually benign, they can result in systemic symptoms, embolic events, malignant arrhythmias, chest pain, and heart failure. Because of these potential complications, it is recommended that cardiac tumors be removed whenever possible. The study most frequently quoted to describe the spectrum of cardiovascular tumors is that of the Armed Forces Institute of Pathology (2) (Table 16–1). From 1957 to 1991, 108 patients at our institution underwent surgical removal of 112 primary intracardiac tumors. The characteristics of these tumors and patient data are presented in Table 16–2 (3).

Myxoma

Myxoma is the most common cardiac tumor and accounts for 20% to 30% of intracardiac tumors (1,4). Its most common location is the left atrium (LA), with the

attachment site at the atrial septum. It has a typical M-mode and two-dimensional (2D) echocardiographic appearance (Fig. 16–1). Other locations and attachment sites have been observed (4,5), including the right atrium (RA), right ventricle (RV), left ventricle (LV), and atrioventricular valve (Figs. 16–2 and 16–3). In 5% of cases, myxoma is multiple. The atypical location of a myxoma is usually associated with a familial pattern in younger patients (along with lentiginosis and endocrine abnormalities). The tumor appears gelatinous and friable, with occasional central necrosis. Embolic events are more frequent with a small myxoma (6). It can produce obstruction of the atrioventricular valve (i.e., similar symptoms as in mitral or tricuspid valve stenosis) and result in a tumor plop on auscultation after the second heart sound (7), which can be misinterpreted as an opening snap. Ventricular myxoma can cause obstruction of the outflow tract (Fig. 16–3A), and outflow murmur is common. Doppler echocardiography is valuable in detecting the extent of valvular obstruction caused by an atrial myxoma (Fig. 16–1D).

Myxoma should be at the top of the list for the differential diagnosis of all intracavitary cardiac tumors. The diagnosis is almost assured if the attachment site to the atrial septum can be established by echocardiography. Rarely, a thrombus can be attached to the atrial septum, even with the formation of neovascularization (8,9). Other differential diagnoses for an atrial tumor (Fig. 16–4) include metastatic tumors (sarcoma and melanoma in the LA and hypernephroma, hepatoma, melanoma, and intravenous leiomyomatosis in the RA). Atrial tumor can be characterized further by percutaneous TEE-guided transvenous biopsy, especially if it is located in the RA (10).

Fibroma

Fibroma usually is located in the LV free wall, in the ventricular septum, or at the apex. It is well demarcated from the surrounding myocardium by multiple calcifications (Fig. 16–5). It occasionally grows into the LV cavity

(text continues on page 209)

TABLE 16-1. *Relative incidence of tumors of the heart*

Type of tumor	No.	%	Type of tumor	No.	%
Benign			Malignant		
Myxoma	130	30.5	Angiosarcoma	39	9.2
Lipoma	45	10.5	Rhabdomyosarcoma	26	6.1
Papillary fibroelastoma	42	9.9	Fibrosarcoma	14	3.3
Rhabdomyoma	36	8.5	Malignant lymphoma	7	1.6
Fibroma	17	4.0	Extraskeletal osteosarcoma	5	—
Hemangioma	15	3.5	Neurogenic sarcoma	4	—
Teratoma	14	3.3	Malignant teratoma	4	—
Mesothelioma of atrioventricular node	12	2.8	Thymoma	4	—
Granular cell tumor	3	—	Leiomyosarcoma	1	—
Neurofibroma	3	—	Liposarcoma	1	—
Lymphangioma	2	—	Synovial sarcoma	1	—
Subtotal	319	75.1	Subtotal	106	24.9
			Total	425	100.0

From ref. 2, with permission.

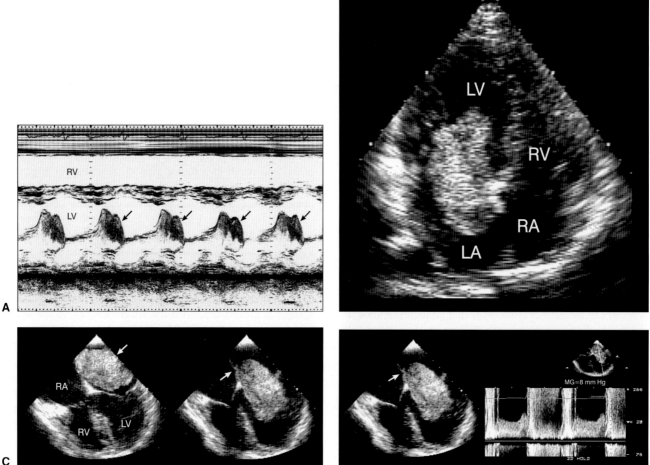

FIG. 16-1. A: M-mode echocardiogram of left atrial (*LA*) myxoma recorded from the parasternal trans-ducer position. During diastole, the mitral orifice is filled with increased echodensity (*arrows*) repre-senting protruding leiomyxoma. **B:** Diastolic frame of apical four-chamber view showing a large LA myxoma protruding into the left ventricular (*LV*) cavity. Because of obstruction of the mitral orifice during diastole, a patient with LA myxoma presents with symptoms similar to those of mitral stenosis. **C:** Systolic **(left)** and diastolic **(right)** frames of transesophageal view of a large LA myxoma (*left arrow*) attached to the atrial septum (*right arrow*). **D:** Continuous-wave Doppler examination of the mitral valve shows an increased pressure gradient due to mitral orifice obstruction by the LA myxoma. The mean gradient (*MG*) is 8 mm Hg, and pressure half-time is prolonged. *Arrow*, attachment of myxoma to the atrial septum.

TABLE 16-2. *Summary of surgically excised benign cardiac tumors at the Mayo Clinic, 1957 through March 1991*

Tumor type	No.	Sex (F:M)	Mean age (yr)	Tumor site and no.
Myxoma	80	51:25[a]	53	LA 64, RA 16
Fibroma	9	5:4	14.2	LV 5, RV 1, VS 2, LA 1
Lipomatous tumor	5	0:5	60.4	RA 4, RV 1
Fibroelastic papilloma	7	4:3	47.4	AV 3, MV 2, LV 1, TV 1
Hamartoma	1	1:0	1.2	LV 1

AV, aortic valve; MV, mitral valve; TV, tricuspid valve; VS, ventricular septum.

[a] Some patients had more than one tumor.

From ref. 3, with permission.

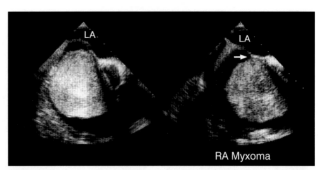

FIG. 16-2. Transesophageal transverse view of a large right atrium (*RA*) myxoma attached to the atrial septum (*arrow*).

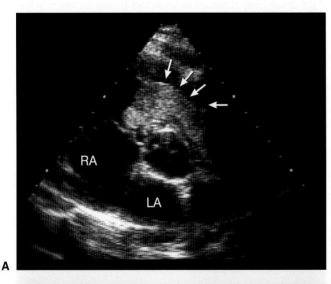

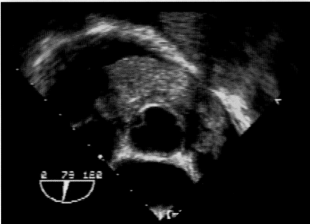

FIG. 16-3. A: Transthoracic parasternal short-axis view showing large mass in the right ventricle (RV) protruding through the pulmonary valve to the main pulmonary artery (*arrows*) in a young woman. **B:** Multiplane transesophageal short-axis view of the same patient. A myxoma in an unusual location usually is related to familial myxoma syndrome in young patients. **C:** Transesophageal long-axis view showing a myxoma in the RV (*arrow*). *Ao,* aorta; *VS,* ventricular septum.

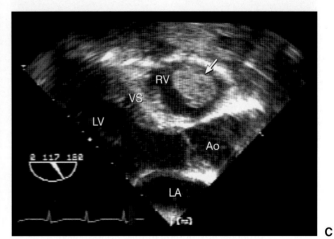

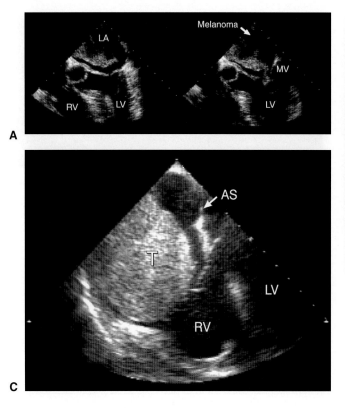

A

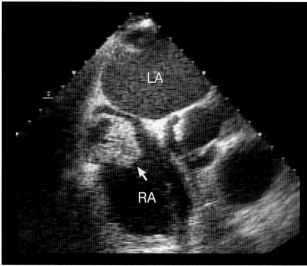

B

C

FIG. 16-4. A: Transverse transesophageal image showing a large left atrial (*LA*) mass in a patient with metastatic melanoma. The mass could be traced to the pulmonary vein. *MV*, mitral valve. **B:** Transverse transesophageal view of right atrial (*RA*) mass. It is attached to the junction of the inferior vena cava and RA (*arrow*), not to the atrial septum. This was a metastatic hepatoma. **C:** An example of metastatic melanoma (*T*) in the RA.

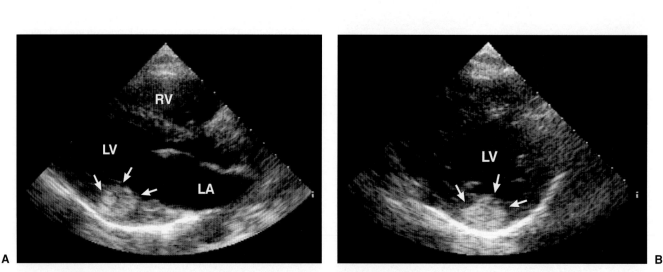

A

B

FIG. 16-5. Parasternal long-axis **(A)** and short-axis **(B)** views of a left ventricular (*LV*) fibroma (*arrows*). It is well-circumscribed in the posterior free wall. It may cause ventricular arrhythmia, but it does not produce any hemodynamic abnormality.

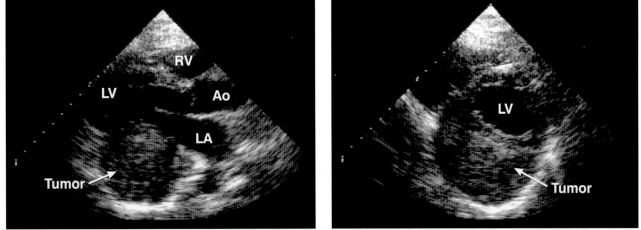

FIG. 16-6. Parasternal long-axis **(A)** and short-axis **(B)** views of a large left ventricular (*LV*) fibroma (*tumor*) occupying a significant portion of the LV cavity and interfering with LV filling. *Ao*, aorta.

and interferes with ventricular filling (Fig. 16–6). Potential problems resulting from fibroma are congestive heart failure and malignant arrhythmias. When located at the apex, it may be misinterpreted by other imaging modalities as apical hypertrophic cardiomyopathy. Echocardiography is helpful in making the diagnosis of fibroma and in following the growth of the tumor in asymptomatic patients.

Rhabdomyoma

Rhabdomyoma is the most common cardiac tumor in children, particularly in those with tuberous sclerosis (11). It is often multiple and present in the RV or RV outflow tract and even in the pulmonary artery (Fig. 16–7). The presence of rhabdomyoma can be diagnosed before birth by fetal echocardiography. This tumor may regress spontaneously after birth.

Papillary Fibroelastoma and Others

Papillary fibroelastomas originate from the cardiac valves or adjacent endocardium. Frequently, they are an incidental finding on a routine echocardiographic examination. These tumors tend to originate from the atrial side of the atrioventricular valve and the ventricular surface of the semilunar valve (Fig. 16–8). Occasionally, it is attached to the ventricular septum or near the LV outflow tract (12). The aortic valve is involved most frequently. The tumor usually is not large. It has an appearance similar to that of Lambl excrescences, although Lambl excrescences are smaller and broader based. The most feared complication of fibroelastoma is an embolic event, such as stroke or coronary embolization. The usual recommendation is to re-

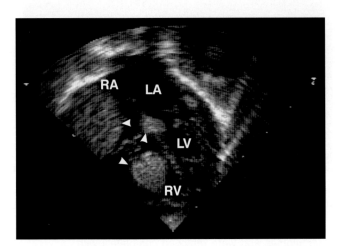

FIG. 16-7. Apex-down four-chamber view demonstrating multiple cardiac tumors (*arrowheads*) on the right side of the heart of a baby with tuberous sclerosis. This is a typical example of rhabdomyoma.

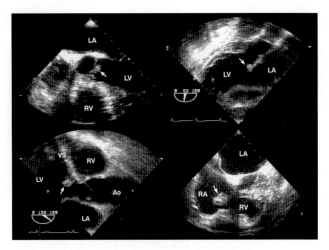

FIG. 16-8. Transesophageal echocardiographic examples of aortic valve **(upper left)**, mitral valve **(upper right)**, left ventricular outflow tract **(lower left)**, and tricuspid valve **(lower right)** papillary fibroelastomas (*arrows*). These tumors were not detected with transthoracic echocardiography. *Ao*, aorta; *VS*, ventricular septum.

move the fibroelastoma even in asymptomatic patients (13). Other unusual benign tumors or masses include hemangioma, hamartoma, and infections such as an echinococcal cyst or tuberculoma (14) (Fig. 16–9).

MALIGNANT TUMORS OF THE HEART

The most frequent malignant primary cardiac tumors are angiosarcoma, rhabdomyosarcoma, and fibrosarcoma. Angiosarcoma occurs most commonly in the RA along with pericardial effusion, whereas rhabdomyosarcoma and fibrosarcoma can occur anywhere in the heart. The prognosis of malignant primary cardiac tumors is grim.

Malignant tumors can metastasize to the heart. Most frequently, they are from the lung, breast, kidney, liver, lymphoma, melanoma, and osteogenic sarcoma. Hypernephroma, hepatoma, and intravenous leiomyomatosis from the uterus tend to metastasize to the inferior vena cava and RA (Fig. 16–10). Whenever an RA mass is detected, the inferior vena cava should be scanned carefully.

OTHER MASSES

The RA also harbors various normal and abnormal structures that appear as a mass on 2D echocardiography. Among these are the eustachian valve, pacemaker wire, balloon or central-line catheter, and thrombus. Each structure has characteristic features, however, and careful examination should be able to differentiate one from the others. Thrombi from lower-extremity deep veins must go through the RA to reach the pulmonary circulation. They are mobile, have a characteristic popcorn or snake-like appearance, and almost always are associated with pulmonary embolism (15) (see Chapter 17). A similar mobile structure may be

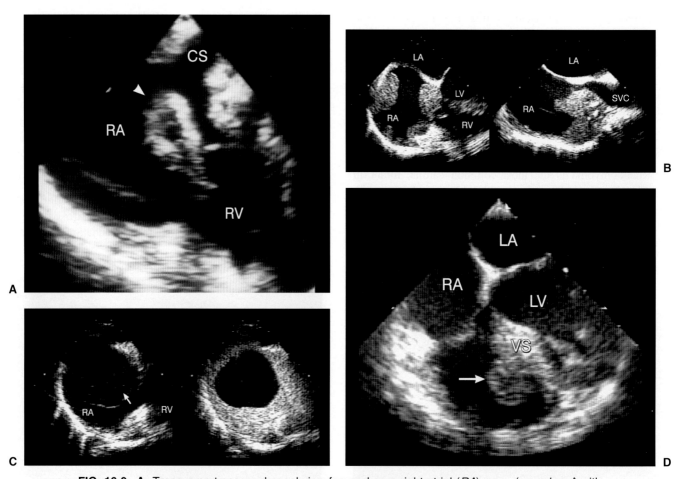

FIG. 16-9. A: Transverse transesophageal view focused on a right atrial (*RA*) mass (*arrowhead*) with a cystic center attached to the tricuspid valve. The mass was removed surgically and found to be a hamartoma. *CS*, coronary sinus. **B:** Transverse **(left)** and longitudinal **(right)** transesophageal views of multiple masses in the RA obstructing the entry of the superior vena cava (*SVC*) into *RA*. The patient had miliary tuberculosis. The masses were tuberculomas and were removed completely with surgical treatment and antituberculosis medication. **C:** Example of a hemangioma, seen as an echolucent mass (*arrow*) in the RA. It is clearly demarcated by contrast injection **(right)**. **D:** An echinococcal cyst (*arrow*) attached to the ventricular septum (*VS*) in a young Middle Eastern woman with chest pain. (**B** courtesy of N. S. Chung and **C** courtesy of D. W. Sohn.)

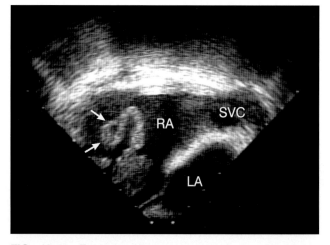

FIG. 16-10. Example of intravenous leiomyomatosis (*arrows*) from a transesophageal long-axis view of the atria. *SVC*, superior vena cava.

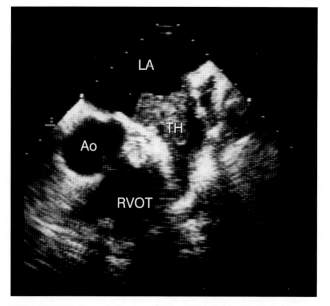

FIG. 16-11. Transverse transesophageal view of the left atrium (*LA*) and its appendage with thrombus (*TH*) in a patient with atrial fibrillation. *Ao*, aorta; *RVOT*, right ventricular outflow tract.

seen in patients with intravenous leiomyomatosis. In patients with mobile RA thrombi, the mortality is high with heparin therapy alone. Although surgical removal has been advocated, these patients can be treated successfully with a bolus of a thrombolytic agent followed by continuous infusion of the agent (250,000 units of streptokinase bolus followed by 100,000 units per hour). LA thrombus is most common in patients with mitral stenosis or atrial fibrillation

(Fig. 16–11) and infrequently occurs as a paradoxical embolus from a RA thrombus passing through a patent foramen ovale (Fig. 16–12). Even in the most ideal case, how-

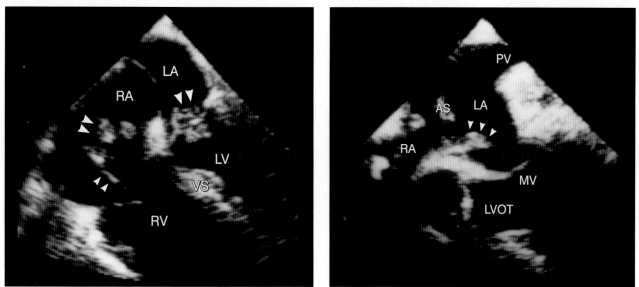

FIG. 16-12. A: Transverse transesophageal view showing biatrial thrombi (*large arrowheads*) in a patient with dyspnea and cold left foot caused by a peripheral embolic event. *Small arrowheads* indicate a pacemaker wire. The atrial septum bulges toward the left atrium (*LA*) because of increased right atrial (*RA*) pressure due to pulmonary embolism. The RA and right ventricle (*RV*) are dilated. *VS*, ventricular septum. **B:** Basal transverse transesophageal view in the same patient showing thrombus (*arrowheads*) traversing the patent foramen ovale. This is a typical example of paradoxical embolism. This patient had undergone hip surgery 1 month before this echocardiographic examination and deep vein thrombosis, pulmonary embolism, and paradoxical embolism developed. *AS*, atrial septum; *LVOT*, LV outflow tract; *MV*, mitral valve; *PV*, pulmonary vein.

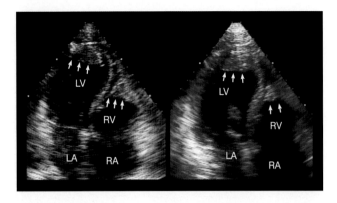

FIG. 16-13. Apical four-chamber view in a patient with hypereosinophilic syndrome. Both ventricular apices are filled with an echodense mass (*arrows*) that obliterates the apices **(left)**. Filling of the apices is better appreciated with B-mode colorization **(right)**. Apical motion in this patient was not impaired.

ever, TTE is limited in detecting thrombus in the LA appendage. The LA appendage is visualized in all patients from a transesophageal window. Ventricular thrombus is easily differentiated from a tumor because the former is almost always associated with akinetic to dyskinetic myocardium underlying the thrombus. An exception is apical thrombus formation in hypereosinophilic cardiomyopathy, which obliterates the ventricular apex (Fig. 16–13). Occasionally, a high-frequency transducer is necessary to delineate the nature of the apical abnormality.

PSEUDOTUMOR AND PITFALLS

Not all masses detected by echocardiography are a thrombus or an intracardiac tumor. The normal appearance of cardiac and extracardiac structures can be misinterpreted as an intracardiac mass. It is extremely important to recognize this pitfall, which has become more common with the introduction of TEE (16). Normal structures that are frequently misinterpreted as an intracardiac mass include a large eustachian valve, hiatal hernia, lipomatous atrial septal hypertrophy,

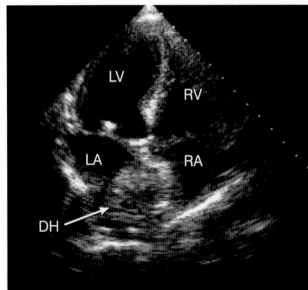

A

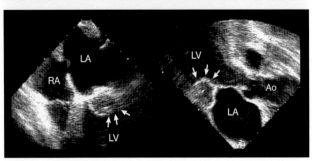

C

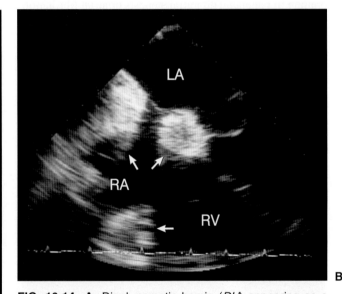

B

FIG. 16-14. A: Diaphragmatic hernia (*DH*) appearing as a mass behind the atria in an apical four-chamber view. This can be diagnosed confidently by demonstrating liquid bubbles after consumption of a carbonated drink. **B:** Transverse transesophageal view of lipomatous hypertrophy of the atrial septum (*double arrows*). It has the characteristic dumbbell appearance. This patient also has fatty infiltration of the tricuspid annulus (*single arrow*), which may be misinterpreted as an intercardiac mass. **C:** Transverse **(left)** and longitudinal **(right)** transesophageal views of the mass in the region of the left atrioventricular groove (*arrows*). It can be misinterpreted as an intercardiac mass, but this is a typical example of calcification of the mitral annulus. *Ao,* aorta.

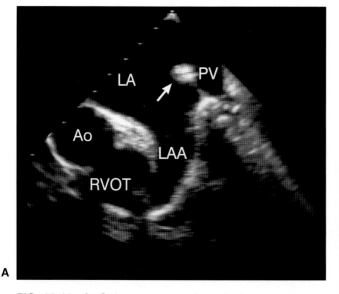

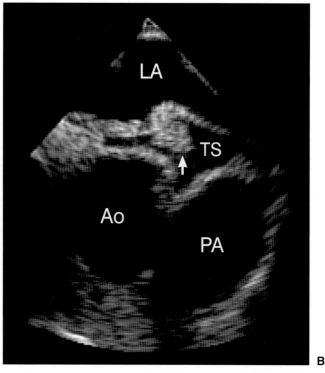

FIG. 16-15. **A:** Q-tip appearance (*arrow*) of a normal structure that separates the left upper pulmonary vein (*PV*) from the left atrial appendage (*LAA*). **B:** Basal transesophageal view of the transverse sinus (*TS*) with fibrin material (*arrow*) and pericardial effusion. *Ao*, aorta; *PA* pulmonary artery; *RVOT*, RV outflow tract.

fatty tricuspid valve annulus, and mitral valve annulus calcification (Fig. 16–14). In TEE, the Q-tip appearance of a globular structure separating the left upper pulmonary vein from the LA appendage and the potential space of the transverse sinus, which may harbor fibrin material in the presence of pericardial effusion, have been misinterpreted as an intracardiac mass (Fig. 16–15). Intracardiac catheters and pacemakers have characteristic appearances on echocardiograms and are not a diagnostic problem.

An extracardiac mass that compresses cardiac structures needs to be differentiated from an intracardiac mass. Extracardiac masses that are occasionally visualized by echocardiography include mediastinal tumor, large hematoma, lung tumor, coronary aneurysm or fistula, and pseudoaneurysm (Fig. 16–16).

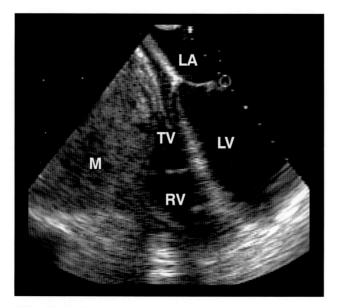

FIG. 16-16. Transverse transesophageal view of a large mass (*M*) compressing the right chambers of the heart. It was identified as a coronary aneurysm with thrombus. *TV*, tricuspid valve.

REFERENCES

1. Schattenberg TT. Echocardiographic diagnosis of left atrial myxoma. *Mayo Clin Proc* 1968;43:620–627.
2. McAllister HA Jr, Fenoglio JJ Jr. Tumors of the cardiovascular system. In: *Atlas of tumor pathology*, Second series, Fascicle 15. Washington DC: Armed Forces Institute of Pathology, 1978.
3. Tazelaar HD, Locke TJ, McGregor CGA. Pathology of surgically excised primary cardiac tumors. *Mayo Clin Proc* 1992;67:957–965.
4. Reynen K. Cardiac myxomas. *N Engl J Med* 1995;333:1610–1617.
5. Harbold NB Jr, Gau GT. Echocardiographic diagnosis of right atrial myxoma. *Mayo Clin Proc* 1973;48:284–286.
6. Fyke FE III, Seqard JB, Edwards WD, et al. Primary cardiac tumors: experience with 30 consecutive patients since the introduction of two-dimensional echocardiography. *J Am Coll Cardiol* 1985;5:1465–1473.
7. Nasser WK, Davis RH, Dillon JC, et al. Atrial myxoma. II. Phonocardiographic, echocardiographic, hemodynamic, and angiographic features in nine cases. *Am Heart J* 1972;83:810–823.
8. Colman T, de Ubago JL, Figueroa A, et al. Coronary arteriography and atrial thrombosis in mitral valve disease. *Am J Cardiol* 1981;47:973–977.
9. Standen JR. Tumor vascularity in left atrial thrombus demonstrated by selective coronary arteriography. *Radiology* 1975;116:549–550.
10. Malouf JF, Thompson RC, Maples WJ, Wolfe JT. Diagnosis of right atrial metastatic melanoma by transesophageal echocardiographic-guided transvenous biopsy. *Mayo Clin Proc* 1996;71:1167–1170.

11. Nir A, Tajik AJ, Freeman WK, et al. Tuberous sclerosis and cardiac rhabdomyoma. *Am J Cardiol* 1995;76:419–421.

12. Klarich KW, Enriquez-Sarano M, Gura GM, Edwards WD, Tajik AJ, Seward JB. Papillary fibroelastoma: echocardiographic characteristics for diagnosis and pathologic correlation. *J Am Coll Cardiol* 1997;30: 784–790.

13. Brown RD Jr, Khandheria BK, Edwards WD. Cardiac papillary fibroelastoma: a treatable cause of transient ischemic attack and ischemic stroke detected by transesophageal echocardiography. *Mayo Clin Proc* 1995;70:863–868.

14. Klodas E, Roger VL, Miller FA Jr, Utz JP, Danielson GK, Edwards WD. Cardiac echinococcosis: Case report of unusual echocardiographic appearance. *Mayo Clin Proc* 1995;70:657–661.

15. Proano M, Oh JK, Frye RL, Johnson CM, Tajik AJ, Taliercio CP. Successful treatment of pulmonary embolism and associated mobile right atrial thrombus with use of a central thrombolytic infusion. *Mayo Clin Proc* 1988;63:1181–1185.

16. Khandheria BK, Seward JB, Tajik AJ. Critical appraisal of transesophageal echocardiography: limitations and pitfalls. *Crit Care Clin* 1996;12:235–251.

CHAPTER 17

Pulmonary Hypertension

Pulmonary hypertension is characterized hemodynamically as systolic pulmonary pressure greater than 35 mm Hg, diastolic pressure greater than 15 mm Hg, and mean pulmonary pressure greater than 25 mm Hg. It is frequently a manifestation of various systemic and cardiac diseases. Various causes of pulmonary hypertension are listed in Table 17-1, according to the pathophysiologic mechanism. Pulmonary hypertension has attracted public attention because of its increased incidence among those taking diet pills (1,2).

Determination of pulmonary artery pressure is a routine part of an echocardiographic examination. Although certain two-dimensional (2D) echocardiographic features suggest pulmonary hypertension, Doppler echocardiography is the primary method for determining actual pulmonary pressures. Systolic and diastolic pulmonary artery pressures are determined from the tricuspid and pulmonary regurgitation velocities, respectively. Transesophageal echocardiography (TEE) provides superb visualization of the main pulmonary trunk, right pulmonary artery, and proximal portion of the left pulmonary artery and, hence, is useful in detecting pulmonary artery thromboembolism. After pulmonary hypertension is diagnosed, echocardiography may be helpful in identifying a cardiovascular cause of pulmonary hypertension.

TWO-DIMENSIONAL ECHOCARDIOGRAPHY

Pulmonary hypertension is easily recognized when the following M-mode and 2D echocardiographic features are present (Fig. 17-1 and 17-2) (3,4):

1. Diminished or absent "a" (atrial) wave of the pulmonary valve
2. Midsystolic closure or notching of the pulmonary valve
3. Enlarged chambers on the right side of the heart
4. D-shaped left ventricular (LV) cavity caused by a flattened ventricular septum

These features, however, are not sensitive for pulmonary hypertension. They are qualitative and do not provide actual hemodynamic data.

DOPPLER ECHOCARDIOGRAPHY

Doppler echocardiography allows estimation of pulmonary artery pressure by measuring tricuspid regurgitation velocity, pulmonary regurgitation velocity, and, rarely, right ventricular (RV) outflow tract flow acceleration time.

Tricuspid Regurgitation Velocity

Tricuspid regurgitation velocity usually is obtained by continuous-wave Doppler (using either an imaging duplex transducer or a nonimaging transducer) from the RV inflow or the apical four-chamber view position. From the apical position, the transducer needs to be angled more medially and inferiorly from the mitral valve signal. Tricuspid regurgitation velocity reflects the pressure difference during systole between the RV and the right atrium (RA) (Fig. 17-3) (5–7). Therefore, systolic RV pressure can be estimated by adding right atrial (RA) pressure to the transtricuspid gradient derived from tricuspid regurgitation velocity, that is,

Transtricuspid pressure gradient

$$= 4 \times \textit{Tricuspid regurgitation velocity}^2$$

The RA pressure can be estimated clinically by measuring jugular venous pressure or by the respiratory motion of the inferior vena cava seen on 2D echocardiograms. When the diameter of the inferior vena cava decreases by 50% or more with inspiration (Fig. 17-3C), RA pressure is usually below 10 mm Hg, and those with less than 50% inspiratory collapse tend to have right RA pressures above 10 mm Hg (8). In the absence of pulmonic stenosis or RV outflow obstruction, RV systolic pressure is equal to pulmonary artery systolic pressure. The normal tricuspid regurgitation velocity is 2.0 to 2.5 m/sec. A higher velocity indicates pulmonary hypertension, RV outflow tract obstruction, or pulmonic stenosis. Four different tricuspid regurgitation velocity recordings are shown in Fig. 17-4. Tricuspid regurgitation velocity may be below 2.0 m/sec when RA pressure is markedly increased because of RV infarct, RV failure, or severe tricuspid regurgitation.

TABLE 17-1. *Etiologic classification of pulmonary hypertension*

Pulmonary venous hypertension
  Thoracic aorta
    Coarctation of the aorta
    Supravalvular aortic stenosis
  Left ventricle
    Aortic stenosis or insufficiency
    Congenital subaortic stenosis
    Hypertrophic cardiomyopathy
    Constrictive pericarditis
    Myocardial disease of various causes
  Left atrium
    Ball-valve thrombus
    Myxoma
    Cor triatriatum
  Pulmonary veins
    Congenital pulmonary vein stenosis
    Mediastinitis or mediastinal fibrosis
    Mediastinal neoplasm
Chronic hypoxia
  Residence at high altitude
  Inadequate respiratory excursion
    Extreme obesity (pickwickian syndrome)
    Severe kyphoscoliosis
    Neuromuscular disorders
    Extreme pleural fibrosis or lung resection
  Chronic upper airway obstruction
    Congenital webs
    Enlarged tonsils
  Chronic lower airway obstruction
    Chronic bronchitis
    Asthmatic bronchitis
    Bronchiectasis
  Cystic fibrosis
    Emphysema

Chronic diffuse pulmonary parenchymal
  disease
  Interstitial fibrosis (idiopathic, chronic
  pneumonitic, toxic, etc.)
  Pneumoconioses (silicosis, asbestosis, etc.)
  Granulomatous diseases (sarcoidosis,
  tuberculosis, etc.)
  Alveolar filling disorders (alveolar proteinosis,
  etc.)
  Connective tissue disorders (rheumatoid
  lung, systemic sclerosis, etc.)
Vascular disorders of the lung
  Primary vascular disease
    Plexogenic pulmonary arteriography (diet
    pills, AIDS)
    Connective tissue disorders (lupus,
    systemic sclerosis, or scleroderma)
Thrombotic disease
  Sickle cell disease
  Pulmonary veno-occlusive disease
Embolic disease
  Persistent large pulmonary emboli
  Recurrent pulmonary emboli
  Tumor emboli (e.g., breast carcinoma)
  Schistosomiasis
Left-to-right shunts
  Extracardiac shunts
    Patent ductus arteriosus
    Aortopulmonary window
    Rupture of aortic sinus
Intracardiac shunts
  Ventricular septal defect
  Atrial septal defect

AIDS, acquired immunodeficiency syndrome.
From McGoon MD, Fuster V, Freeman WK, Edwards WD, Scott JP. Pulmonary hypertension. In: Giuliani ER, Gersh BJ, McGoon MD, Hayes DL, Schaff HV, eds. *Mayo Clinic Practice of Cardiology,* 3rd ed. St. Louis: Mosby, 1996;1815–1836, with permission.

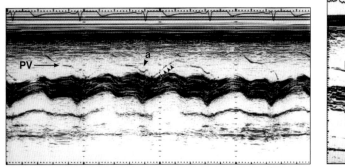
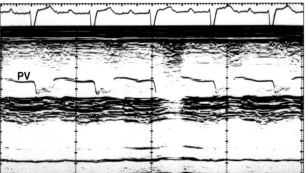

FIG. 17-1. A: Normal M-mode echocardiogram of the pulmonary valve (*PV; arrow* and *arrowheads*) with atrial wave (*a*) deflection. **B:** M-mode of the pulmonary valve in pulmonary hypertension. The atrial wave is absent, and there is midsystolic closure of the valve, giving M-mode of the pulmonary valve the shape of "W" during systole.

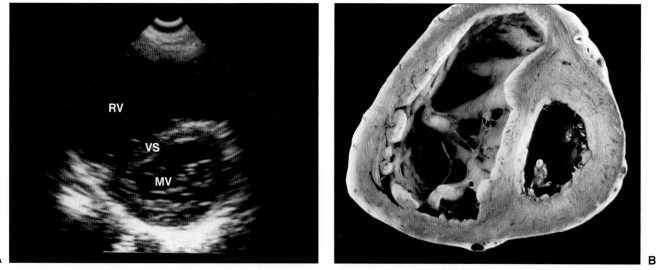

FIG. 17-2. A: Parasternal short-axis view demonstrating the D-shaped left ventricular cavity and enlarged right ventricular (*RV*) cavity in pulmonary hypertension. Similar appearances are present in RV volume overload; however, flattening of the ventricular septum (*VS*) persists during the entire cardiac cycle in RV and pulmonary artery pressure overload, whereas it disappears during systole in RV volume overload. *MV*, mitral valve. **B:** Corresponding pathology specimen.

Tricuspid regurgitation is present in more than 75% of the normal adult population. When the tricuspid regurgitation jet is trivial and its continuous-wave Doppler spectrum is suboptimal, injection of agitated saline solution into an arm vein enhances the tricuspid regurgitation velocity signal (Fig. 17-5).

Technical Caveat

Doppler velocity recordings from patients with aortic stenosis or mitral regurgitation can mimic the tricuspid regurgitant jet. All three Doppler jets move away from the apex, but they can be differentiated by angulation of the transducer, Doppler peak velocity, flow duration, and the accompanying diastolic signal. Tricuspid regurgitation is directed most medially and tricuspid inflow (diastole) velocity is usually below 0.5 m/sec unless the tricuspid regurgitation is severe or the valve is stenotic. Flow duration is shortest in aortic stenosis. Mitral regurgitant jet peak velocity is usually, but not always, greater than 4 m/sec and always greater than that of aortic stenosis in the same patient (see Chapter 9).

Pulmonary Regurgitation Velocity

The end-diastolic velocity of pulmonary regurgitation reflects the end-diastolic pressure gradient between the pulmonary artery and the RV (Fig. 17-6). At end diastole, RV pressure should be equal to RA pressure (RAP). Therefore,

$$PAEDP = 4 \times PREDV^2 + RAP$$

where *PAEDP* is the pulmonary artery end-diastolic pressure, and *PREDV* is the pulmonary regurgitation end-diastolic velocity.

The peak early diastolic pulmonary regurgitation (PR) velocity is useful in estimating mean pulmonary artery pressure. According to Masuyama and colleagues (9), the peak diastolic pressure gradient between the pulmonary artery and RV approximates the mean pulmonary artery pressure (PAP). Therefore,

$$Mean\ PAP = 4 \times Peak\ PR\ velocity^2$$

RV Outflow Tract Flow Acceleration Time

The RV outflow tract flow velocity has a characteristic pattern as pulmonary artery pressure increases (Fig. 17-7). The acceleration phase becomes shorter with increased pulmonary artery pressure. Several investigators have derived regression equations to estimate the mean pulmonary artery pressure (MPAP) from the RV outflow tract acceleration time (AcT) (10,11). Mahan's equation is simplest and preferred for estimating mean pulmonary artery pressure:

$$MPAP = 79 - 0.45\ (AcT)$$

It should be noted that acceleration time is dependent on cardiac output and heart rate (12). With increased output through the cardiac chambers on the right side (as in atrial septal defect), acceleration time may be normal even when pulmonary artery pressure is increased. If the heart rate is lower than 60 beats per minute or greater than 100 beats per minute, acceleration time needs to be corrected for heart rate. This method is rarely used in our practice.

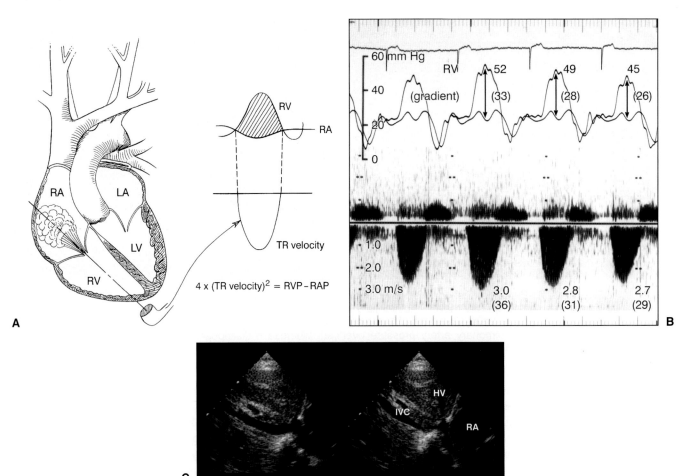

FIG. 17-3. A: Diagram of the chambers on the right side of the heart demonstrating how to measure systolic right ventricular (*RV*) pressure from tricuspid regurgitation (*TR*) velocity. The peak systolic transtricuspid pressure gradient from the RV to the *RA* is represented by 4 × (peak TR velocity)². Therefore, systolic RV pressure is estimated by adding right atrial (*RA*) pressure to the pressure gradient derived from tricuspid regurgitation velocity. *RAP*, RA pressure; *RVP*, RV pressure. **B:** Simultaneous RV and RA pressure tracings and tricuspid regurgitation velocity recording by continuous-wave Doppler echocardiography. Pressure gradients (36, 31, and 29 mm Hg) derived from the peak Doppler velocities of the second, third, and fourth beats (3.0, 2.8, and 2.7 m/sec, respectively) are close to the catheter-derived RV and RA gradients (33, 28, and 26 mm Hg). **C:** Subcostal view of the inferior vena cava (*IVC*), hepatic vein (*HV*), and RA during expiration **(left)** and inspiration **(right)** in a patient with normal RA pressure. The IVC collapses more than 50% with inspiration.

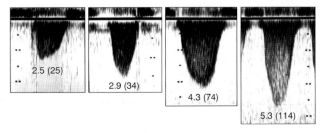

FIG. 17-4. Representative tricuspid regurgitation velocities. The numbers in parentheses are pressure gradients derived from peak velocities using the simplified Bernoulli equation.

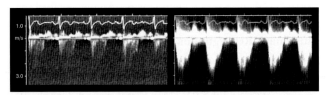

FIG. 17-5. Continuous-wave Doppler recording of tricuspid regurgitation velocity without **(left)** and with **(right)** injection of agitated saline.

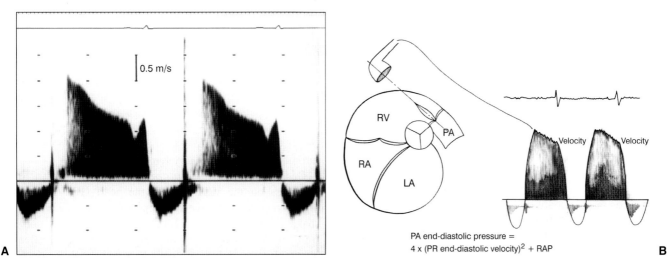

PA end-diastolic pressure =
4 × (PR end-diastolic velocity)^2 + RAP

A

B

FIG. 17-6. A: Continuous-wave Doppler spectrum of pulmonary regurgitation velocity in a patient with normal pulmonary artery pressure. Because the pressure difference between the pulmonary artery and right ventricle (RV) is small during diastole, contraction of the right atrium (RA) (hence, increase in RA and RV pressures) decreases the pulmonary artery-RV pressure gradient, resulting in a dip in pulmonary regurgitation velocity. When pulmonary pressure is high, RA contraction usually does not make a significant change in pulmonary artery-RV pressure gradients; hence, there is no dip in the continuous-wave Doppler signal of pulmonary regurgitation. **B:** Diagram of continuous-wave Doppler interrogation of pulmonary regurgitation (*PR*) from the left parasternal window and the pulmonary regurgitation Doppler spectrum. If end-diastolic pulmonary regurgitation velocity is 3 m/sec, end-diastolic pulmonary artery (*PA*) pressure = 4 × 3^2 + 20 = 56 mm Hg, assuming an RA pressure (*RAP*) of 20 mm Hg.

Using the aforementioned Doppler variables, systolic, diastolic, and mean pulmonary artery pressures can be estimated (Fig. 17-8). Tricuspid and pulmonary regurgitations are present in more than 85% of normal subjects (13). The incidence is higher in those with pulmonary hypertension. The tricuspid regurgitation velocity signal is enhanced by the injection of agitated saline or a contrast agent into the RA through an arm vein (see Fig. 17-5). After echocardiography has established that pulmonary artery pressure is increased, the potential causes of this increase should be evaluated thoroughly with 2D Doppler and color-flow imaging to look for left-sided abnormality [left ventricular (LV) failure, mitral stenosis, mitral regurgitation, etc.], left-to-right shunt, atrial septal defect,

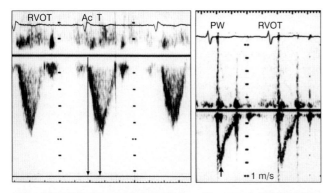

FIG. 17-7. Right ventricular (*RV*) outflow tract (*RVOT*) flow velocity recordings by pulsed-wave Doppler echocardiography. The sample volume is placed in the region of the pulmonary valve annulus. Normal flow pattern **(left).** Acceleration time (*Ac T*) is the time interval between the beginning of the flow and its peak velocity (between the two vertical arrows). It is 130 msec (normal, ≥120 ms). Flow velocity in pulmonary hypertension is shown on the right. AcT is shortened to 40 msec.

Mean pulmonary artery pressure = 79 − (0.45 × 40) = 61 mm Hg using Mahan's regression equation (9). *PW*, pulsed-wave Doppler.

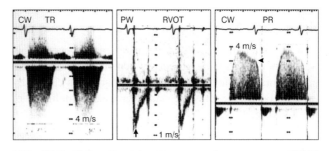
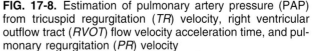

FIG. 17-8. Estimation of pulmonary artery pressure (PAP) from tricuspid regurgitation (*TR*) velocity, right ventricular outflow tract (*RVOT*) flow velocity acceleration time, and pulmonary regurgitation (*PR*) velocity

$$Systolic\ PAP = 4 \times TR^2 + RAP$$
$$= 4 \times 4^2 + 20$$
$$= 84\ mm\ Hg$$

where *RAP*, RA pressure

$$Mean\ PAP = 79 - 0.45 \times 60$$
$$= 52\ mm\ Hg\ (Mahan)$$
$$Mean\ PAP = 4 \times peak\ PR^2$$
$$= 4 \times 3.5^2$$
$$= 49\ mm\ Hg\ (Masuyama)$$

CW, continuous-wave Doppler; *PW*, pulsed-wave Doppler.

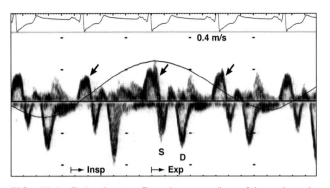

FIG. 17-9. Pulsed-wave Doppler recording of hepatic vein velocities in pulmonary hypertension. There is a prominent atrial flow reversal (*arrows*). *D*, diastolic; *Exp*, expiration; *Insp*, inspiration; *S*, systolic.

ventricular septal defect, cor pulmonale, or pulmonary embolism.

Mitral Inflow Velocity Pattern

Pulmonary pressure usually is increased in patients with increased LV filling pressures. When LV filling pressures are increased, the mitral inflow velocity pattern becomes restrictive (↑E velocity, ↓A velocity, E/A > 2.0, and ↓deceleration time). Therefore, it is safe to assume that pulmonary hypertension is related to a pulmonary process if mitral inflow shows a nonrestrictive diastolic filling pattern (14). RV pressure overload may induce LV filling abnormality because of the shift of the ventricular septum (15). In patients with chronic obstructive pulmonary disease, mitral inflow velocity may demonstrate a respiratory variation similar to the degree of variation seen in constrictive pericarditis; however, the respiratory change in superior vena cava flow velocities is different in those two conditions (see Chapter 14).

Hepatic Vein Velocity Pattern

A characteristic velocity pattern in hepatic venous flow is seen in patients with pulmonary hypertension. There is a prominent atrial flow reversal in the hepatic vein caused by increased diastolic pressure and decreased compliance of the RV (Fig. 17-9).

COR PULMONALE AND PULMONARY EMBOLISM

Transthoracic Echocardiography

It may be difficult to distinguish acute cor pulmonale (i.e., pulmonary embolism) from chronic obstructive lung disease. RV hypertrophy is common in the chronic form. In both forms, the right chambers are dilated, and there is 2D and Doppler evidence of RV pressure overload, as described herein. The LV cavity is relatively small and hyperdynamic unless an abnormality is also present on the left side of the heart. A still frame from the subcostal 2D

echocardiographic image of a patient who had hemodynamic collapse after an orthopedic operation is shown in Fig. 17-10. The chambers on the right side are dilated and the ventricular septum is deviated to the left because of increased RV pressure from acute pulmonary embolism. This RV strain pattern is normalized after regression of pulmonary hypertension with anticoagulation therapy (16). A similar normalization has been noted after pulmonary thromboendarterectomy (17) in patients with chronic thromboembolic pulmonary hypertension.

Occasionally, *thrombi-in-transit* are detected in the chambers on the right side of the heart (18). They are highly mobile and have the appearance of popcorn or a snake (Figs. 17-11 and 17-12). The mobile mass comes from *en bloc* embolization of venous thrombi cast. Patients inevitably have pulmonary embolism and should be treated vigorously with anticoagulation, thrombolytic therapy, or even surgical removal of the embolus. A similar echocardiographic appearance has been noted in patients with intravenous leiomyomatosis that originated from an endometrial tumor (see Fig. 16–10). The same kind of thrombus material is responsible for paradoxical embolus when the foramen ovale is patent (see Fig. 16–12). At the Mayo Clinic, we have successfully treated mobile RA thrombi with the following thrombolytic regimen: streptokinase, 250,000 units by bolus, followed by 100,000 units per hour by continuous infusion. RA thrombi usually dissolve within 24 to 48 hours. Therapeutic results are monitored by repeated echocardiographic examinations. When there are LA thrombi due to paradoxical emboli, thrombolytic therapy is relatively contraindicated; surgical removal is the most effective treatment.

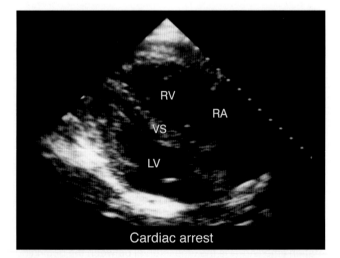

FIG. 17-10. Subcostal two-dimensional echocardiogram demonstrating dilated right ventricle (*RV*) and right atrium (*RA*) with the ventricular septum (*VS*) deviated to the left, in a patient who had cardiac arrest. When the dilated right chambers are detected in the setting of an acute hemodynamic event, pulmonary embolus should be considered. RV infarct is almost always associated with infarction of the left ventricle (*LV*) inferoseptal region.

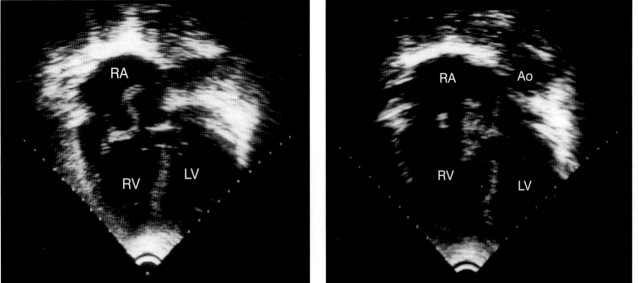

FIG. 17-11. Apex-down apical view demonstrating mobile thrombi in the right chamber. The shape of the mass changes because of its highly mobile nature. **A:** During systole, it has the shape of a snake. **B:** During diastole, the mass assumes the shape of popcorn as it traverses the tricuspid valve. *Ao,* aorta.

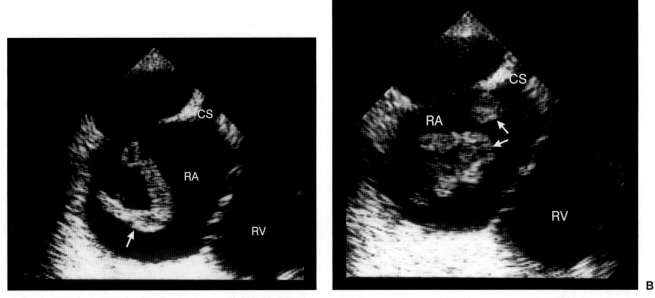

FIG. 17-12. A, B: Separate frames from horizontal transesophageal echocardiographic imaging of mobile right atrial thrombi-in-transit (*arrow* in **A**; *arrows* in **B**). The configuration of the thrombi is dynamic. In all patients with pulmonary embolism, varying degrees of this phenomenon probably exist. When the thrombi are large, the duration of their presence in the right chambers is longer than for similar thrombi. *CS,* coronary sinus.

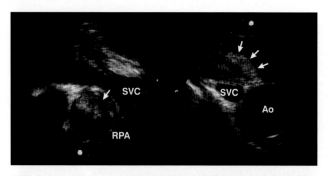

FIG. 17-13. Transesophageal echocardiogram of pulmonary artery thrombus. Longitudinal plane view **(left)** showing the right pulmonary artery (*RPA*) with a large thrombus (*arrow*). Horizontal plane basal view **(right)** showing the right pulmonary artery with thrombus (*arrows*). *Ao,* aorta; *SVC,* superior vena cava.

Transesophageal Echocardiography

The main pulmonary trunk and its bifurcation into the right and left pulmonary arteries are well seen on TEE. Thrombus in the proximal part of the pulmonary artery can be detected easily with TEE (Fig. 17-13). As shown in Fig. 17-12, thrombi-in-transit in the right chambers also arc seen easily with TEE. When transthoracic echocardiography is unable to characterize an intracardiac mass on the right side, TEE should be considered. As shown in one study, TEE detected central pulmonary thromboemboli in 35 of 60 patients (58%) with severe pulmonary embolism, mostly in the right pulmonary artery (19). Although it is more difficult to visualize the left pulmonary artery with TEE, even with the longitudinal plane, the sensitivity of TEE in the detection of pulmonary thrombi is 97%, using pulmonary angiography, computed tomography, autopsy, or surgery as a reference standard.

When RA pressure is increased, there may be a significant right-to-left shunt through the patent foramen ovale, resulting in severe hypoxemia (20). Because the entire atrial septum is clearly seen with TEE, patients with refractory hypoxemia in the setting of increased RA pressure should undergo TEE and color flow imaging.

REFERENCES

1. Abenhaim L, Moride Y, Brenot F, et al. for the International Primary Pulmonary Hypertension Study Group. Appetite-suppressant drugs and the risk of primary pulmonary hypertension. *N Engl J Med* 1996;335:609–616.
2. Mark EJ, Patalas ED, Chang HT, Evans RJ, Kessler SC. Fatal pulmonary hypertension associated with short-term use of fenfluramine and phentermine. *N Engl J Med* 1997;337:602–606.
3. Weyman AE, Dillon JC, Feigenbaum H, Chang S. Echocardiographic patterns of pulmonic valve motion with pulmonary hypertension. *Circulation* 1974;50:905–910.
4. Nanda NC, Gramiak R, Robinson TI, Shah PM. Echocardiographic evaluation of pulmonary hypertension. *Circulation* 1974;50:575–581.
5. Yock PG, Popp RL. Noninvasive estimation of right ventricular systolic pressure by Doppler ultrasound in patients with tricuspid regurgitation. *Circulation* 1984;70:657–662.
6. Currie PJ, Seward JB, Chan KL, et al. Continuous wave Doppler determination of right ventricular pressure: a simultaneous Doppler-catheterization study in 127 patients. *J Am Coll Cardiol* 1985;6:750–756.
7. Hatle L, Angelsen BA, Tromsdal A. Non-invasive estimation of pulmonary artery systolic pressure with Doppler ultrasound. *Br Heart J* 1981;45:157–165.
8. Kircher BJ, Himelman RB, Schiller NB. Noninvasive estimation of right atrial pressure from the inspiratory collapse of the inferior vena cava. *Am J Cardiol* 1990;66:493–496.
9. Masuyama T, Kodama K, Kitabatake A, Sato H, Nanto S, Inoue M. Continuous-wave Doppler echocardiographic detection of pulmonary regurgitation and its application to noninvasive estimation of pulmonary artery pressure. *Circulation* 1986;74:484–492.
10. Mahan G, Dabestani A, Gardin J, Allfie A, Burn C, Henry W. Estimation of pulmonary artery pressure by pulsed Doppler echocardiography. *Circulation* 1983;68(Suppl 3):III–367(abst).
11. Kitabatake A, Inoue M, Asao M, et al. Noninvasive evaluation of pulmonary hypertension by a pulsed Doppler technique. *Circulation* 1983;68:302–309.
12. Chan KL, Currie PJ, Seward JB, Hagler DJ, Mair DD, Tajik AJ. Comparison of three Doppler ultrasound methods in the prediction of pulmonary artery pressure. *J Am Coll Cardiol* 1987;9:549–554.
13. Borgeson DD, Seward JB, Miller FA Jr, Oh JK, Tajik AJ. Frequency of Doppler measurable pulmonary artery pressures. *J Am Soc Echocardiogr* 1996;9:832–837.
14. Enriquez-Sarano M, Rossi A, Seward JB, Bailey KR, Tajik AJ. Determinants of pulmonary hypertension in left ventricular dysfunction. *J Am Coll Cardiol* 1997;29:153–159.
15. Schena M, Clini E, Errera D, Quadri A. Echo-Doppler evaluation of left ventricular impairment in chronic cor pulmonale. *Chest* 1996;109:1446–1451.
16. Fang BR, Chiang CW, Lee YS. Echocardiographic detection of reversible right ventricular strain in patients with acute pulmonary embolism: report of 2 cases. *Cardiology* 1996;87:279–282.
17. Mayer E, Dahm M, Hake U, et al. Mid-term results of pulmonary thromboendarterectomy for chronic thromboembolic pulmonary hypertension. *Ann Thorac Surg* 1996;61:1788–1792.
18. Proano M, Oh JK, Frye RL, Johnson CM, Tajik AJ, Taliercio CP. Successful treatment of pulmonary embolism and associated mobile right arial thrombus with use of a central thrombolytic infusion. *Mayo Clin Proc* 1988;63:1181—1185.
19. Wittlich N, Erbel R, Eichler A, et al. Detection of central pulmonary artery thromboemboli by transesophageal echocardiography in patients with severe pulmonary embolism. *J Am Soc Echocardiogr* 1992;5:515–524.
20. Lin SS, Oh JK, Tajik AJ, Gay PC, Kishon Y, Seward JB. Right-to-left shunts in patients with severe hypoxemia: transesophageal contrast echocardiography study. *J Am Coll Cardiol* 1995;25:17A(abst).

CHAPTER 18

Congenital Heart Disease

Echocardiography has markedly changed the evaluation, diagnosis, and management of congenital heart disease. A complete echocardiographic examination can establish goal-directed management, reduce the need for confirmatory cardiac catheterization, and provide serial evaluation of residua and sequelae of congenital heart disease. For a more comprehensive discussion of the echocardiographic assessment of congenital heart disease, readers are referred to a textbook and atlas on the subject (1–3). This manual presents an abbreviated systematic tomographic two-dimensional (2D) approach to congenital heart disease as encountered in an adult cardiology practice.

SYSTEMATIC TOMOGRAPHIC APPROACH

A systematic approach to a 2D echocardiographic examination is necessary in most patients with congenital heart disease. The format for image orientation should be the same for every form of congenital heart disease. The following step-by-step approach can be applied to all cardiac anomalies and conforms to the recommendations of the American Society of Echocardiography (ASE) and the Society of Pediatric Echocardiography (SOPE).

Short-Axis View

Short-axis views are portrayed as though looking from the apex toward the base of the heart (Fig. 18-1A). From a parasternal or transesophageal transducer position, left-sided structures will be on the right side of the video screen and right-sided structures on the left; sternal (*anterior*) structures will be at the top, and diaphragmatic (*posterior*) structures will be toward the bottom.

Long-Axis View

Long-axis views of the heart, regardless of transducer position or arrangement of the cardiac chambers, are displayed as though looking from left cardiac structures to-

ward the right (Fig. 18-1B). Parasternal and transesophageal long-axis views are portrayed with the basal (*superior*) cardiac structures to the viewer's right, sternal (*anterior*) structures toward the top, and diaphragmatic (*posterior*) structures toward the bottom of the screen.

Four-Chamber View

Four-chamber views or frontal projections of the heart are by convention more commonly displayed with the apex down (ASE option 1) when imaging congenital anomalies (Fig. 18-1C). Apex-down is used because it orients cardiac structures in a manner most closely resembling classic anatomic dissections and surgical approaches to the heart. Thus, four-chamber views orient the heart as though looking from the anterior toward the posterior surface. When looking down on the heart in this manner, left-sided structures are to the viewer's right and right-sided structures to the viewer's left.

TWO-DIMENSIONAL EXAMINATION

The most important prerequisite to a complete examination is knowing how to position the transducer to obtain the appropriate image orientation. Standard anatomic and transducer references should be used to obtain proper display of the image consistently. For a surface echocardiographic examination, it is easiest to understand transducer orientation by beginning with the examination of the upper abdomen.

Step 1: Short-Axis Image of the Upper Abdomen

Place the transducer in the epigastrium in short axis and direct the beam directly posterior. To confirm proper short-axis orientation, tilt the transducer from right to left. If the image is properly oriented, tilting the transducer to the patient's right will bring structures on the right side of the screen toward the midline. If the opposite happens, rotate the transducer 180 degrees or do an electronic side-to-side

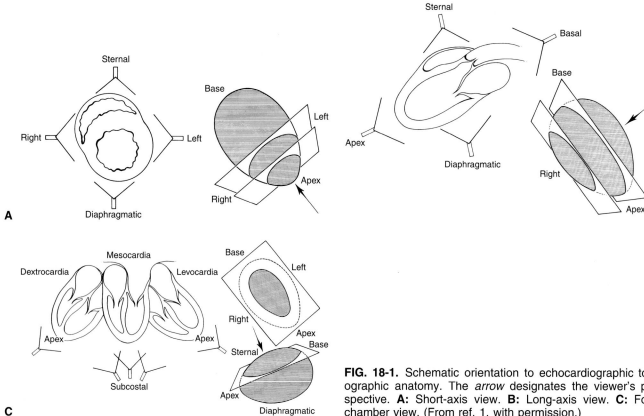

FIG. 18-1. Schematic orientation to echocardiographic tomographic anatomy. The *arrow* designates the viewer's perspective. **A:** Short-axis view. **B:** Long-axis view. **C:** Four-chamber view. (From ref. 1, with permission.)

inversion of the image. A proper short-axis transducer orientation is now confirmed. All subsequent short-axis views, regardless of the precordial transducer position, are obtained with this same left-to-right orientation of the transducer. If disorientation ensues, return to the upper abdomen to confirm a consistent transducer image orientation.

Step 2: Long-Axis Image of the Upper Abdomen

Rotate the transducer 90 degrees clockwise from step 1, or orient the transducer to a proper long-axis orientation. To simply confirm a proper orientation, tilt the transducer toward the patient's head, which should bring the structures on the right side of the video screen toward the middle of the picture. If the opposite occurs, reverse the image 180 degrees. The chest, upper abdomen, and basal cardiac structures should be displayed toward the right side of the video image, and structures toward the feet, lower abdomen, and cardiac apex should be displayed toward the left side of the image. All long-axis views, regardless of heart position, are obtained with this transducer orientation.

Step 3: Four-Chamber Image Beginning in the Upper Abdomen

Initially, orient the transducer in a proper short-axis view of the upper abdomen (see the preceding). Tilt the transducer beam upward toward the chest and the transducer

handle downward toward the feet, parallel with the abdominal wall. The echo of the pulsatile heart will be visible near the bottom of the video screen. Electronically, reorient the image from top to bottom, maintaining the same left-right relationship. The ultrasound burst is now at the bottom of the video screen. To confirm the proper left-right orientation of the image, direct the ultrasonic beam to the patient's right. Right-sided structures should move toward the center of the image. If the opposite occurs, either perform electronic side-to-side reversal of the image or rotate the transducer 180 degrees. To determine the position of the heart confidently, alternately aim the transducer toward the right, midline, and left side of the patient's chest (Fig. 18-1C). Cardiac pulsations will disclose the cardiac position. This maneuver determines whether the cardiac position is *dextrocardia* (cardiac apex in the right side of the chest), *mesocardia* (cardiac apex in the midline), or *levocardia* (cardiac apex in the left side of the chest).

Step 4: Precordial Examination

After the position of the heart in the chest is known, the transducer, in an appropriate short-axis, long-axis, or four-chamber orientation, may be moved from the abdominal position to any place on the precordium. Until familiar with the examination technique or when dealing with complex or unfamiliar anatomy, use the upper abdomen as an easy point of reference for each transducer reorientation.

OVERVIEW OF ADULT CONGENITAL HEART DISEASE

The most commonly encountered congenital heart defect of clinical significance after bicuspid valve is atrial septal defect. Currently, with precordial and transesophageal echocardiography (TEE), both the anatomic and hemodynamic characteristics of this abnormality can be made confidently in virtually all patients (4–6). Some anomalies, such as sinus venosus atrial septal defect, are difficult to diagnose by precordial echocardiography; however, this anomaly and others can be diagnosed confidently with TEE (6). Associated anomalous pulmonary venous connections also can be detected and characterized (7). Hemodynamics, such as pulmonary artery pressure and flow characteristics, can be determined noninvasively (8). A detailed echo/Doppler examination has eliminated the need for cardiac catheterization in most patients with congenital heart disease. Other *acyanotic* congenital cardiac diseases commonly found in adults include small ventricular septal defect, pulmonary stenosis, (residual) coarctation, patent ductus arteriosus, Ebstein anomaly, left ventricular outflow tract (LVOT) obstruction (including discrete subaortic stenosis), and other acyanotic congenital conditions. Currently, a comprehensive echo/Doppler examination is considered the primary means of diagnosing and characterizing most congenital cardiac anomalies.

Many patients with *cyanotic* heart disease are now reaching adulthood because of better medical and surgical management. Tetralogy of Fallot, pulmonary atresia, ventricular septal defect (VSD), and single ventricle are recognized and characterized by echocardiographic morphologic and Doppler hemodynamic observations. Currently, the management of congenital heart disease, including the use of catheterization, is goal directed and largely assisted by comprehensive noninvasive ultrasonographic imaging and hemodynamic examination. Complete, or blind, diagnostic catheterization is no longer necessary or acceptable. Patients operated on for congenital heart disease are usually left with residua and sequelae that require serial follow-up evaluation, which can also be obtained safely using echo/Doppler technology.

Atrial Septal Defect

The four distinct types of atrial septal defect are (a) primum or partial atrioventricular canal, (b) secundum, (c) sinus venosus, and (d) coronary sinus defect. The secundum defect is the most common, followed by the primum, sinus venosus, and coronary sinus defects. The primum defect (partial atrioventricular canal) is associated with a cleft mitral valve. Sinus venosus defect is associated with a high incidence of partial anomalous pulmonary venous connection. Each form of atrial septal defect is normally associated with a left-to-right shunt, which results in right atrial (RA) and right ventricular (RV) volume overload. Pulmonary hypertension of a magnitude that would preclude surgical re-

pair is rare and can be recognized and quantitated by echo/Doppler studies.

Echocardiographic findings of an atrial septal defect usually include RV enlargement and abnormal (paradoxical) ventricular septal motion, which are the signature of volume overload (Fig. 18-2). In addition to visualizing the actual defect with 2D echocardiography, the left-to-right shunt can be visualized with flow imaging [4–7]. A complete transthoracic echocardiographic examination can detect most primum and secundum atrial septal defects; however, sinus venosus defect, which is normally located near the entry of the superior vena cava, is visualized in only about 70% of patients (Fig. 18-3). TEE is exquisitely sensitive for the identification of all types of atrial septal defect (5,6,8) as well as associated anomalous pulmonary venous connections (7,9) (Fig. 18-4 and 18-5).

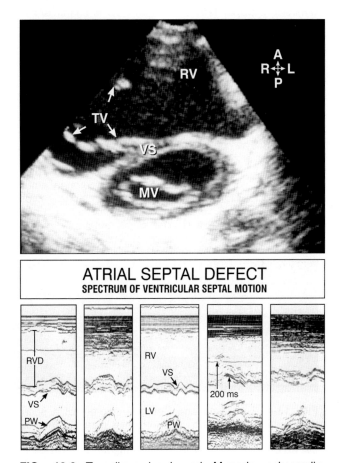

FIG. 18-2. Two-dimensional and M-mode echocardiographic features of atrial septal defect. **Top:** The right ventricle (*RV*) is dilated and the tricuspid valve (*TV*) is enlarged because of RV volume overload. Ventricular septal (*VS*) motion was paradoxical. *MV*, mitral valve. Orientation abbreviations: *A*, anterior; *L*, left; *P*, posterior; *R*, right. **Bottom:** A wide spectrum of VS motion abnormalities in patients with atrial septal defect. From left to right, the first two M-mode echocardiograms show typical paradoxical motion, and the next two show atypical septal motion. Septal motion occasionally may be normal in atrial septal defect, as shown in the far right echocardiogram. *PW*, posterior wall; *RVD*, RV dimension. (From ref. 1, with permission.)

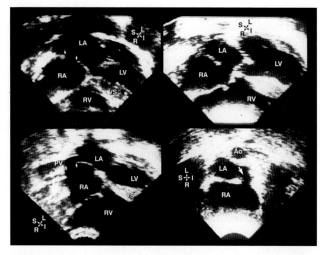

FIG. 18-3. A collage of various forms of atrial septal defect (ASD) seen on subcostal echocardiographic four-chamber examination. **Upper left:** Secundum ASD is characterized by a defect (*arrows*) in the midportion of the atrial septum. **Upper right:** Primum ASD is characterized by a defect in the lower atrial septum and downward displacement of the atrioventricular valves, which insert at the same level on the crest of the ventricular septum. **Lower left:** Sinus venosus ASD is characterized by a defect (*arrows*) in the upper atrial septum just beneath the orifice of the superior vena cava. Frequently, the right upper pulmonary veins (*PV*) anomalously connect to the superior vena cava or right atrium (*RA*). **Lower right:** The coronary sinus ASD is the most rare ASD and is characterized by the absence of the roof of the coronary sinus, which is located in the floor of the LA. Thus, left atrial (*LA*) blood can enter the unroofed coronary sinus (*arrow*) and cross its orifice into the RA (i.e., "coronary sinus ASD"). *Ao*, aorta; *VS*, ventricular septum. Orientation abbreviations: *I*, inferior; *L*, left; *R*, right; *S*, superior.

Outflow Tract Obstruction

Congenital LVOT obstruction can be classified into *subvalvular, valvular,* and *supravalvular* types. A congenitally abnormal aortic valve, usually bicuspid (see Chapter 9), is the most common congenital cardiac anomaly (1% to 2% incidence) (Fig. 18-6). Bicuspid aortic valves can present with aortic stenosis, regurgitation, or both. Symptomatic aortic stenosis due to a bicuspid aortic valve usually occurs before the age of 65 years. Patients with a bicuspid aortic valve also have a higher incidence of proximal aortic dissection and a common association with coarctation of the aorta. Two-dimensional echo/Doppler echocardiographic examination can identify aortic cusp morphology (10) (position of the raphe and commissures) and serially determine the hemodynamic significance of aortic stenosis (11). When a transthoracic examination is not satisfactory for visualizing the aortic cusps, TEE should be satisfactory in all cases (Fig. 18-7).

Subvalvular aortic stenosis may be discrete, fibromuscular, diffuse, or dynamic (Fig. 18-8). Congenital dynamic subpulmonic outflow obstruction is commonly encountered with severe pulmonary stenosis, tetralogy of Fallot, and complete transposition of the great arteries. Dynamic subaortic stenosis is most commonly associated with congenital hypertrophic cardiomyopathy.

Supravalvular aortic stenosis most commonly presents as a fusiform fibrous thickening of the ascending aortic wall (Fig. 18-9). Doppler hemodynamics in fixed or dynamic outflow obstruction can be determined and characterized noninvasively in nearly all cases (Fig. 18-9).

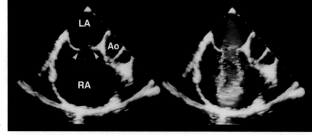

A

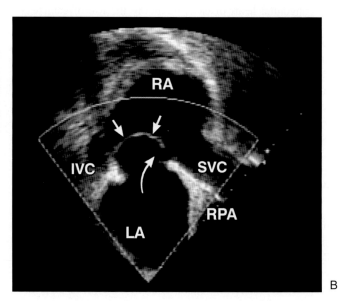

B

FIG. 18-4. Transesophageal echocardiogram of a secundum atrial septal defect. **A:** Horizontal plane in the four-chamber projection. **Left:** The transducer is located within the esophagus posterior to the left atrium (*LA*). The secundum defect (*arrowheads*) is visualized as a communication between the LA and right atrium (*RA*) in the center of the atrial septum. *Ao*, aortic root. **Right:** Color-flow Doppler showing the left-to-right shunt across the defect. **B:** Longitudinal plane in the axis of the superior (*SVC*) and inferior (*IVC*) venae cavae. A secundum atrial septal defect (*large curved arrow*) is seen in the superior aspect of the membranous atrial septum (*small arrows*). The posteriorly located LA communicates with the anteriorly located right atrium (*RA*). This image was obtained with a multiplane probe, with the transducer rotated 90 degrees to obtain a longitudinal view. *RPA*, right pulmonary artery.

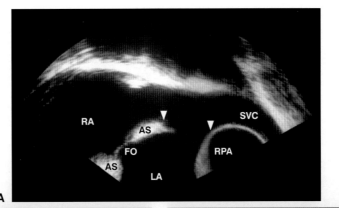

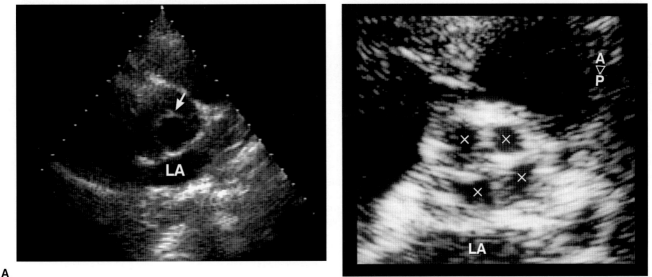

FIG. 18-5. Sinus venosus atrial septal defect (ASD). **A:** Long-axis transesophageal echocardiographic (TEE) examination aligned with the superior vena cava (*SVC*). Note the large atrial septal defect (*arrowheads*) just beneath the SVC, where this vessel enters the right atrium (*RA*). Note the volume-enlarged right pulmonary artery (*RPA*) and that no atrial septal tissues are attached to the wall adjacent to the RPA (absence of the superior limbus of the atrial septum). These features are pathognomonic of sinus venosus ASD. Note the intact membranous portion of the fossa ovalis (*FO*) (i.e., the usual site of secundum ASD). *AS*, atrial septum. **B: Left:** TEE short-axis view at the caval (SVC)-RA junction. Note the ASD (*arrowhead*) just below the SVC, which allows communication between the left atrium (*LA*) and RA. Also note a pulmonary vein anomalously entering the lateral wall of the SVC (*arrow*). **Right:** Color-flow Doppler shows left-to-right shunt flow across the sinus venosus ASD. Also visualized is blood entering the SVC from the anomalously connecting right pulmonary vein (*arrow*). **C: Left:** TEE short-axis view at the level of the right pulmonary artery (RPA), which is displayed in its long axis. The SVC lies anterior to the RPA. Normally, SVC is a circular structure, but in this example, it has a teardrop shape because an anomalous connecting pulmonary vein (*arrow*) enters the lateral wall of the SVC. **Right:** On color-flow Doppler, note blood flow from the anomalously connecting pulmonary vein into the SVC. A sinus venosus ASD is commonly associated with anomalous connection of the right middle and upper pulmonary veins, which enter either the RA or the SVC. (**B** and **C** from ref. 6, with permission.)

FIG. 18-6. Transthoracic parasternal short-axis view at the aortic valve level. **A:** A unicuspid (*arrow*). **B:** A quadricuspid (*x*) aortic valve. *A*, anterior; *P*, posterior.

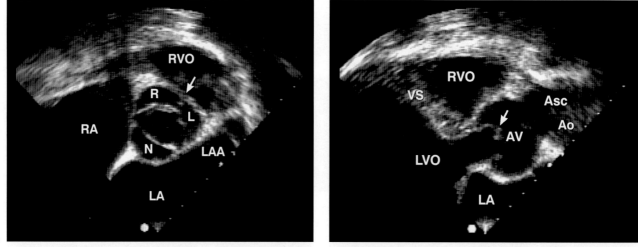

FIG. 18-7. Transesophageal echocardiograms of short-axis **(A)** and long-axis **(B)** views of a bicuspid aortic valve (systolic frame). These images were obtained with a multiplane probe, with the transducer rotated to 45 degrees for the short-axis view and 135 degrees for the long-axis view. In the short-axis view, commissures are seen at the 5 and 9'o clock positions, with the raphe at the 1 o'clock position (*arrow*). In the long-axis view, the doming of the anterior aortic cusps (*arrow*) is well seen. *Asc Ao*, ascending aorta; *AV*, aortic valve; *L*, left coronary cusp; *LAA*, left atrial appendage; *LVO*, left ventricular outflow; *N*, noncoronary cusp; *R*, right coronary cusp; *RVO*, right ventricular outflow; *VS*, ventricular septum.

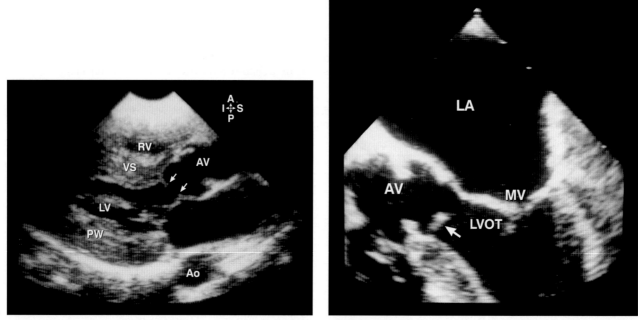

FIG. 18-8. A: Parasternal long-axis view of discrete membranous subaortic stenosis (*arrows*). A discrete subaortic membrane narrows the left ventricular outflow tract (LVOT). Note LV hypertrophy. **B:** Transesophageal four-chamber plane of discrete membranous subaortic stenosis (*arrow*). *A*, anterior; *Ao*, aorta; *AV*, aortic valve; *I*, inferior; *MV*, mitral valve; *P*, posterior; *PW*, posterior wall; *S*, superior; *VS*, ventricular septum.

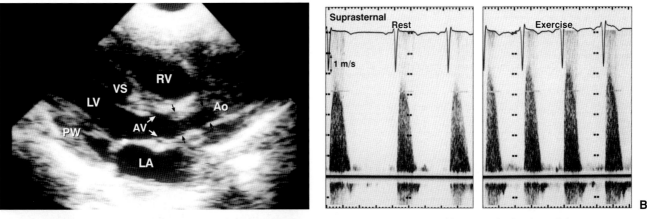

FIG. 18-9. A: Parasternal long-axis view of supravalvular aortic stenosis (AS) due to thickening of the aortic wall (*black arrows*) above the aortic valve (*AV, white arrows*). This would result in the typical appearance of an hourglass deformity on aortic root angiography. *Ao*, aorta; *PW*, posterior wall; *VS*, ventricular septum. **B:** Continuous-wave Doppler across supravalvular AS, from a suprasternal transducer position. At rest, peak velocity reaches 4.5 m/sec, corresponding to a maximal gradient of 81 mm Hg. With exercise, the gradient increases to 5.5 m/sec, equivalent to a maximal gradient of 121 mm Hg.

Internal Cardiac Crux

The internal cardiac crux is a very important echocardiographic anatomic landmark used in the evaluation of many common and complex congenital cardiac anomalies. In the four-chamber plane, the components of the internal crux include the atrial septum, ventricular septum, and septal portions of the mitral and tricuspid valves (Fig. 18-10). The tricuspid valve originates from the crest of the ventricular septum, whereas the septal portion of the mitral valve inserts at a higher level off the lower atrial septum. The portion of ventricular septum between the two valves represents the atrioventricular septum (i.e., a potential communication between the LV and RA). The anatomy of the internal cardiac crux can be used to diagnose both ventricular and atrioventricular valve abnormalities. The higher inserting morphologic mitral valve is predictably committed to the morphologically LV, and the lower inserting morphologic tricuspid valve to the morphologically RV.

The anatomy of the crux is best imaged from a precordial, apical, subcostal, or transesophageal four-chamber view. Many complex anomalies of the heart are diagnosed most confidently by their alteration of the crux anatomy (Ebstein anomaly, atrioventricular canal, tricuspid atresia, corrected transposition, double inlet ventricle, and others) (Fig. 18-11 through Fig. 18-14) (12,13). When the atrioventricular valve is malaligned with respect to the ventricular septum, it is described as *straddling* or *overriding* (see Fig. 18-10). *Straddling* is used to describe the atrioventricular valve whose chordae insert into two ventricular chambers, and *overriding* is used when the annulus is committed to both ventricles. Overriding is considered *minor* when less than 50% of the annulus is committed to the contralateral ventricle and *major* when 50% or more of the annulus is committed to a single ventricular chamber; the abnormality is then called *double-inlet ventricle*. All patients with atrioventricular valve straddling have complex congenital heart disease (13).

Ventricular Septal Defect

In adults, VSD may be found as an isolated defect, or it may be associated with other anomalies, such as tetralogy of Fallot or pulmonary atresia. Depending on the location, VSD is classified as (a) membranous/perimembranous (the most common type), (b) outflow (infundibular/supracrystal), (c) inflow (atrioventricular canal), and 4) muscular (trabecular). A comprehensive echocardiographic examination can identify VSD in more than 90% of cases (Fig. 18-15). Continuous-wave Doppler echocardiography can measure the blood-flow velocity and gradient across the VSD, which then can be used to calculate RV pressure. One way to calculate RV systolic pressure is to subtract the VSD gradient from the assumed or measured LV systolic pressure (Fig. 18-16). A large VSD would have a smaller pressure difference between the ventricles; conversely, a small VSD would have a large gradient (i.e., velocity). The infundibular VSD can be associated with increasing aortic valve regurgitation resulting from variable aortic valve prolapse. Even in the presence of modest aortic valve regurgitation and small VSD flow, this particular defect usually should be closed and the aortic valve repaired to prevent worsening aortic valve regurgitation.

Patent Ductus Arteriosus

In adults, patent ductus arteriosus is usually found as an isolated defect. The more complex congenital heart diseases

(text continues on page 233)

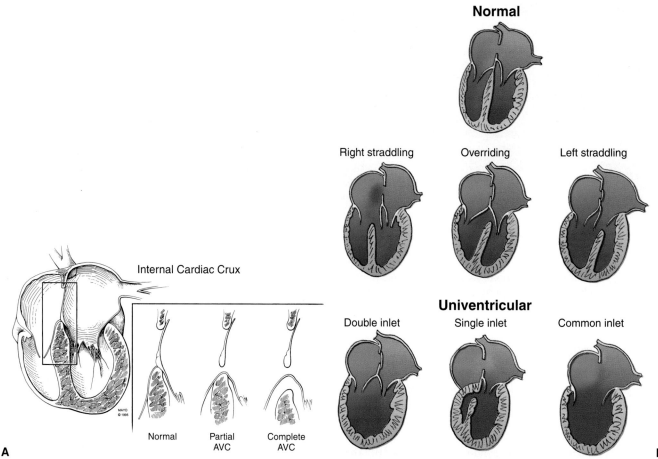

A

B

FIG. 18-10. A: Internal cardiac crux: the joining of the inflow atrial and ventricular septa and respective leaflets of the mitral and tricuspid valves form a cross-like configuration within the heart. This view is predictably obtained with an apical four-chamber view. The normal internal cardiac crux (i.e., cross) is characterized by an apparent lower insertion of the septal leaflet of the morphological tricuspid valve. In fact, this characteristic relationship of crux attachment of the atrioventricular valves can predict not only the morphology of these valves (i.e., tricuspid and mitral) but also ventricular morphology. The morphological tricuspid valve is always committed to the morphologically right ventricle (RV) and the mitral valve to the morphologically left ventricle (LV). Note that with partial (i.e., primum atrial septal defect) and complete (primum atrial septal defect and inflow ventricular septal defect) congenital canal defect (*AVC*) the mitral valve is characteristically displaced downward. This downward displacement and loss of the atrioventricular septum (i.e., potential communication from the LV directly into the right atrium) results in a deficiency of the mitral leaflet (i.e., a cleft) and a potential communication from the LV across the mitral valve cleft directly into the RA. A large number of congenital anomalies are characterized by diagnostic alterations in the internal cardiac crux. **B:** Atrioventricular connections. **Top:** Normal internal cardiac crux. **Middle:** Straddling atrioventricular connection is defined as an atrioventricular valve that has chordal insertions into two ventricles. Overriding atrioventricular connection is defined as an atrioventricular valve whose annulus is committed to two ventricles. These abnormalities can affect either atrioventricular valve (tricuspid or mitral). Straddling and override can exist separately or together in either atrioventricular valve. No other diagnostic technique can appreciate these complex abnormalities with the accuracy of echocardiography. **Bottom:** Both atrioventricular valves can be committed to a single ventricular chamber. This is referred to as *double inlet ventricle.* One atrioventricular valve can be absent (in this example, the right atrioventricular valve is absent, consistent with tricuspid valve atresia). This atrioventricular connection anomaly is termed *single inlet atrioventricular connection* [i.e., a single atrioventricular valve committed to the ventricle(s)]. When only one large atrioventricular valve receives all the venous return (i.e., the atria) and is connected to the ventricular chamber(s), the lesion is called *common inlet atrioventricular connection* [i.e., an atrioventricular valve connecting both atria to the ventricle(s)].

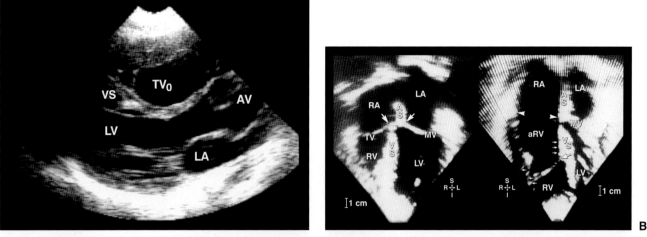

A

B

FIG. 18-11. Ebstein anomaly. A: Transthoracic parasternal long-axis view. Anteriorly, the orifice of the tricuspid valve (TV_o) is reoriented toward the right ventricular (*RV*) outflow tract. *AV*, aortic valve; *VS*, ventricular septum. B: Left: Normal internal cardiac crux. Right: Ebstein anomaly. Normally, the septal leaflet of the tricuspid valve (*TV*) **(left)** inserts lower than the septal attachment of the mitral valve (*arrows*). Note that in Ebstein anomaly **(right)** the downward insertion of the septal TV leaflet is markedly accentuated (*large arrow*). That portion of the RV below the TV annulus (*arrowheads*) and the downwardly displaced septal TV leaflet (*small arrows*) is an atrialized RV (*aRV*). Note that the heart cavities on the right side (RA and RV) become volume overloaded (enlarged) secondary to associated TV regurgitation and the atrial septal defect that is usually present (not shown in this example). *AS*, atrial septum; *MV*, mitral valve. (For orientation abbreviations, see Fig. 18-3.)

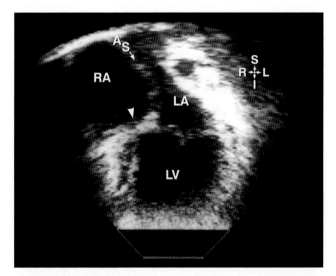

FIG. 18-12. Tricuspid atresia. Apex-down four-chamber view. Note that the tricuspid valve is replaced by a dense fibrous plate (*arrowhead*). Right atrial (*RA*) blood reaches the left atrium (*LA*) via an atrial septal defect (not shown). The left ventricle (*LV*) is the only remaining functional ventricular chamber. *AS*, atrial septum. (For orientation abbreviations, see Fig. 18-3.)

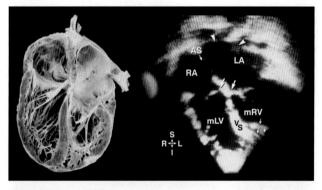

FIG. 18-13. Corrected transposition of the great arteries. The right atrium (*RA*) communicates with a right-sided morphologically left ventricle (mLV), which connects to the pulmonary artery, and the left atrium (*LA*) communicates with a left-sided morphologically right ventricle (mRV), which connects to the aorta. **Left:** Cardiac specimen sectioned in the four-chamber plane. Note that the RA communicates with the mitral valve (inserts higher on the ventricular septum) and the LA communicates with the lower inserting tricuspid valve and mRV. **Right:** Four-chamber echocardiogram showing the reversed relationship of the cardiac crux (i.e., the right-sided mitral valve inserts higher than the left-sided tricuspid valve). The morphologically LV (*mLV*) is to the left below the RA and the morphologically RV (*mRV*) is below the LA. The RV is trabeculated (*arrows*). The pulmonary veins (*arrowheads*) enter the LA. *AS*, atrial septum; *VS*, ventricular septum. (For orientation abbreviations, see Fig. 18-3.)

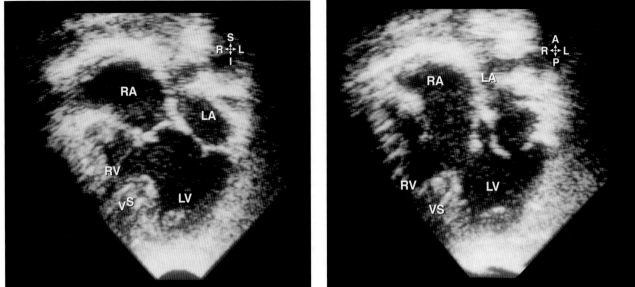

FIG. 18-14. Double-inlet left ventricle (*LV*). **A:** Systole. **B:** Diastole. All the left-sided and >50% of the right-sided atrioventricular valve are committed to the LV. The orifice of the right atrioventricular valve overrides the ventricular septum (*VS*). The right ventricle (*RV*) is small. (For orientation abbreviations, see Figs. 18-2 and 18-3.)

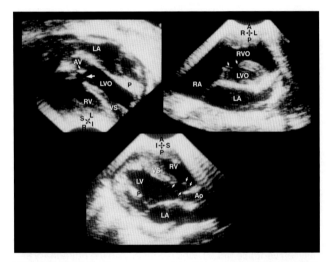

FIG. 18-15. Membranous ventricular septal defect (VSD). **Top left:** Subcostal view. The VSD (*arrow*) is just below the aortic valve (*AV*). **Top right:** Parasternal short-axis view. The VSD (*arrows*) is located on the medial aspect of the left ventricle outflow (*LVO*). **Bottom:** Parasternal long-axis view with medial tilt of the image plane. The VSD (*arrows*) is in the upper ventricular septum (*VS*), just beneath the AV. *Ao,* aorta; *P,* papillary muscle; *RVO,* right ventricular outflow. (For orientation abbreviations, see Figs. 18-2 and 18-3.)

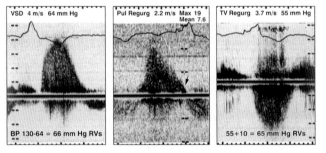

FIG. 18-16. Continuous-wave Doppler recordings in ventricular septal defect (VSD) **(left)**, pulmonary regurgitation (*Pul Regurg*) **(center)**, and tricuspid regurgitation (*TV Regurg*) **(right)** in a patient with VSD. **Left:** Peak velocity across the VSD is 4 m/sec; thus, the left ventricle (LV) to right ventricle (RV) systolic pressure gradient is 64 mm Hg (4×4^2). Systolic blood pressure is 130 mm Hg; thus, RV systolic (*RVs*) pressure is 66 mm Hg (130–64). **Center:** The end-diastolic pulmonary regurgitant signal (*arrow*) is very low constant with low pulmonary artery diastolic pressure. **Right:** Tricuspid regurgitation velocity of 3.7 m/sec equals a gradient of 55 mm Hg [$4 \times (3.7)^2$] from RV to right atrium (RA). Assuming RA pressure is 10, RV systolic pressure equals 65 mm Hg (55+10), which is nearly identical to the RV systolic pressure estimated from VSD Doppler velocity (66 mm Hg).

associated with it are usually discovered early in infancy. In a fetus, the ductus carries blood from the proximal portion of the left pulmonary artery to the descending thoracic aorta. After birth, if the ductus remains patent, the pulmonary pressures will decrease, producing varying degrees of left-to-right shunt (i.e., aorta to pulmonary artery). If the shunt is significant, it ultimately may result in increasing pulmonary hypertension, shunt reversal, and cyanosis. Echocardiographic diagnosis is based on demonstrating a persistent anatomic connection and flow between the descending aorta and pulmonary artery. The best imaging view is a high left parasternal long-axis scan of the RV outflow tract and main pulmonary artery (1). High Doppler velocities across the patent ductus are indicative of low pulmonary artery pressure.

Coarctation

Coarctation of the aorta (see also Chapter 15) represents aortic luminal narrowing, usually just distal to the left subclavian artery. A common association is bicuspid aortic valve. It is also the most common cardiac anomaly seen in patients with Turner syndrome. The area of aortic narrowing often can be seen from the suprasternal or high left parasternal transducer position; however, continuous-wave Doppler echocardiography is the best method for recognizing the presence of coarctation as well as quantitating the magnitude of stenosis. Doppler recordings of hemodynamically significant coarctation are characterized by a continuous abnormal flow velocity throughout diastole. Abdominal aortic flow velocities that appear distorted, extend into diastole, and are of lower amplitude are quite helpful in recognizing (re)coarctation in adults. In older patients and any patient with a repaired coarctation, exercise with continuous Doppler assessment is helpful for recognizing hemodynamically significant (re)coarctation. Magnetic resonance imaging has replaced angiography for definitive diagnosis and overall vascular assessment of surgical coarctation (Fig. 18-17).

Overriding Aorta

Overriding aorta (i.e., aortic valve overriding the VSD) (Fig. 18-18) is associated with (a) tetralogy of Fallot, (b) pulmonary atresia with VSD, and (c) truncus arteriosus. Truncus arteriosus is rarely seen in adults because of the unprotected pulmonary vascular bed. The distinguishing characteristics of these entities include (a) varying degrees of infundibular and pulmonary valvular stenosis in tetralogy of Fallot; (b) atretic pulmonary valve, hypoplastic pulmonary arteries, systemic-to-pulmonary collateral arteries in pulmonary atresia with VSD; and (c) origin of the pulmonary arteries from the ascending aorta in truncus arteriosus.

PEDIATRIC CONGENITAL HEART DISEASE

Echocardiography has markedly affected the indication for cardiac catheterization in children with congenital heart disease. Echocardiography allows early recognition, goal-directed management, and serial hemodynamic assessment of all forms of congenital heart disease. Cardiac catheterization is performed predominantly to assess pulmonary resistance and extracardiac anatomy (i.e., abnormalities of pulmonary arborization and coarctation and collateral vessels). When TEE is used for children younger than about age 9 or 10, general anesthesia usually is required. Thus, TEE is used primarily in the operating room to confirm a surgical result or in a catheterization laboratory to assist with a therapeutic intervention (14,15).

Fetal Congenital Heart Disease

High-resolution echocardiography now can be used to diagnose confidently congenital heart disease in a fetus (Fig. 18-19). This diagnosis allows prenatal counseling and planning of pregnancy, delivery, and neonatal care. Echocardiography is used most effectively to anticipate

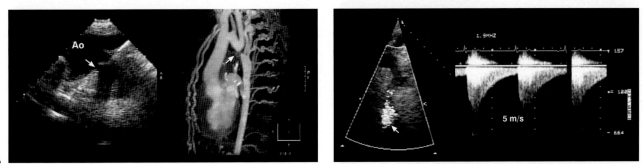

FIG. 18-17. A: Left: Suprasternal view of the aortic arch and the descending thoracic aorta (*Ao*) with coarctation (*arrow*). **Right:** Magnetic resonance imaging of coarctation of the aorta (*arrow*). **B: Left:** Color-flow imaging shows turbulent jet (*arrow*) distal to the coarctation. **Right:** Continuous-wave Doppler recording from the suprasternal notch shows typical Doppler velocity envelope with peak velocity of 4 m/sec and continuous (sawtooth appearing) diastolic flow across the coarctation.

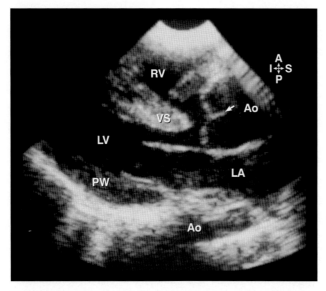

FIG. 18-18. Parasternal long-axis view of an overriding aortic valve in a patient with pulmonary atresia and ventricular septal defect. The aortic valve (*arrow*) and aortic root (*Ao*) override the ventricular septum (*VS*). *Ao*, aortic root **(top)** and descending thoracic aorta **(bottom)**; *PW*, posterior wall. (For orientation abbreviations, see Fig. 18-2.)

fetal or neonatal problems and to plan treatment strategies (16).

Heart Disease in Pregnancy

Congenital heart disease in the mother or fetus is managed most logically with the help of noninvasive echocardiography. Because maternal ultrasonography has no known harmful effects on the fetus, it can be repeated safely. Hemodynamic and morphologic characterization as well as serial evaluation for planning of pregnancy can be done noninvasively (17).

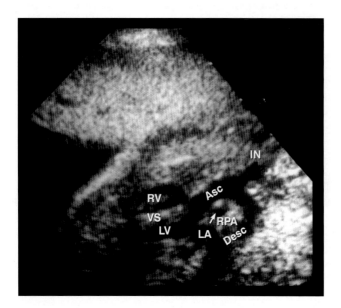

TRANSESOPHAGEAL ECHOCARDIOGRAPHY

Because of its superb visualization of cardiovascular structures, TEE is increasingly being used in the diagnosis of congenital heart disease (14,18). With a smaller probe, it is also possible to perform TEE in infants and small children, although in comparison with adults with congenital heart disease, the need for TEE is less common. TEE is particularly useful in evaluating the atrial septum, cardiac crux, atrial cavities, great arteries and veins of the thorax, and ventricular outflow tracts (Figs. 18-20 and 18-21; also see Figs. 18-4, 18-5, 18-7, and 18-8).

WIDE-FIELD AND THREE-DIMENSIONAL IMAGING

Because most congenital anomalies lie in more than one anatomic plane, wide planes of view are expected to be particularly helpful in understanding these anomalies. By rotating the transducer in the esophagus, wide-field imaging is feasible and allows better appreciation of cardiovascular structural relationships, especially in congenital heart disease (19). Closely aligned sets of 2D images also can be interpreted to produce three-dimensional (3D) images. It is believed that the next era of echocardiography will occur with the advent of true 3D imaging.

INTRAOPERATIVE ECHOCARDIOGRAPHY

Increasingly, echocardiography is being used intraoperatively. No longer is mortality or morbidity an acceptable barometer of surgical success. Instead, the gold standard of care is successful complete repair with a minimal number of residua, which has been accomplished primarily because of the intraoperative confirmation of anatomy, function, hemodynamics, and blood flow using intraoperative echocardiography (14,15).

FIG. 18-19. Fetal echocardiogram (18-week gestation). The echocardiographic examination is of the aortic arch (*Asc*, ascending aorta; *Desc*, descending thoracic aorta). The aorta is connected to the left ventricle (*LV*). Note that the ventricular septum (*VS*) separates the LV from the right ventricle (*RV*). The diameter of the fetal heart was less than 1.5 cm. Other structures visualized included the right pulmonary artery (*RPA*) beneath the ascending aorta, the left atrium (*LA*) at the base of the LV, and the innominate artery (*IN*) arising from the ascending aorta.

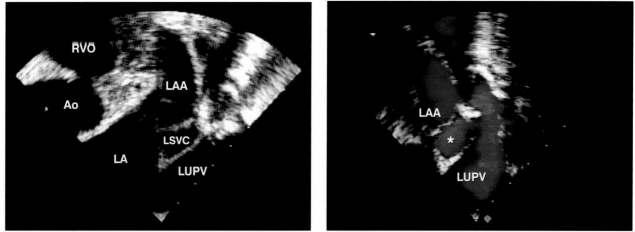

FIG. 18-20. Persistent left superior vena cava (*LSVC*). **A:** Transesophageal echocardiogram (horizontal scan plane in a basal short-axis view). The transducer is posterior to the left atrium (*LA*). In the partition between the orifice of the left upper pulmonary vein (*LUPV*) and the left atrial appendage (*LAA*) courses the persistent LSVC. Anteriorly and medially, the aortic root (*Ao*) and right ventricular outflow (*RVO*) are also visualized. **B:** Color-flow Doppler confirms flow in the LUPV and LSVC (*asterisk*).

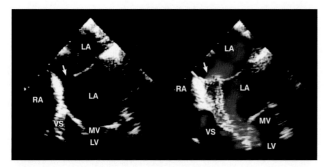

FIG. 18-21. Transesophageal echocardiogram of cor tria-triatum. A horizontal transducer is in the four-chamber plane. The transducer is in the esophagus posterior to the left atrium (*LA*). In the LA cavity is a membrane that divides the LA into two cavities. The posterior cavity contains the pulmonary veins, and the anterior cavity contains the LA appendage (not shown) and mitral valve (*MV*). The two LA cavities communicate through a stenotic orifice (*arrow*) in the membrane. Color-flow Doppler **(right)** shows a turbulent jet across the stenotic membrane. *VS*, ventricular septum.

REFERENCES

1. Seward JB, Tajik AJ, Edwards WD, Hagler DJ. *Two-dimensional echocardiographic atlas*, Volume 1: *Congenital heart disease*. New York: Springer-Verlag, 1987.
2. Snider AR, Serwer GA, Ritter SB. *Echocardiography in pediatric heart disease*, 2nd ed. St. Louis: Mosby, 1997.
3. Silverman NH. *Pediatric echocardiography*. Baltimore: Williams & Wilkins, 1993.
4. Shub C, Dimopoulos IN, Seward JB, et al. Sensitivity of two-dimensional echocardiography in the direct visualization of atrial septal defect utilizing the subcostal approach: experience with 154 patients. *J Am Coll Cardiol* 1983;2:127–135.
5. Morimoto K, Matsuzaki M, Tohma Y, et al. Diagnosis and quantitative evaluation of secundum-type atrial septal defect by transesophageal Doppler echocardiography. *Am J Cardiol* 1990;66:85–91.
6. Pascoe RD, Oh JK, Warnes CA, Danielson GK, Tajik AJ, Seward JB. Diagnosis of sinus venosus atrial septal defect with transesophageal echocardiography. *Circulation* 1996;94:1049–1055.
7. Ammash NM, Seward JB, Warnes CA, Connolly HM, O'Leary PW, Danielson GK. Partial anomalous pulmonary venous connection: diagnosis by transesophageal echocardiography. *J Am Coll Cardiol* 1997;29:1351–1358.
8. Borgeson DD, Seward JB, Miller FA Jr, Oh JK, Tajik AJ. Frequency of Doppler measurable pulmonary artery pressures. *J Am Soc Echocardiogr* 1996;9:832–837.
9. Freeman WK, Seward JB, Khandheria BK, Tajik AJ, eds. *Transesophageal echocardiography*. Boston: Little, Brown and Company, 1994.
10. Brandenberg RO Jr, Tajik AJ, Edwards WD, Reeder GS, Shub C, Seward JB. Accuracy of 2-dimensional echocardiographic diagnosis of congenitally bicuspid aortic valve: echocardiographic-anatomic correlation in 115 patients. *Am J Cardiol* 1983;51:1469–1473.
11. Oh JK, Taliercio CP, Holmes DR Jr, et al. Prediction of the severity of aortic stenosis by Doppler aortic valve area determination: prospective Doppler-catheterization correlation in 100 patients. *J Am Coll Cardiol* 1988;11:1227–1234.
12. Seward JB, Tajik AJ, Hagler DJ, Edwards WD. Internal cardiac crux: two-dimensional echocardiography of normal and congenitally abnormal hearts. *Ultrasound Med Biol* 1984;10:735–745.
13. Rice MJ, Seward JB, Edwards WD, et al. Straddling atrioventricular valve: Two-dimensional echocardiographic diagnosis, classification and surgical implications. *Am J Cardiol* 1985;55:505–513.
14. Practice guidelines for perioperative transesophageal echocardiography. A report by the American Society of Anesthesiologists and the Society of Cardiovascular Anesthesiologists Task Force on Transesophageal Echocardiography. *Anesthesiology* 1996;84:986–1006.
15. O'Leary PW, Hagler DJ, Seward JB, et al. Biplane intraoperative transesophageal echocardiography in congenital heart disease. *Mayo Clin Proc* 1995;70:317–326.
16. Nyberg DA, Mahony BS, Pretorius DH. *Diagnostic ultrasound of fetal anomalies: text and atlas*. St. Louis: Mosby–Year Book, 1990.
17. Connolly HM, Warnes CA. Ebstein's anomaly: outcome of pregnancy. *J Am Coll Cardiol* 1994;23:1194–1198.
18. Seward JB. Biplane and multiplane transesophageal echocardiography: evaluation of congenital heart disease. *Am J Card Imaging* 1995;9:129–136.
19. Seward JB, Belohlavek M, O Leary PW, Foley DA, Greenleaf JF. Congenital heart disease: Wide-field, three-dimensional, and four-dimensional ultrasound imaging. *Am J Card Imaging* 1995;9:38–43.

CHAPTER 19

Intraoperative Echocardiography

Epicardial M-mode echocardiography was used in the operating room as early as 1972 to evaluate the result of open mitral commissurotomy (1), but it was not until the late 1980s, with the widespread use of transesophageal echocardiography (TEE) and the incorporation of color-flow imaging, that intraoperative echocardiography became a routine procedure. Currently, TEE is an important diagnostic and monitoring technique in the operating room that assists with various cardiovascular surgical procedures (2–4). At the Mayo Clinic, intraoperative TEE is used in 50% of all cardiopulmonary bypass operations (5). The gradual increase in the use of intraoperative TEE from 1991 to 1997 at our institution is shown in Fig. 19-1. The case distribution for intraoperative TEE in adult and congenital cardiovascular procedures is shown in Figs. 19-2 and 19-3. The reasons for intraoperative echocardiography are (a) to identify previously undetected but clinically and surgically important lesions, (b) to ensure the optimal result of cardiovascular surgical procedures, (c) to minimize cardiovascular complications during cardiac and noncardiac operations in high-risk patients by monitoring wall motion, air bubbles, or atheromatous plaques in the aorta, and (d) to identify the responsible abnormalities when a patient's condition becomes hemodynamically unstable in the operating room.

IMPLEMENTATION

Intraoperative TEE involves multiple disciplines and requires cooperation among anesthesiologists, cardiologists, and surgeons. Because the anesthesiologist is in charge of the patient's hemodynamic condition and airways, the transesophageal probe is usually inserted by the anesthesiologist. If he or she is comfortable with performing TEE, baseline TEE data can be obtained and reviewed in conjunction with a cardiologist–echocardiographer. Routine monitoring of air in the cardiac chambers or regional wall motion abnormalities is performed mainly by the anesthesiologist. In cases of valve or congenital heart surgery at our institution, the cardiologist–echocardiographer usually is actively involved from the beginning of the operation.

The preoperative TEE findings are discussed with the cardiac surgeon and the anesthesiologist. Identification of the location and extent of morphologic abnormalities of the heart and vascular structures helps the surgeon to direct the necessary attention to problem areas and to formulate a surgical plan.

Echocardiography is repeated immediately after the patient comes off the bypass pump to assess the results of repair. The postoperative echocardiographic findings are discussed with the surgeon. When the structural and hemodynamic results are considered inadequate, the second pump run is initiated to revise the repair, after which the results are again evaluated with echocardiography. It is *not realistic to attempt perfect repair* in all surgical cases, however. If a hemodynamically insignificant lesion remains, it is better to leave it alone than to go back and revise the repair. Sometimes it is difficult to determine the long-term outcome of apparently abnormal structures or functions, shown on intraoperative echocardiography, that are not immediately causing hemodynamic abnormalities. During the early experience, 5% to 10% of cases required a second pump run (4,6,7), and this incidence decreased significantly with more experience (5).

INDICATIONS

The case distribution for adult and congenital cases is shown in Figs. 19-2 and 19-3, respectively. The most common indication for intraoperative TEE in adult cardiovascular procedures is the evaluation of mitral regurgitation for the purpose of mitral valve repair. Evaluation of mitral regurgitation is also a frequent indication in patients undergoing aortic valve replacement or coronary artery bypass surgery, because these patients concomitantly have mitral regurgitation, and more than a moderate degree of mitral regurgitation is usually repaired by ring annuloplasty unless there is a significant structural abnormality of the mitral valve. At our institution, intraoperative TEE is requested for almost all patients undergoing the following cardiovascular procedures: mitral valve repair, suspicion of signifi-

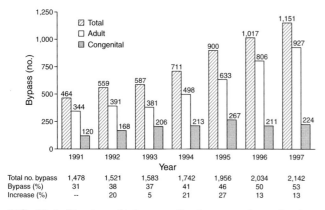

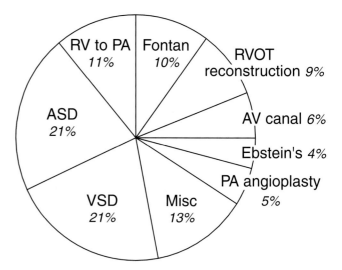

FIG. 19-1. Number of intraoperative transesophageal echocardiographic (TEE) examinations at the Mayo Clinic from 1991 to 1997. Currently, intraoperative TEE is performed in 50% of all cardiopulmonary bypass operations at our institution. Of the total number of intraoperative TEE examinations performed, 20% to 25% are in patients with congenital heart disease.

FIG. 19-3. Primary surgical indications for using intraoperative transesophageal echocardiography at the Mayo Clinic from 1991 to 1996 in cases of congenital heart disease. The most frequent indications were during atrial septal defect (*ASD*) or ventricular septal defect (*VSD*) repair, followed by the right ventricle (*RV*) to pulmonary artery [RV to pulmonary artery (PA)] conduit construction, Fontan, and RV outflow tract obstruction (*RVOT reconstruction*). *AV*, atrioventricular; *Misc*, miscellaneous; *PA*, pulmonary artery. (Courtesy of Congenital Heart Disease Intraoperative TEE Group.)

cant mitral valve regurgitation in those undergoing aortic valve replacement or coronary artery bypass surgery, repair of proximal aortic dissection, myectomy procedure for hypertrophic obstructive cardiomyopathy, repair of intracardiac shunt, removal of intracardiac mass, and repair of congenital heart disease.

MITRAL VALVE REPAIR

Currently at the Mayo Clinic, the mitral valve is repaired rather than replaced in more than 95% of patients with regurgitant mitral valve lesions. Myxomatous degeneration (prolapse, flail with or without ruptured chordae tendineae) is responsible for mitral regurgitation in 70% of the patients undergoing mitral valve repair (4). Other causes include myocardial ischemia, annulus dilatation, papillary muscle dysfunction, cleft mitral leaflet, and, less commonly, rheumatic disease or endocarditis. Valve repair usually is not recommended for an active endocarditic lesion or in a patient with a hemodynamically unstable condition (i.e., a patient with hypotension or in shock with papillary muscle dysfunction or rupture). Compared with mitral valve replacement, repair is associated with lower short- and long-term mortality (8–10). There is no increased need for repeat mitral valve procedure in comparison with mitral valve replacement. In addition, long-term anticoagulation is unnecessary, and there is less risk of infective endocarditis.

Reconstructive cardiac surgery is an individualized procedure, and its outcome is less predictable than that of valve replacement. After the patient is anesthetized, the TEE probe is inserted to obtain baseline data about mitral valve morphology, severity of mitral regurgitation, global systolic function, and other cardiovascular abnormalities (e.g., patent foramen ovale, intracardiac mass, or tricuspid regurgitation). The posterior mitral leaflet is involved more frequently than the anterior leaflet in patients with

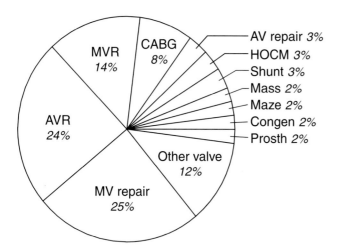

FIG. 19-2. Primary surgical procedures in which intraoperative transesophageal echocardiography (TEE) was used at the Mayo Clinic from 1991 to 1996. The most frequent indication of intraoperative TEE was during mitral valve (*MV*) repair. Other indications included aortic valve replacement (*AVR*), mitral valve replacement (*MVR*), and coronary artery bypass graft (*CABG*). During coronary artery bypass graft and aortic valve replacement, assessment of mitral regurgitation is also an important reason for intraoperative TEE. *AV*, aortic valve; *Congen*, congenital; *HOCM*, hypertrophic obstructive cardiomyopathy for myectomy; *Prosth*, prosthesis. (Courtesy of Dr. Roger L. Click and Intraoperative TEE Group.)

myxomatous degeneration. The success rate for satisfactory mitral valve repair is higher for posterior leaflet prolapse or flail segment than for anterior or bileaflet involvement (4). Intraoperative TEE examples of posterior, anterior, and bileaflet involvement of myxomatous mitral valve are shown in Figs. 19-4, 19-5, and 19-6. For severe mitral regurgitation due to myxomatous degeneration, mitral valve repair consists of (a) quadrangular excision or plication of redundant or flail tissue (especially for the posterior leaflet), (b) reconstruction of a competent mitral leaflet, (c) shortening of the chordae (if elongated) or chordal implantation (for anterior leaflet), and (d) ring annuloplasty (Fig. 19-7). The repair procedure used to correct severe mitral regurgitation depends on the mechanism that causes the regurgitation, for example, perforation, cleft mitral valve, endocarditis, or annulus dilatation.

The echocardiographer responsible for the intraoperative evaluation should be familiar with the TEE views of mitral valve morphology and the repair procedure to assess postoperative results (Figs. 19-8 through 19-10). Immediate feedback about the structural and functional results of a reconstructive procedure before chest closure provides assurance to the surgeon (when the result is good) or an opportunity to revise the repair (when it is not optimal). During the initial experience with intraoperative TEE, revision was necessary in 10 (7%) of 143 patients who underwent mitral valve repair at the Mayo Clinic (4), but this rate decreased significantly afterward. Significant mitral regurgitation still may be present because of systolic anterior motion of the repaired mitral valve, with or without ring annuloplasty (Fig. 19-11), usually in the setting of hypovolemia or hyperdynamic left ventricle (LV) (or both). Systolic anterior motion and mitral regurgitation usually resolve when LV volume is optimally restored. Also, it should be emphasized that the severity of mitral regurgitation after repair needs to be assessed under normal physiologic hemodynamic conditions.

Intraoperative TEE occasionally (<3%) detects clinically

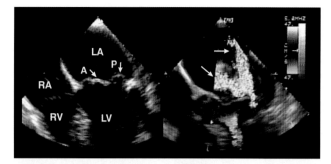

FIG. 19-5. Left: Transesophageal view of the bileaflet of the mitral valve. Both anterior (*A*) and posterior (*P*) leaflets prolapse into the left atrium (*LA*). **Right:** Color-flow imaging showed two jets of mitral regurgitation (*arrows on right side*).

unsuspected abnormalities that alter or add operative procedures (5). Examples include patent foramen ovale, atrial septal defect, cardiac mass (thrombus or tumor), unsuspected valvular regurgitation, and vascular abnormalities.

HYPERTROPHIC OBSTRUCTIVE CARDIOMYOPATHY

Myectomy consists of removing ventricular septal tissue through the aortic valve orifice (Fig. 19-12). Intraoperative TEE is useful preoperatively in determining the site of septal contact by the mitral leaflet (during systolic anterior motion) and the thickness of the ventricular septum, which help a surgeon decide the extent and depth of the myectomy. Evaluation of mitral valve morphology and regurgitation severity is also important because a subset of patients with hypertrophic obstructive cardiomyopathy is prone to develop rupture of the chordae attached to a mitral leaflet (see Fig. 12–17). If a morphologic abnormality of the mitral valve is present, mitral valve repair is indicated in addition to myectomy. Occasionally, the right ventricular (RV) outflow tract also is obstructed by hypertrophy, and it is easily evaluated by TEE. The actual LV outflow tract (LVOT) gradient can be obtained from the transgastric long-axis view (120 to 130 degrees using multiplane TEE), but it may not be feasible in all cases. At our institution, the gradient

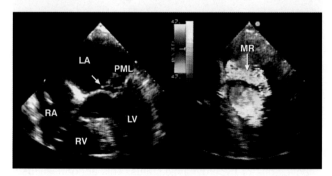

FIG. 19-4. Left: Transverse transesophageal view of flail segment of the posterior mitral leaflet (*PML*) of the mitral valve due to ruptured chordae tendineae (*arrow*). **Right:** Because of the flail posterior leaflet of the mitral valve, color-flow imaging showed a very eccentric mitral regurgitation (*MR*) jet toward the atrial septum (*arrow*) on the right side.

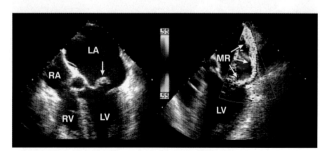

FIG. 19-6. Left: Transverse transesophageal view of the flail anterior mitral leaflet (*arrow*). **Right:** Color-flow imaging showed a very eccentric jet of mitral regurgitation (*MR*) toward the lateral wall of the LA (*arrows*).

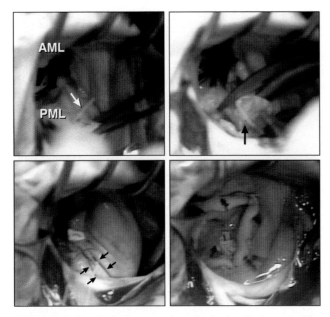

FIG. 19-7. Surgical photographs of mitral valve repair: **Upper left:** Surgeon's view from opened left atrium of the mitral valve with ruptured chordae tendineae (*arrow*) attached to the posterior mitral leaflet (*PML*). On inspection, the anterior mitral leaflet (*AML*) appeared normal. **Upper right:** Quadrangular excision of the redundant posterior mitral leaflet (*arrow*). **Lower left:** Reconstruction of the PML after the quadrangular excision by bringing two edges together (*arrows*). **Lower right:** Ring annuloplasty. In the case shown here, a complete ring was used, but more frequently, a C-shaped ring is used for ring annuloplasty, sparing the anterior portion of the annulus.

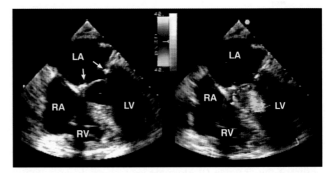

FIG. 19-9. Postoperative transesophageal examination in a patient who had a flail posterior mitral leaflet and underwent mitral valve repair. **Left:** Examination showed evidence of ring annuloplasty (*arrows*). **Right:** Color-flow imaging showed a competent mitral valve with no residual mitral valve regurgitation.

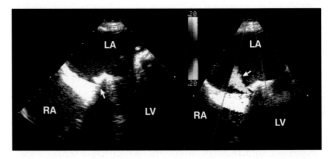

FIG. 19-10. Postoperative transesophageal echocardiographic (TEE) examination in a patient who underwent mitral valve replacement. Mitral valve repair could not be performed because of significant calcification. **Left:** After mitral valve replacement, postoperative TEE demonstrated a gap at the medial sewing ring (*arrow*). **Right:** Color-flow imaging showed periprosthetic mitral regurgitation (*arrow*).

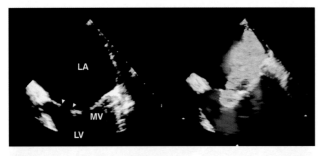

FIG. 19-8. **Left:** Transverse transesophageal imaging of the anterior mitral leaflet with perforation (*arrowheads*). **Right:** Color-flow imaging showed severe mitral valve regurgitation through the perforation. This was repaired by a pericardial patch to the perforated anterior mitral leaflet. *MV*, mitral valve.

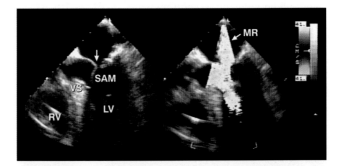

FIG. 19-11. Postoperative transesophageal view of the mitral valve (**left**) with systolic anterior motion (*SAM*) of the anterior mitral leaflet (*arrow*) causing (**right**) significant mitral valve regurgitation (*MR*). It usually occurs in association with hypovolemia or hyperdynamic status. This abnormality usually resolves when left ventricular (*LV*) volume is restored and inotropic support (dopamine) is discontinued. If this persists with optimal hemodynamic conditions and continues to cause severe mitral valve regurgitation, the mitral valve repair needs to be revised or the mitral valve needs to be replaced.

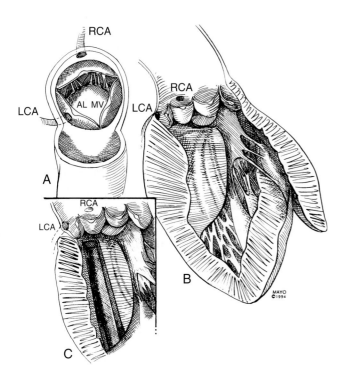

FIG. 19-12. Drawing of the anatomical characteristics of hypertrophic obstructive cardiomyopathy and myectomy. **A:** The surgeon's view through a transverse aortotomy. The right coronary cusp is located anteriorly and the left cusp, posteriorly and to the left. Gentle retraction of the aortic cusps in combination with posterior displacement of the left ventricle (LV) as needed exposes the ventricular septum and anterior leaflet of the mitral valve (*AL MV*). **B:** Sagittal view through the opened LV showing the membranous septum below the commissure between the right and noncoronary cusps, distribution of the left bundle branches, septal hypertrophy, and the anterior leaflet of the mitral valve with its subvalvular apparatus. **C:** The extent of initial septal resection is shown. The resection is then extended leftward to the anterior leaflet of the mitral valve and apically to relieve all midventricular obstruction. *RCA*, right coronary artery; *LCA*, left coronary artery. (From Theodoro DA, Danielson GK, Feldt RH, Anderson BJ. Hypertrophic obstructive cardiomyopathy in pediatric patients: result of surgical treatment. *J Thorac Cardiovasc Surg* 1996;112: 1589–1597, with permission.)

is usually measured by inserting a needle into the aorta and the LV, before and after myectomy. Postoperatively, intraoperative TEE is useful in determining the severity of residual mitral regurgitation (Fig. 19-13) and in assessing potential complications of myectomy, such as ventricular septal defect or aortic regurgitation. It is common for a small shunt to occur between the resected intramyocardial vessel and the LV after myectomy; this should not be confused with ventricular septal defect. Even after a generous myectomy, systolic anterior motion of the mitral valve may persist, although the postoperative LVOT gradient is less. Our follow-up study demonstrated that the systolic anterior motion shown on immediate postoperative TEE disappears in most patients by the time of hospital dismissal (11).

MEASUREMENT OF HOMOGRAFT SIZE

A homograft aortic valve is preferred for patients undergoing aortic valve replacement because of infective endocarditis. The homograft is stored in a freezer and thawed before being used. Intraoperative TEE is able to measure the LVOT diameter for sizing the homograft before the patient is placed on cardiopulmonary bypass, which allows a homograft of correct size to be selected at the beginning of the operation (12). Usually, a homograft that is 1 or 2 mm smaller than the measured LVOT diameter is selected. The homograft aortic valve with a portion of the aortic root is inserted inside the patient's aortic root ["cylinder within cylinder" (see Fig. 10–2)], and the coronary arteries are reimplanted to the donor aortic root (13). Familiarity with

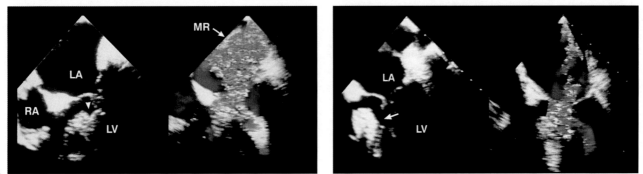

FIG. 19-13. A: After the initial myectomy (*arrowhead*), there was still systolic anterior motion of the mitral valve and severe mitral regurgitation (*MR*). **B:** Because the systolic anterior motion contact was distal to the myectomy site, myectomy was extended further distally (*arrow*). Color-flow imaging after additional myectomy showed only a mild degree of residual mitral regurgitation.

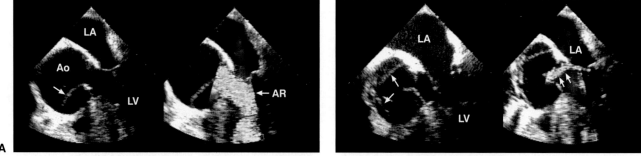

FIG. 19-14. An elderly man with a history of hypertension came to the emergency room with severe back pain, pulse deficit, hypotension, and pulmonary edema. Aortic dissection was suspected, and the patient was taken urgently to the operating room. **A:** Intraoperative transesophageal echocardiography showed proximal aortic dissection with an intimal flap (*arrow*) in the ascending aorta (*Ao*) and severe aortic regurgitation (*AR*) on color-flow imaging. **B:** After repair of the aortic dissection (*arrows on left*), transesophageal echocardiography demonstrated mild residual aortic regurgitation (*arrows on right*).

the surgical procedure allows accurate interpretation of the echocardiographic images of normal and abnormal aortic homografts.

DETECTION OF ATHEROMATOUS PLAQUE IN THE AORTA

Patients with severe atherosclerotic changes in the ascending aorta have an increased risk of stroke after bypass surgery because of dislodgment of an atheromatous plaque by the aortic clamp. Intraoperative TEE can identify atheromatous lesions in the aorta, and the surgical technique can be modified to reduce the risk of embolization (14–16). Epiaortic ultrasonography may be more accurate than TEE for identifying atherosclerosis. The ascending aorta is heavily calcified in some patients with calcific aortic stenosis. Prior knowledge of aortic calcification helps a surgeon to be prepared with an alternative surgical approach.

AORTIC DISSECTION

For proximal aortic dissection, intraoperative TEE evaluates the point of intimal tear, the severity of aortic regurgitation, and the involvement of coronary arteries preoperatively. The aortic valve usually can be resuspended, rather than replaced, and the coronary arteries reimplanted. Postoperatively, the integrity of the aorta, the severity of aortic regurgitation, and ventricular wall motion is evaluated (Fig. 19-14).

INTRAOPERATIVE MONITORING

Intraoperative echocardiography is also useful for monitoring (17,18) intracardiac air during neurosurgical procedures, fat embolism during hip arthroplasty, and regional wall motion abnormalities (as a marker of ischemia) in patients with severe coronary artery disease who are undergoing a noncardiac operation. Intraoperative TEE monitoring is best performed by an anesthesiologist trained in echocardiography. Initially, there was enthusiasm for routine monitoring of regional wall motion abnormalities in patients with suspected or known coronary artery disease during noncardiac operations to detect intraoperative ischemia, but the positive predictive value is low and the correlation between transient wall motion abnormalities and intraoperative infarct is not strong (17). The incremental clinical value of routine intraoperative TEE in a noncardiac operation requires further study, but currently there are no compelling data to support routine TEE monitoring of LV regional myocardial function during noncardiac surgical procedures.

UNSTABLE HEMODYNAMICS

In patients whose condition is unstable perioperatively, intraoperative TEE is useful in the evaluation of structural or hemodynamic problems (19). The problems range from the totally unexpected to the planned surgical procedure to the complication of the surgical procedure, for example, unsuspected cardiac tumor during mitral valve surgery, aortic dissection during coronary artery bypass surgery, and rupture of a cardiac structure after routine valve replacement or bypass surgery. Therefore, intraoperative TEE is valuable in evaluating unstable hemodynamic conditions during or soon after a cardiac or noncardiac surgical procedure.

REFERENCES

1. Johnson ML, Holmes JH, Spangler RD, Paton BC. Usefulness of echocardiography in patients undergoing mitral valve surgery. *J Thorac Cardiovasc Surg* 1972;64:922–934.
2. Task Force on Perioperative Transesophageal Echocardiography. Practice guidelines for perioperative transesophageal echocardiography: a report by the American Society of Anesthesiologists and the Society of Cardiovascular Anesthesiologists Task Force on Transesophageal Echocardiography. *Anesthesiology* 1996;84:986–1006.

3. O'Leary PW, Hagler DJ, Seward JB, et al. Biplane intraoperative transesophageal echocardiography in congenital heart disease. *Mayo Clin Proc* 1995;70:317–326.

4. Freeman WK, Schaff HV, Khandheria BK, et al. Intraoperative evaluation of mitral valve regurgitation and repair by transesophageal echocardiography: incidence and significance of systolic anterior motion. *J Am Coll Cardiol* 1992;20:599–609.

5. Click RL, Abel MD, Sinak LJ, et al. Role of intraoperative TEE and its impact on surgical decisions, prospective review of 2,261 adult cases. *J Am Soc Echocardiogr* 1997;10:396(abst).

6. Stewart WJ, Currie PJ, Salcedo EE, et al. Intraoperative Doppler color flow mapping for decision-making in valve repair for mitral regurgitation: technique and results in 100 patients. *Circulation* 1990;81:556–566.

7. Reichert SL, Visser CA, Moulijn AC, et al. Intraoperative transesophageal color-coded Doppler echocardiography for evaluation of residual regurgitation after mitral valve repair. *J Thorac Cardiovasc Surg* 1990;100:756–761.

8. Orszulak TA, Schaff HV, Danielson GK, et al. Mitral regurgitation due to ruptured chordae tendineae: early and late results of valve repair. *J Thorac Cardiovasc Surg* 1985;89:491–498.

9. Sand ME, Naftel DC, Blackstone EH, Kirklin JW, Karp RB. A comparison of repair and replacement for mitral valve incompetence. *J Thorac Cardiovasc Surg* 1987;94:208–219.

10. Ren JF, Aksut S, Lighty GW Jr, et al. Mitral valve repair is superior to valve replacement for the early preservation of cardiac function: Relation of ventricular geometry to function. *Am Heart J* 1996;131:974–981.

11. Park SH, Click RL, Freeman WK, et al. Role of intraoperative transesophageal echocardiography in patients with hypertrophic obstructive cardiomyopathy. *J Am Coll Cardiol* 1995;25 (Special Issue):82A(abst).

12. Oh CC, Click RL, Orszulak TA, Sinak LJ, Oh JK. The role of intraoperative transesophageal echocardiography in determining aortic annulus diameter in homograft insertion. *J Am Soc Echocardiogr* 1998;11:638–642.

13. Dearani JA, Orszulak TA, Daly RC, et al. Comparison of techniques for implantation of aortic valve allografts. *Ann Thorac Surg* 1996;62:1069–1075.

14. Katz ES, Tunick PA, Rusinek H, Ribakove G, Spencer FC, Kronzon I. Protruding aortic atheromas predict stroke in elderly patients undergoing cardiopulmonary bypass: experience with intraoperative transesophageal echocardiography. *J Am Coll Cardiol* 1992;20:70–77.

15. Davila-Roman VG, Phillips KJ, Daily BB, Davila RM, Kouchoukos NT, Barzilai B. Intraoperative transesophageal echocardiography and epiaortic ultrasound for assessment of atherosclerosis of the thoracic aorta. *J Am Coll Cardiol* 1996;28:942–947.

16. Nihoyannopoulos P, Joshi J, Athanasopoulos G, Oakley CM. Detection of atherosclerotic lesions in the aorta by transesophageal echocardiography. *Am J Cardiol* 1993;71:1208–1212.

17. Eisenberg MJ, London MJ, Leung JM, et al. for the Study of Perioperative Ischemia Research Group. Monitoring for myocardial ischemia during noncardiac surgery: a technology assessment of transesophageal echocardiography and 12-lead electrocardiography. *JAMA* 1992;268:210–216.

18. Ereth MH, Weber JG, Abel MD, et al. Cemented versus noncemented total hip arthroplasty—embolism, hemodynamics, and intrapulmonary shunting. *Mayo Clin Proc* 1992;67:1066–1074.

19. Brandt RR, Oh JK, Orszulak TA, Click RL. Role of emergency intraoperative transesophageal echocardiography. *J Am Soc Echocardiogr (in press)*.

CHAPTER 20

Contrast Echocardiography

Contrast echocardiography represents several different applications using a contrast agent or agitated saline in conjunction with echocardiography. A contrast agent or agitated saline has air-filled microbubbles with acoustic reflectivity, different from that of cardiovascular structures, that allows visualization of intracardiac or vascular structures containing the air bubbles or contrast agent (1). Consequently, contrast echocardiography is useful in the following areas: (a) identification of an intracardiac shunt, (b) identification of unknown cardiovascular structures, (c) improved recording of Doppler flow velocities, (d) visualization of the endocardial border, and (e) demonstration of perfusion in the myocardium.

IDENTIFICATION OF INTRACARDIAC OR PULMONARY SHUNT

The most frequent clinical application of contrast echocardiography is the identification of an intracardiac or pulmonary shunt. If a contrast agent is injected into the right side of the heart through an arm vein, the appearance of contrast bubbles is expected in the superior vena cava, right atrium (RA), right ventricle (RV), and pulmonary artery. Because most of the contrast agents used for this purpose are not able to pass through the pulmonary capillaries, no contrast is expected on the left side. In case of an intracardiac shunt or pulmonary arteriovenous fistula, the contrast agent appears in the left atrium (LA), left ventricle (LV), and aorta. The best example is the identification of a right-to-left shunt through a patent foramen ovale. A patent foramen ovale is present in about 25% of the population, but it is occasionally the conduit for paradoxical embolism. It is not usually visualized with two-dimensional (2D) echocardiography, even with color-flow imaging unless the size and the amount of shunt are large. A contrast study is a routine part of transesophageal echocardiography, especially during the evaluation of a potential cardiac source of embolism (Fig. 20-1). For this purpose, a three-way stopcock is connected to an intravenous catheter in the forearm. Saline (10 mL) is agitated back and forth between two syringes before being injected forcefully into an arm vein,

followed by elevation and squeezing of the arm. Before the use of color-flow imaging, contrast echocardiography also was used to detect left-to-right shunts, as in atrial septal defect, by demonstrating a negative contrast effect (i.e., displacement of contrast in the RA by the shunt), but it has been replaced completely by color-flow imaging. Another important example is the detection of pulmonary arteriovenous fistulas. Contrast appears in the LA through the pulmonary vein; hence, the appearance of contrast agent in the LA is delayed three to five cardiac cycles after it appears in the RA. If a shunt is present at the level of the atrium, however, contrast agent is seen in the LA immediately after being seen in the RA. The origin of a pulmonary arteriovenous fistula can be identified with a contrast study using transesophageal echocardiography, which can visualize all four pulmonary veins (Fig. 20-2).

IDENTIFICATION OF UNKNOWN INTRACARDIAC OR VASCULAR STRUCTURES

When only M-mode echocardiography was available, intracardiac structures were identified using contrast injection (2). Even with 2D echocardiographic visualization of cardiovascular structures, contrast injection is helpful in identifying unusual or uncommonly encountered structures, such as a left-sided superior vena cava, azygous vein (see Fig. 15–11), innominate vein, and anomalous pulmonary venous connections. It is also helpful in confirming the position of a needle in the pericardium during pericardiocentesis. Opacification of the pericardium after injection of agitated saline or indocyanine green helps to ensure that the needle is in the pericardial cavity and not in the RV or another cardiac chamber.

ENHANCEMENT OF DOPPLER FLOW VELOCITY SIGNAL

Faint Doppler-flow velocity signals can be enhanced by contrast injection. If the contrast bubbles are injected into an arm vein, tricuspid and pulmonary flow signals are en-

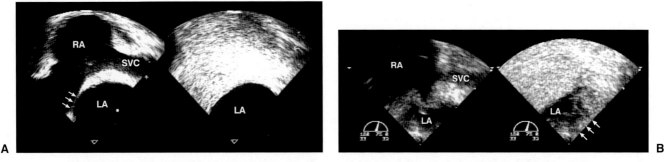

FIG. 20-1. A: Transesophageal longitudinal view of the atrial septum (*arrows*) before **(left)** and after **(right)** contrast injection in a patient with no intra-atrial shunt. **B:** Transesophageal echocardiographic demonstration of a right-to-left shunt in a 29-year-old woman with a stroke and patent foramen ovale using an injection of agitated saline. Contrast appears in the left atrium (*LA*) (*arrows*) immediately after being seen in the right atrium (*RA*). *SVC,* superior vena cava.

hanced (3). This ability is particularly useful in detecting tricuspid regurgitation velocity, which is essential in determining RV or pulmonary artery systolic pressure (see Fig. 17–5). If the contrast agent can pass through the pulmonary capillaries to the left side of the heart, mitral valve and aortic valve signals can be enhanced (4,5).

VISUALIZATION OF THE ENDOCARDIAL BORDER

Visualization of the endocardial border was the first clinical indication for which commercially available contrast agents (Albunex and Optison) were approved for use in humans. Under optimal conditions, these contrast agents opacify the LV cavity, which allows the border between the myocardium and blood flow to be identified (6,7). Adequate visualization of the endocardial border is the ''Achilles heel'' of assessing global and regional LV systolic function and of stress echocardiography. Currently, detection of the endocardial border by contrast echocardiography requires further clinical evaluation and refinement. New imaging methods for contrast, such as second harmonic imaging, may improve this potentially important application of contrast echocardiography.

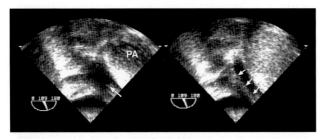

FIG. 20-2. Transesophageal echocardiographic demonstration of an arteriovascular fistula in the lung by contrast echocardiography. Bubbles are seen (*arrows on right*) coming out of the left upper pulmonary vein (*single arrow on left*) after agitated saline was injected into an arm vein. *PA*, pulmonary artery.

DETECTION OF MYOCARDIAL PERFUSION

Of the potential clinical applications being explored for contrast echocardiography, the identification and quantification of myocardial perfusion are the most exciting. Extensive research efforts by investigators in this field have brought this application close to a clinical reality (8–10). The myocardium has a dense microvascular circulation whose blood supply depends on the large epicardial coronary arteries. If a contrast agent can pass through the myocardial blood vessels, the degree of the acoustical reflectivity from the bubbles within the microvascular circulation detected by 2D echocardiography should correlate with the extent of coronary blood flow. An ideal agent should have the following characteristics: (a) is not harmful to humans, (b) is able to pass through the pulmonary capillaries, (c) does not change intracardiac hemodynamics, (d) can be imaged well with 2D echocardiography, and (e) should be resistant to change in size when it comes in contact with blood because ultrasound backscatter is related to the sixth power of bubble radius. Other desired physical characteristics include low solubility and nondiffusibility. Numerous agents are being developed to fulfill these requirements and are undergoing various phases of clinical testing (Table 20-1). If contrast echocardiography demonstrates myocardial perfusion reliably, it will become an integral part of echocardiography practice in the following clinical areas: (a) determination of myocardium at risk in patients with chest pain or acute myocardial infarction, (b) determination of myocardial salvage after reperfusion therapy, (c) determination of reperfusion status, (4) determination of myocardial viability, and (e) detection of ischemia during stress echocardiography.

Optimal detection of contrast in the intracardiac cavity and in the myocardium requires an understanding of the backscatter properties of microbubbles and the physics of ultrasound. Microbubbles are destroyed by constant exposure to an ultrasound beam (11). Intermittent ultrasound imaging at a certain interval minimizes the destruction of microbubbles (12). Another important backscatter property of microbub-

TABLE 20-1. *Echocardiographic contrast agents*

Agent	Diameter (μm)	Concentration, $\times 10^{-9}$	Shell composition	Gases
AFO150	5.0	0.5	Surfactant stabilized	Air and perfluorohexane
Albunex	4.3	0.5	Denatured albumin	Air
BRI	2.5	0.2	Lipids and surfactant	Air and H_2SF_6
Echogen	3–5		Surfactant stabilized	Dodecafluoropentane
Levovist	2–4		Palmitic acid stabilized	Air
MRX-115			Lipids and surfactants	Air and perfluoropropane
Optison	3.9	0.8	Denatured albumin	Air and perfluoropropane
PESDA	4–5	1.5	Denatured albumin	Decaperfluorobutane
Quantison	3.2	1.5	Denatured albumin	Air
Sonovist	1–2		Cyanoacrylate	Air

PESDA, perfluorocarbon-exposed sonicated dextrose albumin.

bles is their ability to resonate at frequencies that are multiples of the transmitted frequency (2*f*, 3*f*, 4*f*). Because other surrounding structures (myocardium and valves) emit only the original transmitted frequency (1*f*), imaging at a frequency twice (2*f*) the transmitted frequency identifies the structures containing the microbubbles (increased signal-to-noise-ratio). For example, if the transmitted frequency is 1.8 MHz, the backscatter of 3.6-MHz frequency is imaged. This has been termed *second harmonic imaging* (13), in contrast to fundamental imaging that identifies structures with backscatter of the transmitted frequency (1*f*). The combined approach of second harmonic imaging and transient intermittent gating improves the detection of microbubbles in the cardiac chambers and myocardium (Fig. 20-3).

Visualization of the Coronary Artery

Intramyocardial coronary arteries can be opacified by second harmonic imaging of an echocardiographic contrast

agent. Mulvagh et al. (14) at the Mayo Clinic were the first to demonstrate discrete contrast-containing intramyocardial linear branching structures in the basal and midseptal region after intravenously injecting Imagent (AFO 145) in dogs. A Doppler study with a sample volume in the sample vessels demonstrated a typical coronary flow signal at baseline and appropriately increased flow velocity after the intracoronary administration of adenosine. Hence, contrast echocardiography has the potential for evaluating coronary flow reserve if the above findings can be validated in humans.

Evaluation of Myocardial Perfusion

The ultimate goal of contrast echocardiography is the evaluation of myocardial perfusion. Currently, myocardial perfusion is evaluated by thallium or sestamibi radionuclide imaging. Intracoronary or intraaortic root injection of contrast agent can identify reliably perfusion defects created experimentally in animals and in patients with acute myo-

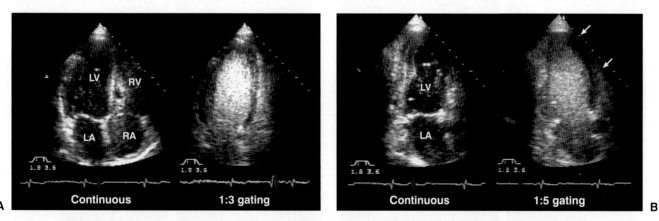

FIG. 20-3. Transient-response second harmonic imaging of the left ventricle (*LV*) with continuous infusion of perfluorocarbon-exposed sonicated dextrose albumin (*PESDA*) in a patient with an acute anterior wall myocardial infarction treated with angioplasty. **A:** Apical four-chamber view of second harmonic imaging during infusion of PESDA. **Left:** Continuous imaging shows contrast in the chambers on the right side of the heart but not much in the LV and myocardium. **Right:** 1:3 gating transient-response imaging shows contrast in the ventricular septum and lateral myocardium as well as in the LV cavity. **B:** Two-chamber view. **Left:** Continuous imaging does not demonstrate contrast in the myocardium or in the LV cavity. **Right:** 1:5 gating transient-response imaging shows contrast in the LV cavity and the inferior wall, but the defect is in the anterior wall (defined by *arrows*) despite TIMI III flow on coronary angiogram.

cardial infarction (15,16); however, fundamental imaging has not been successful in demonstrating myocardial perfusion after intravenous injection of contrast agent. The combination of second harmonic imaging and transient-response imaging improved visualization of contrast agent in the myocardium (Fig. 20-3). This improvement was demonstrated initially by Porter and Xie (12), who used intravenous injections of perfluorocarbon-exposed sonicated dextrose albumin (PESDA) microbubbles, and similar improvement was noted with other agents. The location of myocardial perfusion abnormalities and their physiologic relevance (reversible or irreversible) demonstrated by second harmonic transient-response imaging with the use of FS-069, perfluorocarbon albumin microbubbles, correlates well with that provided by thallium sestamibi single-photon emission computed tomography (SPECT) (Fig. 20-4) (17,18). Although several technical aspects need to be refined to make contrast echocardiography a clinical reality, it appears promising for evaluating myocardial perfusion abnormalities, which will be useful in the diagnosis of acute myocardial infarction, evaluation of coronary artery disease, estimation of myocardial risk area, evaluation of reperfusion therapy, and determination of myocardial viability. Myocardial function may not return after successful

acute reperfusion therapy if there is no reflow (patent epicardial artery with no perfusion in the myocardium). This phenomenon also can be demonstrated by contrast perfusion imaging (16).

Evaluation of Myocardial Viability

Because myocardial contractility ceases when >20% of myocardial thickness is involved with ischemia/infarction, akinetic myocardium demonstrated with 2D echocardiography may contain viable tissue. Determining whether akinetic myocardium contains viable tissue or only a necrotic scar requires information about myocardial metabolism, microvascular integrity, or contractile reserve. Positron emission tomography detects myocardial viability by demonstrating a mismatch between myocardial metabolism (glucose uptake) and myocardial perfusion (ammonium tracer). Contractile reserve is best evaluated by using low-dose dobutamine echocardiography (see Chapter 8). Demonstration of an intact microvascular circulation in akinetic myocardium is good evidence for myocardial viability and presently is evaluated with thallium SPECT. Similarly, contrast echocardiography also can identify intact microvascular circulation in the myocardium. Several studies have

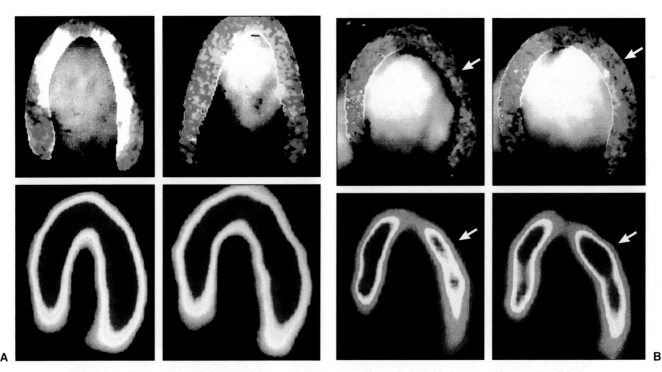

A **B**

FIG. 20-4. Comparison of a second harmonic contrast echocardiographic image with a sestamibi single-photon emission computed tomographic (*SPECT*) image. **A:** Example of normal perfusion in a four-chamber view after dipyridamole infusion **(left panels)** and at baseline **(right panels)** with myocardial contrast echocardiography **(top panels)** and SPECT **(bottom panels)**. **B:** Example of a large, fully reversible defect in the lateral wall (*arrows*) in an apical four-chamber view on myocardial contrast echocardiography **(top panels)** and SPECT **(bottom panels)**. The postdipyridamole images are on the left, and the baseline images are on the right. The lateral defect in the postdipyridamole images **(left panels)** are no longer seen in the baseline images **(right panel)**. The apical defect, however, remains irreversible. (From ref. 17, with permission.)

demonstrated that contrast echocardiography is more sensitive for detecting myocardial viability but less specific in predicting recovery of LV systolic function after revascularization in comparison with low-dose dobutamine stress echocardiography (19,20). A combination of low-dose dobutamine and contrast echocardiography holds promise for detecting, with optimal sensitivity and specificity, viable akinetic myocardium that has the potential for recovering its function after revascularization.

REFERENCES

1. Gramiak R, Shah PM. Echocardiography of the aortic root. *Invest Radiol* 1968;3:356–366.
2. Seward JB, Tajik AJ, Spangler JG, Ritter DG. Echocardiographic contrast studies: initial experience. *Mayo Clin Proc* 1975;50:163–192.
3. Hagler DJ, Currie PJ, Seward JB, Tajik AJ, Mair DD, Ritter DG. Echocardiographic contrast enhancement of poor or weak continuous-wave Doppler signals. *Echocardiography* 1987;4:63–67.
4. von Bibra H, Sutherland G, Becher H, Neudert J, Nihoyannopoulos P, for the Levovist Cardiac Working Group. Clinical evaluation of left heart Doppler contrast enhancement by a saccharide-based transpulmonary contrast agent. *J Am Coll Cardiol* 1995;25:500–508.
5. Nakatani S, Imanishi T, Terasawa A, Beppu S, Nagata S, Miyatake K. Clinical application of transpulmonary contrast-enhanced Doppler technique in the assessment of severity of aortic stenosis. *J Am Coll Cardiol* 1992;20:973–978.
6. Crouse LJ, Cheirif J, Hanly DE, et al. Opacification and border delineation improvement in patients with suboptimal endocardial border definition in routine echocardiography: results of the Phase III Albunex Multicenter Trial. *J Am Coll Cardiol* 1993;22:1494–1500.
7. Schröder K, Agrawal R, Völler H, Schlief R, Schröder R. Improvement of endocardial border delineation in suboptimal stress-echocardiograms using the new left heart contrast agent SH U 508 A. *Int J Card Imaging* 1994;10:45–51.
8. Kaul S, Kelly P, Oliner JD, Glasheen WP, Keller MW, Watson DD. Assessment of regional myocardial blood flow with myocardial contrast two-dimensional echocardiography. *J Am Coll Cardiol* 1989;13:468–482.
9. Porter TR, D'Sa A, Turner C, et al. Myocardial contrast echocardiography for the assessment of coronary blood flow reserve: validation in humans. *J Am Coll Cardiol* 1993;21:349–355.
10. Schrope BA, Newhouse VL. Second harmonic ultrasonic blood perfusion measurement. *Ultrasound Med Biol* 1993;19:567–579.
11. Villarraga HR, Foley DA, Aeschbacher BC, Mulvagh SL. Power output-dependent destruction of echocardiographic contrast agents by conventional ultrasound imaging systems. *J Am Coll Cardiol* 1996;27 [Suppl A]:127A(abst).
12. Porter TR, Xie F. Transient myocardial contrast after initial exposure to diagnostic ultrasound pressures with minute doses of intravenously injected microbubbles: demonstration and potential mechanisms. *Circulation* 1995;92:2391–2395.
13. Schrope B, Newhouse VL, Uhlendorf V. Simulated capillary blood flow measurement using a nonlinear ultrasonic contrast agent. *Ultrason Imaging* 1992;14:134–158.
14. Mulvagh SL, Foley DA, Aeschbacher BC, Klarich KK, Seward JB. Second harmonic imaging of an intravenously administered echocardiographic contrast agent: visualization of coronary arteries and measurement of coronary blood flow. *J Am Coll Cardiol* 1996;27:1519–1525.
15. Kaul S, Glasheen W, Ruddy TD, Pandian NG, Weyman AE, Okada RD. The importance of defining left ventricular area at risk *in vivo* during acute myocardial infarction: an experimental evaluation with myocardial contrast two-dimensional echocardiography. *Circulation* 1987;75:1249–1260.
16. Ito H, Tomooka T, Sakai N, et al. Lack of myocardial perfusion immediately after successful thrombolysis: a predictor of poor recovery of left ventricular function in anterior myocardial infarction. *Circulation* 1992;85:1699–1705.
17. Kaul S, Senior R, Dittrich H, Raval U, Khattar R, Lahiri A. Detection of coronary artery disease with myocardial contrast echocardiography: Comparison with ^{99m}Tc-sestamibi single-photon emission computed tomography. *Circulation* 1997;96:785–792.
18. Cheirif J, Desir RM, Bolli R, et al. Relation of perfusion defects observed with myocardial contrast echocardiography to the severity of coronary stenosis: correlation with thallium-201 single-photon emission tomography. *J Am Coll Cardiol* 1992;19:1343–1349.
19. Nagueh SF, Vaduganathan P, Ali N, et al. Identification of hibernating myocardium: comparative accuracy of myocardial contrast echocardiography, rest-redistribution thallium-201 tomography and dobutamine echocardiography. *J Am Coll Cardiol* 1997;29:985–993.
20. Meza MF, Kates MA, Barbee RW, et al. Combination of dobutamine and myocardial contrast echocardiography to differentiate postischemic from infarcted myocardium. *J Am Coll Cardiol* 1997;29:974–984.

CHAPTER 21

Comprehensive Examination According to the Referral Diagnosis

Echocardiography has become an extension of the physical examination in cardiovascular practice. Frequently, it is used to confirm a clinical diagnostic suspicion. Another important role is to detect the underlying cardiovascular lesion to explain a patient's symptom complex or an abnormality found on chest radiography, electrocardiography (ECG), or cardiac enzyme tests. Patients are referred to the echocardiography laboratory because of their symptoms or nonspecific laboratory abnormalities, and echocardiographers are expected to provide a definite diagnosis or a diagnostic clue. This chapter describes the comprehensive diagnostic approach according to the referral diagnosis.

EVALUATION OF VENTRICULAR FUNCTION

Knowledge of ventricular function is the basic step in the evaluation of patients with cardiovascular abnormalities. The general status of left ventricular (LV) function is usually evident from the history and physical examination; however, quantitation of LV function is important to explain a patient's symptoms, to select the optimal therapeutic option, to select the optimal surgical timing, or to monitor the efficacy of therapy. When a patient is referred for evaluation of ventricular function, the following information about systolic and diastolic function should be provided:

LV cavity and wall dimensions, LV mass index
LV ejection fraction
Description of regional wall motion abnormalities
Wall motion score index (especially in patients with ischemic heart disease)
Right ventricular (RV) cavity and wall dimensions
Description of RV function
Stroke volume and cardiac output
Diastolic filling pattern and estimation of LV filling pressure

EVALUATION OF DYSPNEA OR HEART FAILURE

Dyspnea is a clinical manifestation of various cardiac and noncardiac disorders. This referral diagnosis requires a complete evaluation of the following:

Ventricular systolic and diastolic function as described above
Valvular anatomy and function
Exclusion of intracardiac shunt
Respiratory variation in transvalvular and central venous flow (? constrictive pericarditis)
Evidence of cardiomyopathy
Pulmonary artery pressure
Dynamic LV outflow tract (LVOT) obstruction

Stress echocardiography should be considered if the dyspnea is thought to be angina-equivalent or is exertional in nature. Measurement of valvular hemodynamics, diastolic filling pattern, and pulmonary pressure needs to be repeated with exercise if resting data do not explain the patient's exertional dyspnea.

MURMUR OR MITRAL VALVE PROLAPSE

Although various bedside maneuvers are helpful in determining the cause of murmur by auscultation, it is often necessary to confirm a clinical suspicion or to characterize the morphologic and hemodynamic abnormalities responsible for the murmur. Another frequent reason for referral to echocardiography is mitral valve prolapse. It is still the most common cause for severe mitral regurgitation and mitral valve repair (or replacement), but most patients with mitral valve prolapse are relatively free of symptoms. Because of the medical, financial, and psychologic impact of the diagnosis of mitral valve prolapse, strict diagnostic criteria should be used (see Chapter 9) (1): (a) thickened or myxomatous mitral leaflets, (b) systolic displacement of the mitral leaflet into the left atrium (LA) at least 3 mm or more beyond the mitral annulus in the parasternal or apical long-axis view, and (c) mitral regurgitation.

Two-dimensional (2D) echocardiography should be able to detect abnormal cardiac valve morphology such as a bicuspid valve or pulmonic stenosis. After the abnormal valve has been identified, its hemodynamic severity should be established with Doppler and color-flow imaging. If 2D echocardiography does not identify the source of a cardiac murmur, continuous-wave Doppler interrogation of all four valves and the septa (atrial and ventricular) should be performed. Occasionally, color-flow imaging can provide the first clue about an abnormal valve: trivial-to-mild aortic regurgitation from a bicuspid aortic valve or turbulent pulmonary artery flow from the pulmonic stenosis. Dynamic LVOT obstruction should be looked for, especially in elderly patients who have a thickened basal septum with or without hypertension. Also, look for congenital heart lesions in adults, such as atrial septal defect, small ventricular septal defect, or patent ductus arteriosus.

NONSPECIFIC ELECTROCARDIOGRAPHIC ABNORMALITIES

Although electrocardiography (ECG) is useful when it is diagnostic for certain cardiac lesions (e.g., ST-segment elevation for transmural myocardial infarction, diffuse ST-segment elevation for pericarditis), many ECG abnormalities are not specific or diagnostic. T-wave inversion may be a result of myocardial ischemia, electrolyte abnormalities, apical hypertrophic cardiomyopathy, or subarachnoid hemorrhage, or it may even be a normal variation. Because an ECG abnormality can indicate a serious underlying cardiovascular condition, an abnormal finding raises concern. Similarly, a nonspecific ECG abnormality may develop after a surgical or interventional procedure and raise concern about procedure-related myocardial ischemia or infarction.

Echocardiography is the next logical diagnostic step because it can clarify the significance of ECG abnormalities by assessing the following:

Regional wall motion abnormalities
Cardiomyopathy
Pericardial effusion
Intracardiac mass
Pulmonary embolism
LV hypertrophy
Valvular heart disease

Transient myocardial dysfunction, along with ECG repolarization changes, has been noted after electroconvulsive therapy or subarachnoid hemorrhage (2,3). Most likely, it is related to a catecholamine surge, and gradual resolution of wall motion abnormalities has been documented by serial echocardiographic examination (3).

CHEST PAIN

Echocardiography is helpful in the evaluation of chest pain, especially when it is not accompanied by a diagnostic ECG change. In a significant proportion of patients with acute myocardial infarction, the initial ECG is nondiagnostic. The diagnostic value is greatest if the study is performed during the episode of chest pain. If the pain is of ischemic cause, regional wall motion abnormalities are usually present, sometimes even before typical ECG changes occur. The presence of regional wall motion abnormalities is not specific for acute ischemia, but their absence strongly suggests a nonischemic cause. Other cardiac reasons for chest pain can be readily detected by echocardiography. The following diagnoses should be considered when patients with nonspecific chest pain are evaluated:

Ischemia or infarction
Aortic dissection
Pericarditis
Valvular heart disease, especially aortic stenosis
Cardiomyopathies, especially hypertrophic cardiomyopathy
Pulmonary embolism
Intracardiac or extracardiac mass

CARDIAC SOURCE OF EMBOLI

The cardiac sources of systemic or cerebral embolism include intracardiac thrombus, mass, vegetation, atrial septal aneurysm, paradoxical embolism via a patent foramen ovale, and ulcerated plaques in the aorta (4–6). Transthoracic echocardiography (TTE) alone is inadequate to evaluate all the above lesions. The LA appendage (LAA) is not well visualized with TTE, and a patent foramen ovale is not recognized in almost one-half of patients on a TTE examination. Therefore, for comprehensive evaluation of the cardiac source of emboli, transesophageal echocardiography (TEE) should be performed. In fact, this is the most common indication for performing TEE at the Mayo Clinic.

Evaluation by TTE should include the following:

Evaluate LV function
Evaluate the anatomic substrate for thrombi formation, such as aneurysm, dyskinetic segments, LA enlargement, mitral valve disease, hypereosinophilic syndrome, and atrial septal aneurysm
Look for vegetation
Look for a cardiac tumor

Evaluation by TEE should include the following:

Search for intracardiac mass or thrombi
Thrombus in the LAA or LA
Scan the atrial septum for patent foramen ovale or atrial septal aneurysm
Contrast echocardiography for detection of a right-to-left shunt by injection of agitated saline via an arm vein at rest and with release of the Valsalva maneuver
Thoracic aorta for atheromatous plaque

HYPOTENSION, SYNCOPE, OR CARDIOGENIC SHOCK

Echocardiography is the most valuable bedside diagnostic tool to evaluate a patient who has hypotension or shock syndrome. If the symptoms are of cardiac origin, echocardiography should be able to identify the responsible cause. The following should be evaluated by echocardiography:

LV and RV function

Valvular abnormalities (severe aortic stenosis, mitral regurgitation, aortic regurgitation, endocarditis, etc.)

Cardiac tamponade (search for localized regional tamponade in postoperative patients)

Dynamic LVOT obstruction

Hypovolemia (small LV cavity size with hypercontractile walls)

Pulmonary embolism (acute RV dilatation with generalized RV hypokinesis)

Cardiac shunt (e.g., infarct ventricular septal rupture)

Aortic dissection

Cardiac rupture (after acute myocardial infarction)

Patients in an intensive care unit who are critically ill have multiple monitoring and lifesaving devices, and it may not be possible to perform echocardiography from the transthoracic window; however, TEE can be performed safely and provide diagnostic-quality images in these patients (7,8). For TEE in a critically ill patient, do the following:

Sedate the patient well (midazolam, meperidine hydrochloride [Demerol], or pancuronium for severely agitated patients on a ventilator)

Administer glycopyrrolate (0.2 mg intravenously) for secretion control

Monitor oxygen saturation and blood pressure during the examination

Perform a comprehensive examination expeditiously

No need to remove the nasogastric tube for satisfactory TEE examination

CARDIAC CONTUSION, DONOR HEART EVALUATION, AND CARDIAC TRANSPLANTATION

Cardiovascular lesions resulting from chest trauma are potentially fatal, but frequently are not recognized because they occur in the setting of multiple organ system injury. Clinical examination, cardiac enzyme measurements, chest radiography, and ECG may not be sensitive or specific for cardiac contusion or other cardiovascular structural abnormalities. Potential cardiac complications of chest trauma include ventricular dysfunction (especially contusion of the RV because it is close to the chest wall), cardiac tamponade, cardiac rupture, valvular rupture (especially the tricuspid valve), aortic rupture, and intracardiac thrombus. These cardiovascular lesions can be detected promptly at the bed-

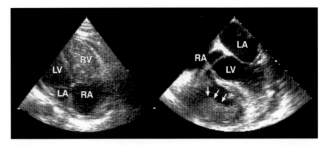

FIG. 21-1. Left: Transthoracic four-chamber view. **Right:** Transverse transesophageal view of a dilated right ventricle (*RV*) filled with thrombus (*arrows*). These images are from a young man with chest trauma caused by a fall from a ladder.

side with 2D or Doppler echocardiography (Fig. 21-1). TEE is especially helpful in the evaluation of aortic lesions, cardiac or valvular rupture, and in patients with a suboptimal transthoracic window because of chest injury or motor vehicle accident (Fig. 21-2) (9). Detection or exclusion of cardiac contusion is crucial when victims of motor vehicle accidents are evaluated as potential cardiac donors, to minimize donor-heart failure rate.

Echocardiography is also important after cardiac transplantation. Because the patient's atria are sutured to the atria of the donor heart, the atria appear enlarged (Fig. 21-3). The LV wall thickness increases soon after transplantation. Because of repeated RV biopsies, the tricuspid leaflet may be injured, resulting in significant tricuspid regurgitation. If rejection occurs, ventricular systolic function decreases. The age of donor hearts differs; therefore, it is not reliable to use the diastolic filling pattern on Doppler echocardiography to detect rejection. Interpretation of mitral and pulmonary vein flow velocities is also hampered by independent contraction of the patient's atria and those of the donor heart.

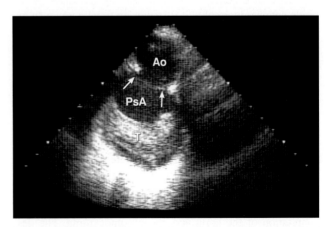

FIG. 21-2. Transesophageal view of a ruptured aorta that resulted in a pseudoaneurysm (*PsA*) with thrombus (*T*). This image is from a patient who was in a motor vehicle accident 3 years before this imaging study. A large tear (*arrows*) of the aortic arch (*Ao*) is clearly seen.

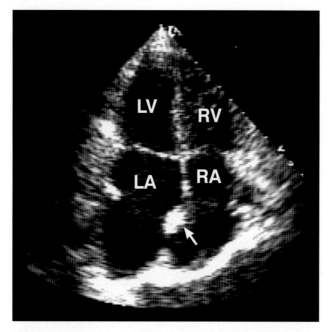

FIG. 21-3. Apical four-chamber view of a transplanted heart. The atria are enlarged, resembling the appearance of restrictive cardiomyopathy (see Fig. 12-19). The increased echodensity (*arrow*) of the atrial septum corresponds to the site of anastomosis.

SYSTEMIC HYPERTENSION

Hypertension is a common condition that contributes significantly to cardiovascular morbidity and mortality. LV hypertrophy is a characteristic response to systemic hypertension and is an independent prognostic indicator. Two-dimensional and M-mode echocardiography can measure LV wall thickness and estimate LV mass, both of which are indices of LV hypertrophy.

LV mass is derived from 2D-guided M-mode echocardiography of the LV from a parasternal short-axis view, as described in Chapter 4. When measuring LV mass by M-mode echocardiography, it is important to take into account patient age, body surface area, and sex (10,11). The values for the upper-normal LV mass index, as determined from M-mode echocardiography, are shown in the Appendix.

Not uncommonly, global systolic LV function in hypertensive patients is hyperdynamic because of a hyperadrenergic state and intravascular volume contraction, resulting from diuretic therapy. Hypercontractile systolic function in the setting of LV hypertrophy may result in dynamic LVOT obstruction, which produces a characteristic systolic late-peaking, dagger-shaped, continuous-wave Doppler signal (see Chapter 12).

Infrequent but important causes for hypertension are coarctation of the aorta and pheochromocytoma. The descending thoracic aorta should be interrogated from the suprasternal notch with continuous-wave Doppler echocardiography. Often, it is difficult to visualize coarctation on TEE.

Diastolic function is another important variable that can be measured by 2D Doppler echocardiography in patients with systemic hypertension. The prominent diastolic abnormality in hypertension is a relaxation abnormality, and Doppler shows prolonged LV isovolumic relaxation time, reduced mitral inflow E velocity, increased mitral inflow A velocity, reduced E/A ratio, and prolonged mitral inflow deceleration time (DT). The diastolic filling pattern becomes pseudonormalized or restrictive when congestive heart failure develops during an end-stage hypertensive state or hypertensive crisis, however. A triphasic mitral inflow velocity pattern may develop because of impaired relaxation (see Chapter 5).

In patients with hypertension and chronic renal failure, myocardial texture may become abnormal, simulating the appearance of cardiac amyloidosis, but usually it is accompanied by a marked increase in QRS voltage on the ECG, compared with low voltage in cardiac amyloidosis. Therefore, the following information needs to be assessed and evaluated in patients with systemic hypertension:

LV cavity and wall dimensions
LV mass index
LV systolic and diastolic function
Dynamic LVOT obstruction
Evaluation for coarctation of the aorta

ATRIAL FIBRILLATION

Atrial fibrillation is an arrhythmia commonly encountered in clinical practice. This arrhythmia generates a large referral for echocardiography and, at the same time, creates problems in the analysis of echocardiographic data. In patients with atrial fibrillation, echocardiography is helpful in determining the cause and in identifying the subset of patients at high risk for thromboembolism. TEE provides superb visualization of the LA and LAA, and when no thrombus is seen, cardioversion can be performed with minimal embolic risk in patients with atrial fibrillation.

Identification of Underlying Cause

Atrial fibrillation usually is related to a cardiac functional or structural abnormality such as mitral valve disease, cardiomyopathy, or atrial septal defect or other congenital heart disease. Because atrial fibrillation may be the first manifestation of these treatable or repairable diseases, echocardiography is one of the most commonly used initial diagnostic tests in patients with atrial fibrillation. Stroke Prevention in Atrial Fibrillation (SPAF) investigators studied 568 patients with nonrheumatic atrial fibrillation and showed that LV dysfunction and LA size (>2 cm/m^2) were the strongest independent predictors of subsequent thromboembolism (12b). The presence of three clinical variables—congestive heart failure, history of hypertension, and previous thromboembolism—were significantly and independently associated with substantial risk for thromboembolism (12a). These variables defined patients with the rate of embolism of 2.5% per year (no risk factor), 7.2% per year (one risk factor), and 17.6% (two or three risk factors); however, 38% of the patients with atrial fibrillation classified as low risk by the aforementioned clinical variables were found to be at higher risk on the basis of additional echocardiographic data (LV systolic dysfunction and enlarged LA size).

Evaluation of Systolic and Diastolic Function in Atrial Fibrillation

Global systolic function frequently appears reduced in patients with rapid ventricular response to atrial fibrillation. The features of dilated cardiomyopathy may develop if tachycardia persists for a long time (tachycardia-induced cardiomyopathy) (13). Varying lengths of cardiac cycle make the evaluation of diastolic filling difficult. If the diastolic filling period is too short, E velocity becomes prematurely terminated and its DT is shortened. Therefore, it is recommended that E velocity and DT be measured from cardiac cycles that permit completion of LV diastolic filling before the onset of QRS. In patients with atrial fibrillation, the peak acceleration rate of E velocity was found to correlate best with LV filling pressure (13), but it is difficult to measure. DT is still a good factor to estimate LV filling pressure, especially in patients with atrial fibrillation and decreased LV systolic function (14). DT <130 msec usually indicates restrictive filling and increased filling pressure (15).

Precardioversion TEE

Atrial fibrillation is associated with increased thromboembolism and decreased cardiac output resulting from loss of atrial contractility. Usually, an attempt is made to cardiovert this arrhythmia to sinus rhythm if possible. Conventionally, patients with atrial fibrillation receive anticoagulation treatment with warfarin (Coumadin) for 3 weeks before cardioversion and for another 4 weeks after cardioversion to minimize thromboembolism (16). Because TEE is able to visualize the LA and LAA with diagnostic accuracy in nearly all patients, many medical centers, including our own, recommend cardioversion if TEE shows no thrombus in the LA and LAA (17,18); however, embolic events have occurred after cardioversion in patients whose transesophageal echocardiographic findings are negative, usually when they were not therapeutically anticoagulated at the time of cardioversion (19). Therefore, if TEE is to be used as part of the management strategy for atrial fibrillation, patients need to receive anticoagulation treatment with heparin, usually 6 to 12 hours before the DC cardioversion, and the risk for thromboembolism will be minimal if TEE shows no thrombus. It also is recommended that the warfarin treatment be started at the same time as the heparin therapy and be continued for 4 weeks after successful cardioversion, because atrial stunning occurs with DC cardioversion and it takes atrial function a few weeks to recover. A pilot study called ACUTE (Assessment of Cardioversion Using Transesophageal Echocardiography) compared this strategy of cardioversion using TEE with the conventional strategy of chronic anticoagulation in cardioversion; in this study, no patient had an embolic event after negative TEE findings and cardioversion (20), although one patient in the conventionally treated group had an embolic event 3 days after cardioversion. A substantial proportion of patients achieved spontaneous cardioversion to sinus rhythm while receiving anticoagulation therapy in the conventionally treated group. Therefore, currently, it appears that both the TEE strategy and the conventional strategy are acceptable for cardioversion in stable patients with atrial

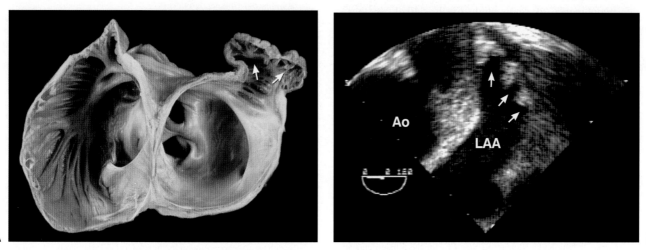

FIG. 21-4. Left: Pathology specimen of a left atrial (LA) appendage with multiple lobes (*arrows*). (Courtesy of Dr. William D. Edwards.) **Right:** Transesophageal view of multilobed (*arrows*) LA appendage (*LAA*). *Ao*, aorta.

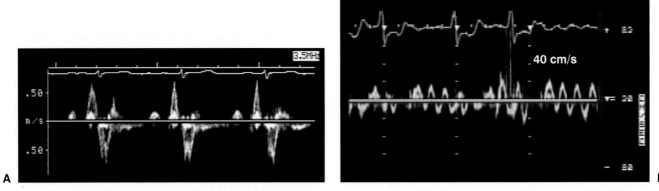

FIG. 21-5. Pulsed-wave Doppler recording of left atrial appendage flow velocity in a patient with sinus rhythm **(A)** and in a patient with atrial fibrillation **(B)**.

fibrillation as long as the anticoagulation treatment is adequate at the time of cardioversion and for 4 weeks afterward. An optimal cardioversion strategy should be selected according to the patient's needs and the clinical circumstances. The TEE strategy requires complete visualization of the LAA. The LAA has two or more lobes in most patients (Fig. 21-4). To evaluate LAA thrombus, all the lobes should be inspected. The pectinate muscles of the LAA may be mistaken for LAA thrombus. They are located along the wall of the LAA and have the same density as the surrounding tissue.

LAA FLOW VELOCITIES

Contraction and relaxation of the LAA produce flow velocities that can be detected at the mouth of the appendage (i.e., at the entry to the main body of the LA). The velocities are normally >50 cm/sec. With the loss of sinus rhythm, these flow velocities become smaller (Fig. 21-5). Studies have indicated that patients with LAA velocities <20 cm/sec are more likely to develop LAA thrombus or systemic thromboembolism (or both). Also, cardioversion to or maintenance of sinus rhythm is less likely in these patients.

REFERENCES

1. Shah PM. Echocardiographic diagnosis of mitral valve prolapse. *J Am Soc Echocardiogr* 1994;7:286–293.
2. Zhu WX, Olson DE, Karon BL, Tajik AJ. Myocardial stunning after electroconvulsive therapy. *Ann Intern Med* 1992;117:914–915.
3. Fine DG, Oh JK, Edwards WD, et al. Electrocardiographic, echocardiographic, and pathological correlation in patients with subarachnoid hemorrhage. *J Am Coll Cardiol* 1990;15(Suppl A):215A (abst).
4. DeRook FA, Comess KA, Albers GW, Popp RL. Transesophageal echocardiography in the evaluation of stroke. *Ann Intern Med* 1992;117:922–932.
5. Amarenco P, Duyckaerts C, Tzourio C, Henin D, Bousser MG, Hauw JJ. The prevalence of ulcerated plaques in the aortic arch in patients with stroke. *N Engl J Med* 1992;326:221-225.
6. Laperche T, Laurian C, Roudaut R, Steg PG, for the Filiale Echocardiographie de la Société Française de Cardiologie. Mobile thromboses of the aortic arch without aortic debris: a transesophageal echocardiographic finding associated with unexplained arterial embolism. *Circulation* 1997;96:288–294.
7. Sohn DW, Shin GJ, Oh JK, et al. Role of transesophageal echocardiography in hemodynamically unstable patients. *Mayo Clin Proc* 1995;70:925–931.
8. Heidenreich PA, Stainback RF, Redberg RF, Schiller NB, Cohen NH, Foster E. Transesophageal echocardiography predicts mortality in critically ill patients with unexplained hypotension. *J Am Coll Cardiol* 1995;26:152–158.
9. Smith MD, Cassidy JM, Souther S, et al. Transesophageal echocardiography in the diagnosis of traumatic rupture of the aorta. *N Engl J Med* 1995;332:356–362.
10. Shub C, Klein AL, Zachariah PK, Bailey KR, Tajik AJ. Determination of left ventricular mass by echocardiography in a normal population: Effect of age and sex in addition to body size. *Mayo Clin Proc* 1994;69:205–211.
11. Gardin JM, Siscovick D, Anton-Culver H, et al. Sex, age, and disease affect echocardiographic left ventricular mass and systolic function in the free-living elderly. The Cardiovascular Health Study. *Circulation* 1995;91:1739–1748.
12. The Stroke Prevention in Atrial Fibrillation Investigators. Predictors of thromboembolism in atrial fibrillation: I. Clinical features of patients at risk. II. Echocardiographic features of patients at risk. *Ann Intern Med* 1992;116:a, 1–5; b, 6–12.
13. Grogan M, Smith HC, Gersh BJ, Wood DL. Left ventricular dysfunction due to atrial fibrillation in patients initially believed to have idiopathic dilated cardiomyopathy. *Am J Cardiol* 1992;69:1570–1573.
14. Nagueh SF, Kopelen HA, Quinones MA. Assessment of left ventricular filling pressures by Doppler in the presence of atrial fibrillation. *Circulation* 1996;94:2138–2145.
15. Hurrell DG, Oh JK, Mahoney DW, Miller FA Jr, Seward JB. Short deceleration time of mitral inflow E velocity: prognostic implication with atrial fibrillation versus sinus rhythm. *J Am Soc Echocardiogr* 1998;11:450–457.
16. Laupacis A, Albers G, Dunn M, Feinberg W. Antithrombotic therapy in atrial fibrillation. *Chest* 1992;102(Suppl 4):426S–433S.
17. Manning WJ, Silverman DI, Gordon SP, Krumholz HM, Douglas PS. Cardioversion from atrial fibrillation without prolonged anticoagulation with use of transesophageal echocardiography to exclude the presence of atrial thrombi. *N Engl J Med* 1993;328:750–755.
18. Stoddard MF, Dawkins PR, Prince CR, Ammash NM. Left atrial appendage thrombus is not uncommon in patients with acute atrial fibrillation and a recent embolic event: a transesophageal echocardiographic study. *J Am Coll Cardiol* 1995;25:452–459.
19. Black IW, Fatkin D, Sagar KB, et al. Exclusion of atrial thrombus by transesophageal echocardiography does not preclude embolism after cardioversion of atrial fibrillation: a multicenter study. *Circulation* 1994;89:2509–2513.
20. Klein AL, Grimm RA, Black IW, et al. Cardioversion guided by transesophageal echocardiography: the ACUTE Pilot Study. A randomized, controlled trial: assessment of cardioversion using transesophageal echocardiography. *Ann Intern Med* 1997;126:200–209.

Appendix

APPENDIX 1. *Normal values from M-mode echocardiography[a]*

	Men (n = 288)		Women (n = 524)	
	Mean	SD	Mean	SD
Age (yr)	35.7	6.1	35.9	5.5
Height (m)	1.77	0.06	1.63	0.06
Weight (kg)	74.1	6.9	59.3	6.1
Body mass index (kg/m²)	23.5	1.6	22.1	1.7
Body surface area (m²)	1.91	0.11	1.64	0.10
Systolic blood pressure (mm Hg)	117.0	9.1	110.0	10.5
Diastolic blood pressure (mm Hg)	74.8	6.8	70.9	7.5
LV diastolic dimension (mm)	50.8	3.6	46.1	3.0
LV systolic dimension (mm)	32.9	3.4	28.9	2.8
LV wall thickness (mm)[b]	18.1	2.0	15.5	1.5
LA dimension (mm)	37.5	3.6	33.1	3.2

LA, left atrium; LV, left ventricle.

[a] These reference values were derived from a healthy subset of the Framingham Heart Study. These values were obtained by M-mode measurement with two-dimensional echocardiographic guidance.

[b] LV wall thickness is the sum of the ventricular septum and posterior wall thickness.

From Lauer MS, Larson MG, Levy D. Gender-specific reference M-mode values in adults: population-derived values with consideration of the impact of height. *J Am Coll Cardiol* 1995;26:1039–1046, with permission.

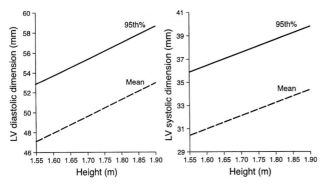

Appendix 2. Nomogram plots of mean and 95th percentile value for left ventricular end-diastolic and end-systolic dimensions as a function of height for healthy men. (From Lauer MS, Larson MG, Levy D. Gender-specific reference M-mode values in adults: population-derived values with consideration of the impact of height. *J Am Coll Cardiol* 1995;26:1039–1046, with permission.)

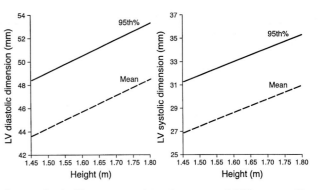

Appendix 3. Nomogram plots of mean and 95th percentile value for LV end-diastolic and end-systolic dimensions as a function of height for healthy women. (From Lauer MS, Larson MG, Levy D. Gender-specific reference M-mode values in adults: population-derived values with consideration of the impact of height. *J Am Coll Cardiol* 1995;26:1039–1046, with permission.)

APPENDIX 4. *Normal heart chamber measurements by two-dimensional echocardiography*[a]

View	Normal range (cm) (mean ± 2 SD)	Mean (cm)	Index range (cm/m²)	Absolute range (cm)
Apical four-chamber				
LVED major	6.9–10.3	8.6	4.1–5.7	7.2–10.3
LVED minor	3.3–6.1	4.7	2.2–3.1	3.8–6.2
LVES minor	1.9–3.7	2.8	1.3–2.0	2.1–3.9
LVFS (%)	27–50	38.0	—	26–47
RV major	6.5–9.5	8.0	3.8–5.3	6.3–9.3
RV minor	2.2–4.4	3.3	1.0–2.8	2.2–4.5
Parasternal long-axis				
LVED	3.5–6.0	4.8	2.3–3.1	3.8–5.8
LVES	2.1–4.0	3.1	1.4–2.1	2.3–3.9
FS (%)	25–46	36.0	—	0.26–0.45
RV	1.9–3.8	2.8	1.2–2.0	1.9–3.9
Parasternal short-axis				
Chordal level				
LVED	3.5–6.2	4.8	2.3–3.2	3.8–6.1
LVES	2.3–4.0	3.2	1.5–2.2	2.6–4.2
LVFS (%)	27–42	34.0	—	27–41
Papillary muscle level				
LVED	3.5–5.8	4.7	2.2–3.1	3.9–5.8
LVES	2.2–4.0	3.1	1.4–2.2	2.5–4.1
LVFS (%)	25–43	34.0	—	25–43

ED, end-diastole; ES, end-systole; FS, fractional shortening.

[a] Although it is a common and useful practice in adult cardiology to correct values for body surface area, for pediatric applications or for smaller or larger than average subjects, charts based on subjects of a wide range of body sizes should be consulted.

From Schiller NB, Shah PM, Crawford M, et al. Recommendations for quantitation of the left ventricle by two-dimensional echocardiography. American Society of Echocardiography Committee on Standards, Subcommittee on Quantitation of Two-Dimensional Echocardiograms. *J Am Soc Echocardiogr* 1989;2: 358–367, with permission.

APPENDIX 5. *LV volumes (normal values)*

Methods	End-diastole (mL)		End-systole (mL)	
	Mean ± SD	Range	Mean ± SD	Range
Four-chamber area length				
Men	112 ± 27	65–193	35 ± 16	13–86
Women	89 ± 20	59–136	33 ± 12	13–59
Two-chamber area length				
Men	130 ± 27	73–201	40 ± 14	17–74
Women	92 ± 19	53–146	31 ± 11	11–53
Biplane disk summation (modified Simpson's rule)				
Men	111 ± 22	62–170	34 ± 12	14–76
Women	80 ± 12	55–101	29 ± 10	13–60

Modified from Wahr DW, Wang YS, Schiller NB. Left ventricular volumes determined by two-dimensional echocardiography in a normal adult population. *J Am Coll Cardiol* 1983;1:863–868, with permission.

APPENDIX 6. *Echocardiographic data for 111 normal subjects, stratified by age and sex*

Group	No. of subjects	Measurements (mean ± SD)[a,b,c]				
		LV mass/BSA (g/m²)	LV mass/height (g/m)	Septum (mm)	LVPW (mm)	LVID (mm)
Male subjects						
Total	47	99 ± 15 (129)	108 ± 17 (143)	10.2 ± 1.2 (12.6)	9.9 ± 1.0 (11.9)	51 ± 3 (57)
Age (yr)						
<50	27	97 ± 14 (124)	107 ± 15 (136)	10.1 ± 0.9 (11.8)	9.6 ± 0.8 (11.3)	52 ± 3 (57)
≥ 50	20	102 ± 17 (135)	111 ± 20 (151)	10.4 ± 1.5 (13.4)	10.2 ± 1.1 (12.4)	51 ± 3 (56)
Age (yr)						
20–39	19	97 ± 14 (124)	106 ± 14 (134)	9.9 ± 0.9 (11.6)	9.6 ± 0.8 (11.3)	52 ± 3 (57)
40–59	16	99 ± 12 (123)	110 ± 14 (139)	10.6 ± 1.3 (13.2)	9.8 ± 0.8 (11.5)	51 ± 2 (56)
≥ 60	12	103 ± 20 (144)	110 ± 25 (160)	10.1 ± 1.4 (12.9)	10.3 ± 1.3 (13.3)	50 ± 3 (57)
Female subjects						
Total	64	88 ± 15 (118)	89 ± 17 (123)	9.2 ± 1.0 (11.3)	8.9 ± 0.9 (10.6)	47 ± 4 (55)
Age (yr)						
< 50	34	82 ± 13 (108)	83 ± 14 (111)	8.6 ± 0.7 (10.0)	8.6 ± 0.7 (10.0)	47 ± 3 (54)
		$p = 0.004$	$p = 0.002$	$p < 0.0001$	$p = 0.004$	
≥ 50	30	93 ± 16 (124)	96 ± 18 (132)	9.8 ± 0.9 (11.7)	9.2 ± 0.9 (10.6)	47 ± 4 (55)
Age (yr)						
20–39	24	83 ± 13 (108)	83 ± 14 (110)	8.6 ± 0.7 (10.0)	8.5 ± 0.7 (9.9)	48 ± 4 (55)
		$p = 0.008$	$p = 0.009$	$p < 0.001$	$p = 0.05$	
40–59	20	85 ± 11 (107)	88 ± 13 (113)	9.0 ± 0.9 (10.8)	9.0 ± 0.7 (10.4)	47 ± 4 (55)
		$p = 0.04$		$p < 0.001$	$p = 0.02$	
≥ 60	20	96 ± 18 (132)	98 ± 21 (140)	10.1 ± 0.9 (11.9)	9.2 ± 1.0 (11.2)	47 ± 4 (55)

BSA, body surface area; ht, height; LV, left ventricular; LVID, LV internal dimension; LVPW, LV posterior wall thickness.

[a] Numbers in parentheses are upper 95% confidence limits.

[b] P values are based on two-sample t tests between pairs of age groups; brackets indicate groups compared.

[c] LV mass was calculated with the cube function formula from the two-dimensional guided M-mode echocardiogram.

From Shub C, Klein AL, Zachariah PK, Bailey KR, Tajik AJ. Determination of left ventricular mass by echocardiography in a normal population: effect of age and sex in addition to body size. *Mayo Clin Proc* 1994;69:205–211, with permission.

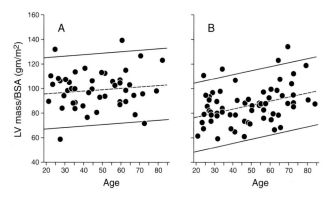

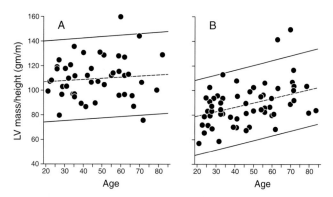

Appendix 7. Left ventricular mass in normal subjects of various ages, normalized by body surface area (*BSA*). **A:** Men. **B:** Women. *Solid lines*, 95% confidence limits; *dashed lines*, mean values. (From Shub C, Klein AL, Zachariah PK, Bailey KR, Tajik AJ. Determination of left ventricular mass by echocardiography in a normal population: effect of age and sex in addition to body size. *Mayo Clin Proc* 1994;69:205–211, with permission.)

Appendix 8. Left ventricular mass in normal subjects of various ages, normalized by height. **A:** Men. **B:** Women. *Solid lines*, 95% confidence limits; *dashed lines*, mean values. (From Shub C, Klein AL, Zachariah PK, Bailey KR, Tajik AJ. Determination of left ventricular mass by echocardiography in a normal population: effect of age and sex in addition to body size. *Mayo Clin Proc* 1994;69:205–211, with permission.)

APPENDIX 9. *Echocardiographic reference values for aortic root size[a,b]*

Variable	Men (n = 1,433)	Women (n = 1,816)
Age (yr)	46 ± 13	47 ± 13
Weight (kg)	80 ± 11	62 ± 10
Height (m)	1.75 ± 0.07	1.61 ± 0.06
Body surface area (m²)	1.95 ± 0.15	1.64 ± 0.13
Systolic blood pressure (mm Hg)	120 ± 10	115 ± 12
Diastolic blood pressure (mm Hg)	76 ± 7	72 ± 7
Aortic root (mm)	32 ± 3	28 ± 3

[a] Values are mean ± SD.

[b] Aortic root measurements were obtained by M-mode echocardiography by a leading-edge to lending-edge technique. Obtained from healthy participants in the Framingham Heart Study and Framingham offspring study.

From Vasan RS, Larson MG, Benjamin EJ, Levy D. Echocardiographic reference values for aortic root size: the Framingham Heart Study. *J Am Soc Echocardiogr* 1995;8:793–800, with permission.

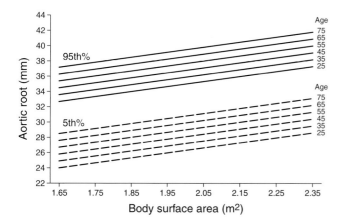

Appendix 10. Predicted upper and lower normal limits of aortic root diameter in men as function of age and body surface area. (From Vasan RS, Larson MG, Benjamin EJ, Levy D. Echocardiographic reference values for aortic root size: the Framingham Heart Study. *J Am Soc Echocardiogr* 1995;8:793–800, with permission.)

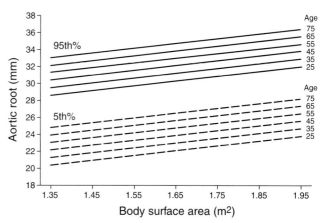

Appendix 11. Predicted upper and lower normal limits of aortic root diameter in women as function of age and body surface area. *Note:* To obtain appropriate values, select appropriate set of lines according to the age. Draw a perpendicular line to X-axis at appropriate body surface area. Y-axis value at the intersection indicates limit of aortic root dimension. (From Vasan RS, Larson MG, Benjamin EJ, Levy D. Echocardiographic reference values for aortic root size: the Framingham Heart Study. *J Am Soc Echocardiogr* 1995;8:793–800, with permission.)

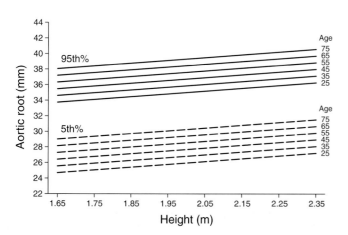

Appendix 12. Predicted upper and lower normal limits of aortic root diameter in men as function of age and height. (From Vasan RS, Larson MG, Benjamin EJ, Levy D. Echocardiographic reference values for aortic root size: the Framingham Heart Study. *J Am Soc Echocardiogr* 1995;8:793–800, with permission.)

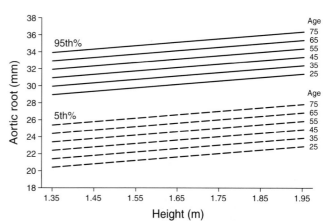

Appendix 13. Predicted upper and lower normal limits of aortic root diameter in women as function of age and height. (From Vasan RS, Larson MG, Benjamin EJ, Levy D. Echocardiographic reference values for aortic root size: the Framingham Heart Study. *J Am Soc Echocardiogr* 1995;8:793–800, with permission.)

APPENDIX 14. *Mitral inflow velocities and diastolic parameters in normal subjects[a]*

Variable	Decade of life					
	3rd (n = 23)	4th (n = 20)	5th (n = 18)	6th (n = 20)	7th (n = 21)	≥ 8th (n = 15)
Peak E (cm/sec)	75 ± 12	67 ± 14	72 ± 14	62 ± 10	62 ± 13	64 ± 19
Peak A (cm/sec)	36 ± 9	39 ± 10	46 ± 9	49 ± 8	62 ± 11	67 ± 17
E/A ratio	2.2 ± 0.7	1.7 ± 0.4	1.6 ± 0.4	1.3 ± 0.2	1.0 ± 0.2	1.0 ± 0.4
DT (msec)	182 ± 19	176 ± 19	177 ± 23	201 ± 22	214 ± 41	219 ± 42
IVRT (msec)	71 ± 11	79 ± 8	79 ± 13	88 ± 18	94 ± 17	86 ± 15

A, filling wave due to atrial contraction; DT, deceleration time; E, early rapid filling wave; IVRT, isovolumic relaxation time.

[a] Sample volume at leaflet tip.

From Klein AL, Burstow DJ, Tajik AJ, Zachariah PK, Bailey KR, Seward JB. Effects of age on left ventricular dimensions and filling dynamics in 117 normal persons. *Mayo Clin Proc* 1994;69:212–224, with permission.

APPENDIX 15. *Mitral inflow velocities in 117 normal subjects, stratified by phase of respiration*

Variable	Inspiration	Expiration	Apnea
Peak E (cm/sec)	67 ± 14[a]	68 ± 15[b]	68 ± 15
Peak A (cm/sec)	48 ± 16	50 ± 16[b]	49 ± 15
E/A ratio	1.5 ± 0.6	1.5 ± 0.7	1.7 ± 0.6
DT (msec)	195 ± 34	192 ± 33	194 ± 35
IVRT (msec)	83 ± 16	83 ± 16	82 ± 16

A, filling wave due to atrial contraction; DT, deceleration time; E, early rapid filling wave; IVRT, isovolumic relaxation time.

[a] Significantly different ($p < 0.05$) from apnea.

[b] Significantly different ($p < 0.05$) from inspiration.

From Klein AL, Burstow DJ, Tajik AJ, Zachariah PK, Bailey KR, Seward JB. Effects of age on left ventricular dimensions and filling dynamics in 117 normal persons. *Mayo Clin Proc* 1994;69:212–224, with permission.

APPENDIX 16. *Mitral inflow velocities at leaflet tips and mitral annulus in 117 normal subjects*

Variable	Leaflet tips	Annulus
Peak E (cm/sec)	66 ± 15[a]	53 ± 13
Peak A (cm/sec)	52 ± 16	50 ± 15
E/A ratio	1.4 ± 0.5[a]	1.1 ± 0.4
DT (msec)	197 ± 33[a]	163 ± 36

A, filling wave due to atrial contraction; DT, deceleration time; E, early rapid filling wave.

[a] Significantly different ($p < 0.001$) from annulus.

From Klein AL, Burstow DJ, Tajik AJ, Zachariah PK, Bailey KR, Seward JB. Effects of age on left ventricular dimensions and filling dynamics in 117 normal persons. *Mayo Clin Proc* 1994;69: 212–224, with permission.

APPENDIX 17. *Pulmonary venous flow velocities in 85 normal subjects, stratified by age in decades*

Variable	3rd (n = 18)	4th (n = 15)	5th (n = 11)	6th (n = 16)	7th (n = 16)	≥ 8th (n = 9)
			Decade of life			
Peak velocity (cm/s)						
Systolic	47 ± 9	45 ± 7	54 ± 9	59 ± 10	62 ± 8	62 ± 10
Diastolic	56 ± 10	46 ± 8	47 ± 10	42 ± 7	34 ± 5	38 ± 13
PVa	19 ± 5	18 ± 2	21 ± 4	22 ± 3	23 ± 4	23 ± 4
FTVI (cm)						
Systolic	11 ± 3	12 ± 2	14 ± 2	14 ± 2	15 ± 2	15 ± 4
Diastolic	11 ± 3	10 ± 2	9 ± 2	9 ± 2	7 ± 2	8 ± 3
PVa	1.8 ± 0.9	1.7 ± 0.5	2.0 ± 0.6	2.0 ± 0.6	2.0 ± 0.7	1.9 ± 0.3
FTVI systole (%)	51 ± 7	55 ± 9	60 ± 4	61 ± 5	69 ± 5	66 ± 7
Reverse TVI as % of FTVI	8.6 ± 4.7	8.1 ± 2.9	8.4 ± 2.8	9.0 ± 2.8	11.0 ± 3.6	8.7 ± 2.5

FTVI, forward flow time velocity integral; PVa, pulmonary vein atrial flow reversal; TVI, time velocity integral.

From Klein AL, Burstow DJ, Tajik AJ, Zachariah PK, Bailey KR, Seward JB. Effects of age on left ventricular dimensions and filling dynamics in 117 normal persons. *Mayo Clin Proc* 1994;69:212–224, with permission.

APPENDIX 18. *Pulmonary venous flow velocities in 85 normal subjects, stratified by phase of respiration*

Variable	Inspiration	Expiration	Apnea
Peak velocity (cm/sec)			
Systolic	55 ± 11	54 ± 11	54 ± 11
Diastolic	43 ± 11[a]	46 ± 12	44 ± 11[b]
PVa	20.2 ± 4.4	21.1 ± 4.6[c]	20.6 ± 4.3[b]
Forward time velocity integral (cm)			
Systolic	14 ± 3[a]	13 ± 3[c]	13 ± 3
Diastolic	8.8 ± 2.6[a]	9.4 ± 2.7[c]	9.1 ± 2.6[b]
PVa	1.9 ± 0.6	2.0 ± 0.8	2.0 ± 0.1
FTVI systole (%)	61 ± 9[a]	59 ± 10[c]	60 ± 9
Reverse TVI as % of FTVI	8.8 ± 3.2	9.2 ± 4.0	9.1 ± 3.7

FTVI, forward flow time velocity integral; PVa, pulmonary vein atrial flow reversal; TVI, time velocity integral.

[a] Significantly different ($p < 0.05$) from apnea.
[b] Significantly different ($p < 0.05$) from expiration.
[c] Significantly different ($p < 0.05$) from inspiration.

From Klein AL, Burstow DJ, Tajik AJ, Zachariah PK, Bailey KR, Seward JB. Effects of age on left ventricular dimensions and filling dynamics in 117 normal persons. *Mayo Clin Proc* 1994;69:212–224, with permission.

APPENDIX 19. *Normal Doppler data (n = 223): mitral valve flow variables and left ventricular isovolumic relaxation time, stratified by age-group*

Factor	3–8 yr (n = 75) Mean	1 SD	9–12 yr (n = 72) Mean	1 SD	13–17 yr (n = 76) Mean	1 SD
E velocity (cm/sec)	92	14	86	15	88	14
E TVI (cm)	12.0	2.6	12.3	2.9	14.0	2.9
A velocity (cm/sec)	42	11	41	9	39	8
A TVI (cm)	3.7	1.1	3.7	1.0	3.7	1.1
A duration (msec)	136	22	142	21	141	22
E at A velocity (cm/sec)	16	7	14	5	12	4
E to A velocity ratio	2.4	0.7	2.2	0.6	2.3	0.6
E to A TVI ratio	3.7	2.0	3.7	1.5	4.2	1.7
Deceleration time (msec)	145	18	157	19	172	22
End mitral A to R wave interval (msec)	34	16	29	15	27	19
LV IVRT (msec)	62	10	67	10	74	13

A, atrial filling wave; E, early filling wave; IVRT, isovolumic relaxation time; LV, left ventricular; SD, standard deviation; TVI, time velocity integral.

From O'Leary PW, Durongpisitkul K, Cordes TM, Bailey KR, Hagler DJ, Tajik AJ, Seward JB. Diastolic ventricular function in children: a Doppler echocardiographic study establishing normal values and predictors of increased ventricular end-diastolic pressure. *Mayo Clin Proc* 1998;73:616–628, with permission.

APPENDIX 20. *Normal Doppler data (n = 223): pulmonary vein flow variables*

Factor	3–8 yr (n = 75) Mean	1 SD	9–12 yr (n = 72) Mean	1 SD	13–17 yr (n = 76) Mean	1 SD
Systolic velocity (cm/sec)	46	9	45	9	41	10
Systolic TVI (cm)	11.1	2.3	11.5	2.2	10.8	2.8
Diastolic velocity (cm/sec)	59	8	54	9	59	11
Diastolic TVI (cm)	8.8	1.8	9.2	2.5	12.1	3.1
Ratio of systolic to diastolic velocity	0.8	0.2	0.8	0.2	0.7	0.2
Ratio of systolic to diastolic TVI	1.3	0.3	1.3	0.4	0.9	0.3
Atrial reversal velocity (cm/sec)	21	4	21	5	21	7
Atrial reversal duration (msec)	130	20	125	20	140	28
Atrial reversal TVI (cm)	1.7	0.5	1.6	0.6	2.0	0.9

SD, standard deviation; TVI, time velocity integral.

From O'Leary PW, Durongpisitkul K, Cordes TM, Bailey KR, Hagler DJ, Tajik AJ, Seward JB. Diastolic ventricular function in children: a Doppler echocardiographic study establishing normal values and predictors of increased ventricular end-diastolic pressure. *Mayo Clin Proc* 1998;73:616–628, with permission.

APPENDIX 21. *Normal Doppler data (n = 223): comparisons of the pulmonary vein atrial reversal to the mitral valve atrial wave*

Factor	3–8 yr (n = 75)		9–12 yr (n = 72)		13–17 yr (n = 76)	
	Mean	1 SD	Mean	1 SD	Mean	1 SD
Ratio data						
PVAR/MV A reversal duration	0.96	0.19	0.88	0.16	0.98	0.23
PVAR/MV A reversal TVI	0.52	0.25	0.46	0.22	0.60	0.43
Difference data						
PVAR duration—MV A duration (msec)	−8	26	−17	24	−6	33
Alternative method for calculating						
"PVAR duration—MV A duration" (msec)	16	20	4	27	−1	32

A, atrial wave; MV, mitral valve; PVAR, pulmonary vein atrial reversal; SD, standard deviation; TVI, time velocity integral.

From O'Leary PW, Durongpisitkul K, Cordes TM, Bailey KR, Hagler DJ, Tajik AJ, Seward JB. Diastolic ventricular function in children: a Doppler echocardiographic study establishing normal values and predictors of increased ventricular end-diastolic pressure. *Mayo Clin Proc* 1998;73:616–628, with permission.

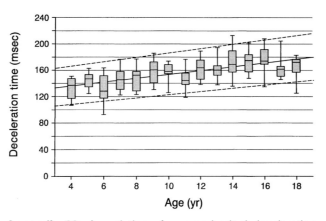

Appendix 22. Association of age and mitral deceleration time. *Solid line,* predicted mean, as determined by linear regression. *Dashed lines,* 90% confidence limits for overall group. *Boxes,* values ranging from the 25th to the 75th percentile for each age group, by years. *Line within each box,* median value for that age group. *Vertical lines extending from each box,* 95% confidence intervals for that specific age group. Subjects younger than 5 years old were pooled into the 4-year-old category. (From O'Leary PW, Durongpisitkul K, Cordes TM, Bailey KR, Hagler DJ, Tajik AJ, Seward JB. Diastolic ventricular function in children: a Doppler echocardiographic study establishing normal values and predictors of increased ventricular end-diastolic pressure. *Mayo Clin Proc* 1998;73:616–628, with permission.)

Subject Index

Note: Page numbers followed by f *indicate figures; those followed by* t *indicate tables.*

267